END OF LIFE NURSING CARE

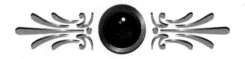

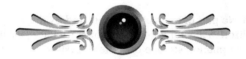

END OF LIFE NURSING CARE

Belinda Poor
RN, MSN, OCN

Gail P. Poirrier
RN, DNS

JONES AND BARTLETT PUBLISHERS
Sudbury, Massachusetts
BOSTON   TORONTO   LONDON   SINGAPORE

National League for Nursing

World Headquarters
Jones and Bartlett Publishers
40 Tall Pine Drive
Sudbury, MA 01776
978-443-5000
www.jbpub.com
info@jbpub.com

Jones and Bartlett Publishers Canada
2406 Nikanna Road
Mississauga, ON L5C 2W6
CANADA

Jones and Bartlett Publishers International
Barb House, Barb Mews
London W6 7PA
UK

Library of Congress Cataloging-in-Publication Data
Poor, Belinda
   End of life nursing care / Belinda Poor, Gail P. Poirrier.
      p. cm.
   Includes bibliographical references and index.
   ISBN 0-7637-1421-6 (alk. paper)
   1. Terminally ill.   2. Death.   3. Terminal care.   I. Poirrier, Gail P.
II. Title.
   R726.8 .P65 2000
   362.1'75—dc21   00-047351

Production Credits
Acquisitions Editor: Penny Glynn
Associate Editor: Christine Tridente
Production Editor: AnnMarie Lemoine
V.P., Manufacturing and Inventory Control: Therese Bräuer
Cover Design: AnnMarie Lemoine
Design and Composition: Carlisle Communications, Ltd.
Printing and Binding: Malloy Lithographing
Cover Photograph © Photodisc

Printed in the United States of America
03 02 01 00   10 9 8 7 6 5 4 3 2 1

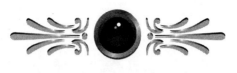

DEDICATION

This book is dedicated to the thousands of multidisciplinary health care workers, health care educators, and employers, whose efforts support quality of life at the end of life. Your unconditional caring at the darkest moment in life is overwhelming, soul wrenching, positive, and special. Thank you for the nurturing.

This is also dedicated to the many patients whose courage and honesty are to be envied. Your stories and life events are very dear, moving, and meaningful for professional growth of health care providers. Thank you for the humbling experiences.

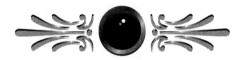

CONTENTS

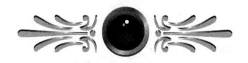

Acknowledgements

EDITORS

Belinda S. Poor, RN, MSN, OCN
Instructor and Coordinator, Continuing Education Nursing Program
College of Nursing and Allied Health Professions
University of Louisiana at Lafayette
Lafayette, LA

Gail P. Poirrier, RN, DNS
Acting Dean and Professor
College of Nursing and Allied Health Professions
University of Louisiana at Lafayette
Lafayette, LA

CONTRIBUTING AUTHORS

Tonia Dandry Aiken, RN, BSN, JD
Nurse Attorney
New Orleans, LA

Pat Andrus, MS
Director, The Mourning After Program, Martin & Castille Funeral Homes, Inc.
Executive Director
The Grief Center of Southwest Louisiana
Lafayette, LA

Gary J. Arnold, MD, FACS
Associate Professor
University of Louisiana at Lafayette
College of Nursing and Allied Health Professions
Lafayette, LA

Michael Blanchard, BA, MA
Executive Director, Director of Community Education
Hospice of Acadiana
Lafayette, LA

Karen Borne
Stephen Minister, Former Lay Chaplain
Texas Children's Hospital
Houston, TX

Randy Bond, RN, MSN, APRN, CFNP
Case Manager
Lafayette General Medical Center
Lafayette, LA

Sarah Brabant, PhD, CCS
Professor of Sociology
University of Louisiana at Lafayette
Lafayette, LA

Tyla Ann Burger, RN, CRNH
Partner, Senior Consultant
Palliative Resources
Philadelphia, PA

Camille Pavy Claibourne, RN, MSN
Chief Nurse Officer
Lafayette General Medical Center
Lafayette, LA

Michelle Crain, RN, MSN, CS, FNP-C
Family Nurse Practitioner
Our Lady of Lourdes Regional
Medical Center
Lafayette, LA

Marlene Foreman, RNCS, MN, CHPN
Professor of Nursing
Louisiana State University at Eunice
Eunice, LA

Gretchen Gaines, MTS, MSW
Bereavement Coordinator
Hospice of Northern Virginia
Falls Church, VA

Elizabeth Gary, RN, BSN
Nurse Manager OPS/PACU
Lafayette General Medical Center
Lafayette, LA

Julie Griffie, RN, MSN, CS, AOCN
Clinical Nurse Specialist, Palliative Care
Froedtert Hospital
Milwaukee, WI

J. Brooke Hamilton III, BA, MA, MBA, PhD
*J.J. Burdin, MD and Helen B. Burdin
Professor of Professional Ethics
and Associate Professor of Management*
University of Louisiana at Lafayette
Lafayette, LA

Patricia A. LaBrosse, RN, MS, CS, CNAA
Instructor
College of Nursing and Allied Health
Professions

University of Louisiana at Lafayette
Lafayette, LA

Heidi T. Landry, RN, MN
Instructor
College of Nursing and Allied Health
Professions
University of Louisiana at Lafayette
Lafayette, LA

Michael T. Landry, RN, MN
Instructor
College of Nursing and Allied Health
Professions
University of Louisiana at Lafayette
Lafayette, LA

Mary B. Neiheisel, RN, EdD, CNS, FNP
*University of Louisiana Foundation
Distinguished Professor
Professor of Nursing, LGMC Regents
Professor 1994–2000
Pfizer-Ardoin Regents Professor 2001*
University of Louisiana at Lafayette
College of Nursing and Allied Health
Professions
Lafayette, LA

Melinda G. Oberleitner, RN, DNS
*Associate Professor and Acting Department
Head*
College of Nursing and Allied Health
Professions
University of Louisiana at Lafayette
Lafayette, LA

Sudha C. Patel, RN, DNS
Assistant Professor
College of Nursing and Allied Health
Professions
University of Louisiana at Lafayette
Lafayette, LA

Regina L. Payne, RN, EdD, CWOCN
Professor of Nursing
Florida Gulf Coast University
College of Health Professions
Fort Myers, FL

Demetrius J. Porche, RN, DNS, FNP, CS
Associate Professor
Louisiana State University Health Sciences Center
New Orleans, LA

Susan M. Randol, RN, MS
Instructor and Freshmen/Sophomore Coordinator
College of Nursing and Allied Health Professions
University of Louisiana at Lafayette
Lafayette, LA

Douglas C. Smith, M.DIV., MA, MS
Author, Lecturer, Consultant
Madison, WI

Thomas J. Smith, RNC, PhD, APRN
BSN *Program Director*
Department of Nursing
Nicholls State University
Thibodaux, LA

Phyllis B. Taylor, RN, BA
Registered Nurse, Counselor, Educator
Philadelphia, PA

Velma Westbrook, RN, DNS
Administrator of Academic Unit and Faculty/Department Head
Department of Nursing
Nicholls State University
Thibodaux, LA

Evelyn M. Wills, RN, PhD
Associate Professor
College of Nursing and Allied Health Professions
University of Louisiana at Lafayette
Lafayette, LA

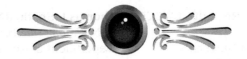

FOREWORD

It is an honor to pen a few words to be included in a book with so many outstanding authors. The academicians, including nurse educators, sociologists, and philosophers, have joined with clinicians, including administrators, staff nurses, advanced practice nurses, ministers, social workers, and hospice and hospital personnel, to produce a timely textbook for undergraduate and graduate student health care providers. The book contains valuable content for anyone facing his or her own death, or the death of a family member, friend, or significant other. The information, the facts, the thought-provoking ideas related by these authors are long overdue for the classroom setting and for the public as well.

The organization of the book flows smoothly from historical perspectives to caring for the caregiver and includes theories, holistic models, the grief process and responses to loss, ethical and legal considerations, patient-centered care, communication, management of specific terminal illnesses, and issues across the lifespan. The content includes the encircling, meaningful parameters of history, sociology, psychology, pathophysiology, philosophy, and the law. Not until we can speak of death in each of these spheres and include death as another step in the developmental process will we achieve acceptance and understanding of end of life care. The behavioral learning objectives, critical thinking activities, and teaching-learning exercises will guide the students and faculty through the content toward scholarship. Critical thinking activities are essential in the learning process of students, and critical thinking is, of course, an essential skill for nursing students. Discussion of alternate solutions will increase the students' understanding of the meaning of death and the importance of quality of care for the dying. These situations will improve the critical thinking abilities of the students. Using the stated objectives and the critical thinking skills, students will be able to apply previous knowledge and gain new knowledge and understanding as they arrive at decisions required in each scenario. Students can evaluate their own decision-making abilities, choices, and outcomes, and then can employ these new skills and knowledge for the benefit of future patients and decisions. As a result, students will be prepared for encountering people who are dying and will approach them with meaningful, compassionate, empathetic caring.

In the 1940s, a young child watched her father and mother grieving over the death in infancy of their last child. The mother, Jane, verbally expressed her grief to her young daughter after receiving no solace from her health care providers or her religion. The father, certainly typical of that generation, was strong, silent, and tearless "for his family." His strength endured for four weeks until he suffered a myocardial infarction at the age of 35—his grief and tearlessness finally expressed with a broken heart. This child, who has lost her father and is herself inconsolable, again becomes the sounding board and "grief counselor" for Jane. During the next few years, death is a regular visitor to this household, but it is a quarter of a century before Jane, who had experienced death as a mother and daughter, finally comes to terms with being a grief-stricken wife. Consolation resources had proven inadequate. These events are not unique. There are millions of similar families who suffer emotional and physical needs in the most traumatic moments of their lives and find few or no comforting resources. This textbook will assist the health care provider in bringing aid and comfort to the dying person and his caregivers in these situations.

To reduce the stress and stressors of dying and death, man must learn early in life that death is part of the circle of life and life is not complete without the end, the final breath. As the great poet, John Donne, said: "Every man's death diminishes me, but does it not also enrich me?" We are "involved in mankind" but we are also involved in the life and death of every human being. Sarah Brabant expresses this in her chapter, "Extending the Circle of Care When Death is Imminent," involving loved ones in the care of the dying. The friend or loved one who avoids "talking to" the dying person will learn from Karen Borne's chapter on communication that the priority is attentive listening. The clarity and importance of listening, caring, therapeutic touch, and the power of maintaining dignity in dying is expressed beautifully by many of the writers and is comprehensible to the layperson as well as the health care providers.

Discussing end of life issues and expressing (verbally and in writing) personal desires regarding dying, death, and burial or cremation will eliminate decision making and subsequent feelings of guilt for survivors. Chapters by Hamilton, Aiken, Andrus, Blanchard, Claibourne, and others will assist the heath care provider and the layperson in coping with these concerns. Making financial arrangements will eliminate the mortician's question, "Is there a problem paying for this?" I was asked this at the time of my own husband's death. In the absence of burial insurance and because this was my first contact with this person, it is probably a legitimate and common inquiry by a good businessman. This incident makes clear the fact that death has become a commercial event for all of us and a financial calamity for many. Heeding the Jewish practice of maintaining simplicity and modesty at funerals was universal only a few decades ago. However, elaborate, expensive funerals have replaced the simplicity, and the epilogue following the death of a loved one has expanded to include closure, memorials, paperwork, legal notices, and the reading of the will. These changes are, to many, unnecessary and unkind.

This textbook is globally significant. It is relevant to every person, to every culture, and to every walk of life. We are involved; no man is an island, and nowhere can you find the man who has not asked for help. Educators—whether in sociology, philosophy, nursing, medicine, or psychology—and clinicians—whether in rural or urban practice, private, home health, hospital, or hospice settings—should welcome and require this book in their curriculum or in their practice. Dying and death belong to us all, and the comprehension of that involvement exemplified in this textbook is a coordinated, harmonious lesson in dying well.

Dr. Mary B. Neiheisel

UNIT I

INTRODUCTION

Learning Objectives

1. Define palliative care
2. Discuss importance of palliative care
3. Define quality of life
4. Describe dignified death
5. Describe physical, psychological, social, and spiritual well-being

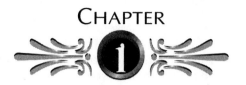

PALLIATIVE CARE AND QUALITY OF LIFE IN CARING FOR THE DYING

Belinda Poor

*"Do not go gently into that good night
Rage, rage against the dying of the light."*

Dylan Thomas, 1951

What's wrong with the poetry cited here? There's nothing wrong with it; in fact, it is excellent poetry. However it is very bad medical advice. Thomas addressed this poem in 1951 to his father who was becoming blind and slowly dying. He encourages his father not to die peacefully but to fight with anger against death. Although Thomas was anguished at the failing independence of his father when he wrote this poem, advice to die angry is not what is wanted for anyone who is dying. It is a simple fact that every person will die. Death is a part of life, a very important part. It is the end, the natural outcome of life. The way that death has been perceived has changed many times through the years.

At the turn of the century, medicine was limited. There were many incorrect diagnoses, with restricted therapies and relatively short life expectancies. People died at home without a medical physician or nurse to provide assistance. People died of infections sometimes in epidemic proportions. Technology was minimal. The first antibiotic, penicillin, was not discovered until the late 1920s.

Advances in medical technology increased the ability to provide better care, administer more advanced therapies for diseases, and significantly increase the life expectancy. It also revolutionized the ability to understand sudden and unexplainable causes of deaths; chronic illnesses, such as chronic obstructive lung disease, renal failure, all types of cancers, diabetes mellitus, and neurological diseases could now be linked to the causes of death.

The way society views death at this time is a concern, as reflected in the SUPPORT (a study to understand prognoses and preferences for outcomes and risks of treatment) Study (1995). At present, there is a tremendous amount of work being done to recognize the needs of the dying and to provide interventions to improve end of life. Health care providers are scrambling to develop methods to enhance end of life care that would provide the setting to be able to die well. But the SUPPORT Study showed health care providers were still significantly deficient in the delivery of care to the dying. This study spanned four years and included more than 9,000 adult patients who were hospitalized with one or more life-threatening illnesses and had an overall six-month mortality prognosis. Despite the fact that the patients were seriously ill and were expected to die within six months, health care providers did not discuss the prognosis or assist patients with important decisions. The study also found that half of the patients who were able to communicate in their last few days spent most of the time, according to their families, in moderate to severe pain.

These findings are not acceptable in health care today. It is imperative that patients and families confronted with a terminal illness be included in discussions about expected outcomes of treatments available, goals of care, and methods of controlling pain and other symptoms. Physicians are ethically and morally responsible for communicating with patients concerning their prognosis and plan of care as well as to answer all questions posed by the patient (SUPPORT, 1993).

Another study presented at the American Academy of Hospice and Palliative Medicine involved 30 internal medicine residency programs across the United States. Residents in these programs answered a questionnaire. The following were the most common misconceptions found:

- excessive concern about morphine-induced respiratory depression
- lack of knowledge concerning opioid dose conversions
- omission of drug therapy for opioid constipation
- regarding clinical depression as a normal event in the dying
- inability or unwillingness to discuss a short prognosis directly with a cancer patient
- confusing opioid toxicity with assisted suicide

These results indicate a need for improvement of education including attitudes, knowledge, and skills about end of life issues for faculty and residents in internal medicine residency programs. (Weissman, Mullan, Ambuel, Gunten, and Hallenback 2000).

Nurses are also responsible for effectively communicating with dying patients as well as managing pain and other symptoms of the dying. But nurses cannot practice what they are not knowledgeable about. A study examining end of life content in nursing textbooks was conducted (Ferrell, Virani, and Grant 1999), and the findings were troubling. A total of 50 textbooks were reviewed. Of the 1,750 chapters in these books, only 24 were related to end of life issues. This represents 1.4% of all of the chapters. The total number of pages in the textbooks was 45,683 with only 901.9 pages, or 2%, relating to end of life.

Curricula for registered nurses devote an entire semester or quarter to maternity nursing yet only a very few hours to end of life care. End of life care is as important as beginning of life care. There have been advances in controlling pain during labor and delivery of an infant, but until recently very little attention has been devoted to controlling pain at the end of life. Since death is the expected and natural outcome of life, why has it not been given the attention needed to make it comfortable and peaceful?

Byock (1996) stated that it is essential that clinicians possess a fundamental knowledge of the issues involved with end of life care and basic competence in pain and symptom management. The End-of-Life Nursing Education Consortium (ELNEC) developed a 3 1/2-year project as a partnership of the American Association of Colleges of Nursing (AACN) and the City of Hope (COH) in Duarte, California. This project is a comprehensive national education program to improve end of life care by nurses and is being funded by a grant from the Robert Wood Johnson Foundation. Courses for nursing faculty will provide information and resources to expand the scope of end of life nursing care in nursing curricula. In conjunction with this project, research scientists at the City of Hope National Medical Center developed content guidelines for end of life care to assist authors/editors of nursing textbooks to cover essential, consistent end of life information (End-of-Life Nursing Education Consortium 2000). Curriculum change is necessary at the level of undergraduate medical and nursing education.

To society and health care professionals, death is seen as failure. Because of this attitude, health care professionals and society in general are hesitant about allowing people to die natural deaths. Advanced medical technology has been able to prolong life without consideration of how people are living. Medical physicians are specialized and seem to focus on their specialties. Consider the following:

A 78-year-old man is admitted to the hospital with a complaint of chest pain. An ECG reveals an acute myocardial infarction. This patient was taken to the cardiac lab and a heart catheterization was performed. It was decided that the patient requires coronary bypass surgery for a triple vessel bypass. The surgery was performed and the patient was admitted to the intensive care unit. The patient developed acute respiratory distress syndrome and a pulmonologist was consulted. The patient developed a gastric bleeding ulcer and a gastroenterologist was consulted. The patient then developed renal failure, a nephrologist was consulted, and hemodialysis was started. After several weeks the patient developed sacral decubiti and a skin care nurse was consulted. After six weeks of intensive care, the patient died of sepsis.

What's wrong with this picture? The patient had a cardiologist, cardiovascular surgeon, pulmonologist, nephrologist, gastroenterologist, skin care nurse, radiologists, and pathologists managing his care, yet he died of massive infection. This scenario is all too common in health care today. Patients have the very best available health care specialists to care for each problem that develops, but is anyone looking at the whole picture? Who is the primary physician? What are the patients' requests for end of life? Is the family well informed of the entire picture or only of what each specialist is reporting? Can the pieces of this puzzle be put together by the family, so they can make accurate and informed decisions?

Billions of dollars are spent in health care annually on situations just like this. The above patient not only died a painful and tragic death, but in the last few weeks of his life there was poor quality of life. Therefore we must address key questions. Have we become so specialized that we cannot care for the whole patient but rather only one particular problem that the patient is experiencing? Is it fair to deprive patients of the best quality of life at the end of their life because we cannot stop this cascade of events? Is medical and nursing education contributing to these scenarios and missing important aspects of the end of life experience? How can we enhance the quality of life for a patient such as this one?

PALLIATIVE CARE

Palliative care is the comprehensive care for patients with a terminal illness who are nearing the end of life. Several definitions of palliative care have been introduced. It is important to understand the difference between palliative care and curative care.

In 1990, the World Health Organization (WHO) defined palliative care as "the active total care of patients whose disease is not responsive to curative treatment. Control of pain, of other symptoms, and of psychological, social, and spiritual problems is paramount. The goal of palliative care is achievement of the best possible quality of life for patients and their families" (WHO 1990, 11–12). Table 1–1 includes characteristics of palliative care as defined by WHO.

Palliative care encompasses care of the body, mind, and spirit, and therefore represents a holistic approach to providing care. This approach means that one part of the body, mind, or spirit cannot be healed without the other (Brant 1998).

TABLE 1–1   CHARACTERISTICS OF PALLIATIVE CARE DEFINED BY THE WORLD HEALTH ORGANIZATION

- affirms life and regards dying as a normal process
- neither hastens death nor prolongs life
- provides relief from pain and other distressing symptoms
- integrates psychological and spiritual aspects of patient care
- offers a support system to help patients live as actively as possible until death
- offers a support system to help the family cope during the patient's illness and their own bereavement

---

Billings (1998, 80) defined palliative care as "comprehensive, interdisciplinary care, focusing primarily on promoting quality of life for patients living with a terminal illness and for their families." The interdisciplinary care in this definition includes elements of physical comfort, psychological comfort, social comfort, and spiritual support for the patient and the family.

Last Acts Task Force (1997) developed five precepts of palliative care, which incorporate these elements. They are

- respecting patient goals, preferences, and choices;
- comprehensive caring;
- utilizing the strengths of interdisciplinary resources;
- acknowledging and addressing caregiver concerns;
- building systems and mechanisms of support.

To achieve this focus in care, a multidisciplinary team approach is required. This team works collectively to meet patient challenges. Members of the team include physicians, nurses, social workers, counselors, chaplains, pharmacists, dieticians, physical therapists, occupational therapists, and volunteers. Patients and family members become members of the team and help to develop the plan of care. Palliative care can be provided in a variety of settings, such as hospitals, nursing homes, and patient homes. The most common form of palliative care is hospice. The hospice movement began in the United States in the 1960s. It has become accepted as a home care–based program that provides palliative care for dying patients and their families.

It still remains that nurses spend most of the time with the patient. Their role as coordinator of care includes assessing patients and referring identified problems to appropriate team members. This role is crucial to the success of the team approach. Communication is the foundation of the success for the team to provide care for the patient and family (Brant 1998).

QUALITY OF LIFE

The purpose of palliative care is to provide the best quality of life for the patient and family. Quality of life is a term used to describe the physical, psychosocial, and spiritual dimensions of a person's life.

At the beginning of this chapter, a medical case concerning a 78-year-old man was presented. In reviewing this case, the following questions must be asked: What quality of life did the patient have for the last few weeks? Was he physically comfortable? Were his psychosocial needs met? Were his spiritual needs met?

An obstetrician once said that he wholeheartedly supported epidural pain management during labor, so the mother could read a good book while laboring for the birth of her child. Most women would agree with this obstetrician, because by eliminating the associated pain, the experience would become more pleasant and comfortable. Would this same concept apply to the dying?

Byock (1996) ascertains that end of life offers an opportunity for tremendous growth and development. Although this period of growth may be difficult and require a great deal of effort and work on the part of the dying patient, it can lead to a profound benefit for the patient and family. Table 1–2 depicts developmental landmarks and tasks for the end of life. Patients and families can achieve the best quality of life during this time with help and support from palliative care teams. It is an ethical and moral obligation of health care providers to develop standards of care for the dying and to ensure that these standards are used to provide the best possible care. It is a privilege for a nurse to be able to provide and manage care of the dying. If the quality of life is the best possible, the nurse can achieve a wonderful sense of satisfaction.

SUMMARY

Caring for the dying is difficult, but it can also be a rewarding experience for the nurse as well as the patient and family. The palliative care team approach has proven to be the best method of assisting patients to a peaceful, comfortable death. Achieving developmental tasks can provide for the best quality of life for dying patients and their families. It is important for the nurse to consider not that patients have died, but that they died comfortably and peacefully.

"... I have learned that dying does not have to be agonizing. Physical suffering can always be alleviated. People need not die alone; many times the calm, caring presence of another can soothe a dying person's anguish. I think it is realistic to hope for a future in which nobody has to die alone and nobody has to die with their pain untreated. But comfort and companionship are not all there is. I have learned from my patients and their families a surprising truth about dying: this stage of life holds remarkable possibilities. Despite the arduous nature of the experience, when people are relatively comfortable and know that they are not going to be abandoned, they frequently find ways to strengthen bonds with people they love and to create moments of profound meaning in their final passage. ...

Being present as someone is dying tears the boundaries between the personal and professional realms of my being. The experience of a patient dying challenges me to accept a more intimate, and yet more deeply respectful relationship with that person. I do not know how it could be otherwise. While I may bring clinical skills and years of experience to the task, ultimately I am simply present, offering to help and wanting to learn."

Ira Byock, MD, author of *Dying Well*

TABLE 1–2 DEVELOPMENTAL LANDMARKS AND TASKS FOR THE END OF LIFE

- To control pain and other associated symptoms certainly improves the quality of life of a dying patient. Once the physical symptoms are controlled, the patient can then focus on psychosocial and spiritual aspects of life. Sense of completion with worldly affairs.
- Transfer of fiscal, legal, and formal social responsibilities.
- Sense of completion in relationships with community.
- Closure of multiple social relationships (employment, commerce, organizational, congregational). Components include: expressions of regret, expressions of forgiveness, acceptance of gratitude and appreciation.
- Leave taking; the saying of goodbye.
- Sense of meaning about one's individual life.
- Life review.
- The telling of "one's stories."
- Transmission of knowledge and wisdom.
- Experience love of self.
- Self-acknowledgment.
- Self-forgiveness.
- Experience love of others.
- Acceptance of worthiness.
- Sense of completion in relationships with family and friends.
- Reconciliation, fulness of communication and closure in each of one's important relationships. Component tasks include: expressions of regret, expressions of forgiveness and acceptance, expressions of gratitude and appreciation, acceptance of gratitude and appreciation, expression of affection.
- Acceptance of finality of life, of one's existence as an individual.
- Acknowledgment of the totality of personal loss represented by one's dying and experience of personal pain of existential loss.
- Expression of the depth of personal tragedy that dying represents.
- Decathexis (emotional withdrawal) from worldly affairs and cathexis (emotional connection) with an enduring construct.
- Acceptance of dependency.
- Sense of a new self (personhood) beyond personal loss.
- Sense of meaning about life in general.
- Achieving a sense of awe.
- Recognition of a transcendent realm.
- Developing and achieving a sense of comfort with chaos.
- Surrender to the transcendent, to the unknown—"letting go."

Note: From I. Byock, "The Nature of Suffering and the Nature of Opportunity at the End of Life," *Clinics in Geriatric Medicine* 12 (2) (1996): 237–250.

REFERENCES

Billings, J. A. (1998). What is palliative care? *Journal of Palliative Medicine.* 1(1):73–81.

Brant, J. (1998). The art of palliative care: Living with hope, dying with dignity. *Oncology Nursing Forum.* 25(6): 995–1004.

Byock, I. (1997). *Dying Well: The Prospect for Growth at the End of Life.* New York: Riverhead Books.

Byock, I. (1996). The nature of suffering and the nature of opportunity at the end of life. *Clinics in Geriatric Medicine.* 12(2):237–252.

End-of-Life Nursing Education Consortium (ELNEC). (2000). *Advancing end-of-life nursing care.* Washington, DC: Association of Colleges of Nursing.

Ferrell, B., Virani, R., & Grant, M. (1999). Analysis of end of life content in nursing textbooks. *Oncology Nursing Forum.* 26(5):869–876.

Last Acts Task Force. (1997). *Precepts of Palliative Care.* Princeton, N.J.: Author.

SUPPORT Study Principle Investigators. (1995). A controlled trial to improve care for seriously ill hospitalized patients: A study to understand prognoses and preferences for outcomes and risks of treatments. *Journal of the American Medical Association.* 274: 1591–1598.

Weissman, D., Mullan, P., Ambuel, B., Gunten, C.V., & Hallenback, J. (2000, June). *What do internal medicine faculty and residents know about end of life care?* Paper presented at the 12th Annual Assembly of the American Academy of Hospice and Palliative Medicine, Atlanta, GA.

World Health Organization (WHO). (1990). *Cancer pain relief and palliative care.* Technical Report Series 804. Geneva, Switzerland: Author.

Unit I

Introduction

Critical Thinking Activities

1. List 10 interventions to help enhance quality of life at the end of life
2. Differentiate the principles of palliative care from the traditional medical model
3. Discuss the need for focus on palliative care amidst the increased use of high technology medicine
4. List expected outcomes of palliative care

Teaching-Learning Exercises

1. Define quality of life among in-class discussion groups and compare ideas
2. Develop a nursing care plan utilizing principles of palliative care

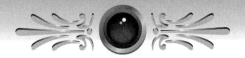

UNIT II

THEORETICAL FOUNDATIONS

Learning Objectives
1. Describe theories that relate to death and dying
2. Discuss application of nursing theories to palliative care
3. Define holistic models relative to end of life care

CHAPTER

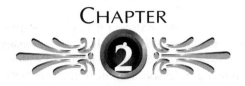

INTRODUCTION TO THEORETICAL FOUNDATIONS

Dr. Evelyn M. Wills

INTRODUCTION AND DEFINITIONS

Facing death brings people to either the pinnacle or the abyss of their lives. For most of us, death is an abstract notion. It gives rise to several other concepts: loss, grief, bereavement, mourning, and separation. As children we may live through the death of a beloved pet. This death gives rise to experiencing the emotions of loss and grief. Bereavement is the state of having lost someone beloved, and mourning takes place while individuals and families adjust to the loss. Until these are experienced firsthand they are abstract terms, the nature of which we have only a limited definition.

The work of Kubler-Ross in the late 1960s heralded the study of death and dying, and thanatology, as the realm of study came to be called (Rhodes and Vedder 1983), assumed theoretical importance. Theories for helping professions began to fill the need for structure in an area that had been avoided in the medical and nursing literature and given short shrift in the literature of other disciplines. The current resurgence of interest in theories of death and dying is welcome. As the so-called baby boom generation enters the phase of life in which the likelihood of death increases, the social changes that accompanied their generation may have changed the care of the dying. It is time for helping professionals to rethink the way we organize care for our ill, aging, and dying people and to study this important dimension of life.

Theories of death and dying help health care workers to explain what it is that the family and the loved ones are experiencing. Theories suggest ways to deal with the situation—how, as caregivers, we can care for our clients. Admittedly, if one has never experienced loss through death, theories are only guidelines, because the process remains a hypothetical one. This unit is about holistic models and applied theories of the processes of death and dying. Some of these theories were developed through deduction using established theories or conceptual models (Bowlby 1961; Dossey, Keegan, Kolkmeier, and

Guzzetta 1989; Lindemann 1944; Watson 1988), whereas others were the result of inductive methods through field data collection and analysis using qualitative methods (Kubler-Ross 1969). Some are included within models and theories developed in nursing (Erickson, Tomlin, and Swain 1983; Henderson 1966; Newman 1994; Watson 1988).

Definitions

Anticipatory grief is that suffering in expectation of the death of someone with whom one has a close relationship. It can soften the blow at the time of death and is preparation for the loss of the beloved one (DeVries 1997, Prigerson et al. 1997, Rando 1984).

Bereavement is the loss of a loved one, the state of no longer having the beloved one available, and is accompanied by pain, loss, and suffering (Rando 1984, Raphael 1983).

Death is the end of life. Many definitions exist for death and usually take the form of the science that is studying it (Rhodes and Vedder 1983). Medically it is the cessation of life functions supported by physiological tests that prove their absence both for medical as well as legal purposes. Although life ends for the client, it may mark a new era of learning for family members, but death may be greatly feared (Rando 1984).

Grief is a period of ambivalence after a death. It is a process of breaking the ties with the departed and reintegration through letting go of the lost one. There are stages of grief accompanied by varying levels of pain (Backer, Hannon, and Russell 1982; Prigerson, et al. 1997) and seeking for the lost one (Bowlby 1961).

Loss is the feeling of incompleteness left when a valued possession or person is no longer available. Loss is part of the grief pattern and requires that the person restructure life in ways that compensate for those valued things that the lost one brought to the relationship (Lundquist 1993).

Mourning is a natural occurrence among those who loved the individual who has died (Bowlby 1961, Rando 1984, Raphael 1983). It is a state of sorrow after a death and a public expression of grief, accompanied by prescribed rituals specific to each culture (Irish, Lundquist, and Nelson, 1993).

Pain is a physical component to the emotional reaction to the death of a loved one. These are natural consequences of the death and can be assuaged but cannot be eliminated (Prigerson et al. 1997, Rando 1984).

Separation after death is the natural consequence between two or more people who have developed a bond or an attachment through their relationship (Bowlby 1961, Rapheal 1983). It is accompanied by intense grief, mourning, sadness, crying, and pain (Rando 1984, Schorr 1983).

All of these and other terms may appear in theories of death. Understanding these concepts of the theories of death may lead to a better understanding of the topic and of the process.

REFERENCES

Backer, B. A., Hannon, N., & Russell, N. A. (1982). *Death and dying: Individuals and institutions*. New York: John Wiley & Sons.

Bowlby, J. (1961). Processes of mourning. *International Journal of Psychoanalysis, 42,* 317–340.

DeVries, B. (1997). Kinship bereavement in later life: Understanding variations in cause, courses, and consequences. *Omega, 35*(1), 141–157.

Dossey, B. M., Keegan, L., Kolkmeier, L. G., & Guzzetta, C. E. (1989). *Holistic health promotion: A guide for practice*. Rockville, MD: Aspen Publishers, Inc.

Erickson, H. C., Tomlin, E. M., & Swain, M. A. (1983). *Modeling and role modeling: A theory and paradigm for nursing*. Englewood Cliffs, NJ: Prentice Hall.

Henderson, V. (1966). *The nature of nursing: A definition and its implications for practice, research, and education*. New York: Macmillan.

Irish, D. P., Lundquist, K. F., & Nelson, V. J. (1993). *Ethnic variations in dying, death, and grief*. Washington, DC: Taylor & Francis.

Kubler-Ross, E. (1969). *On death and dying*. New York: Macmillan.

Lindemann, E. (1944). Symptomatology and management of acute grief. *American Journal of Psychiatry, 101,* 141–148.

Lundquist, K. F. (1993). Personal reflections on death, grief, and cultural diversity. In D. P. Irish, K. F. Lundquist, & V. J. Nelson (Eds.), *Ethnic variations in dying, death, and grief*. (pp. 29–47). Washington, DC: Taylor & Francis.

Newman, M. (1994). *Health as expending consciousness* (2nd ed.). New York: National League for Nursing Press.

Prigerson, H. G., Wolfson, L., Shear, M. K., Hall, M., Bierhals, A. J., Zonarich, D. L., Pilkonis, P. A., & Reynolds, C. F. (1997). Case histories of traumatic grief. *Omega, 35*(1), 9–24.

Rando, T. A. (1984). *Grief, dying and death: Clinical interventions for care givers*. Champagne, IL: Research Press, Inc.

Rapheal, B. (1983). *The anatomy of bereavement*. New York: Basic Books, Inc.

Rhodes, C., & Vedder, C. B. (1983). *An introduction to thanatology: Death and dying in American Society*. Springfield, IL: Charles C. Thomas.

Schorr, J. A. (1983). Manifestations of consciousness and the developmental phenomenon of death. *Advances in nursing science 6*(1), 26–35.

Watson, J. (1988). *Nursing: Human science and human care: A theory of nursing*. New York: National League for Nursing Press.

REFERENCES

CHAPTER

HOLISTIC MODELS

Dr. Evelyn M. Wills

Models of nursing that structure the requisites of the clients such that no dimension of care is omitted are labeled holistic; whether physical, psychological, emotional, spiritual, or cultural, holistic care is a value. Controversies exist as to whether true holistic care is possible (Fuller 1978, Silva and Rothbart 1984); nevertheless, the nurse strives to care for the client as completely as possible.

Nightingale (1969) stated that nursing's function was to help the client get to the point where nature could take its course in healing that person. Henderson (1966) added that nurses assist clients sick or well with activities that they would do for themselves—whether they contribute to health or a peaceful death—if they had the necessary means. Both of these early nurse educators considered the client a whole person to the extent that they understood that concept in their respective eras.

Holistic models of nursing have explicitly guided nursing education, research, and practice for more than four decades. Prior to this time, nurses worked as handmaidens to physicians and therefore accepted the medical model of health and disease, and the medical, surgical, and pharmacological cures available at that time (Chinn and Kramer 1999).

Nightingale defined nursing as a profession separate from and not under the control of medicine. Nursing in 1860 was concerned with the functions of sanitation and nurturance of the whole person including physical, emotional, and social needs (Chinn and Kramer 1999; Nightingale 1969). Abdallah and Henderson, two early nurse educators, wrote that the patient was a person who had biological and psychological needs and Abdallah and Henderson recognized social and spiritual needs (Alexander et al. 1998, Haltermann et al. 1998). Later theorists developed these ideas to produce true holistic models and theories of nursing.

Rogers (1970, 1980, 1990) in her enlightened theory identified man as a unitary human being, as more and greater than the sum of parts, increasing in complexity, and in continuous interaction with the environment. The theory of unitary man became the science of unitary human beings and is the basis of other open system theories (Newman 1994, Parse 1987). Dying was conceptualized by Rogers (1980, 335) as a "rhythmical developmental process" of the human-environmental energy field, and in this transformation the four-dimensional nature of human energy fields is readily apparent. McEvoy's (1990) research indicated that paranormal events—including out-of-body and apparitional experiences—may accompany dying. Many people have recounted their life-threatening experiences after resuscitation as near-death experiences (Kubler-Ross 1982). Most of these experiences provided the individuals with a sense of comfort and hope, with a firm resolve to make the most of their remaining time. No theoretical stance in nursing literature explains these near-death experiences except that defined by Rogers in the science of unitary human beings.

At the end of life, holistic models and theories allow humanistic consideration of multiple dimensions of client care. The more elements of care that are included, the more comfort is possible for client and family. In the wisdom of several nursing theorists (Erickson, Tomlin, and Swain 1983; King 1981; Watson 1988), the nurse's process is also considered important. Death is as powerful a process for the nurse as it is for the client and family, although in differing ways.

HOLISTIC NURSING MODELS AND END OF LIFE CARE

To many practitioners, the science of unitary human beings (Rogers 1990) is abstract enough that application to practice remains difficult. Rogers probably did not mean for the science of unitary human beings to apply to day-to-day health care, rather to instruct the health care giver's vision of what it means to be human. The human-focused theorists (Erickson, Tomlin, and Swain 1983; Watson 1988) have made holistic nursing usable in practice.

Watson's (1988, 58) elucidation of caring as a transpersonal interaction in which the nurse and client are united in the moment of care is termed "the caring occasion." Both client and nurse are composites of spiritual, emotional, and physical dimensions, and are mentally and emotionally present to each other in the caring moment. Watson's ideal is that the nurse attends to the dignity of the person in the "caring occasion," which she labels "transpersonal care," and this is the true essence of nursing. The full participation of both the client and nurse as persons requires a knowledge of the needs, strengths, and limitations of clients and the meaning of the situation for them. The nurse requires a full knowledge of comforting measures and the intention to care and is encouraged to bring knowledge of self and willingness to be authentic in the presence of the client.

The interventions in this model are referred to as carative factors, (Watson 1988, 75) of which there are 10:

1. humanistic-altruistic system of values
2. faith and hope
3. sensitivity to self and others
4. helping, trusting, human care relationship

5. expressing positive and negative feelings
6. creative problem solving
7. transpersonal teaching and learning
8. supportive, protective, or corrective environment
9. human needs assistance
10. existential-phenomenological-spiritual forces

The outcome of transpersonal care is that both the client's and nurse's dignity and integrity are preserved and that the occasion in which care occurs involves a relationship between client and nurse.

Watson's transpersonal caring model is in use with clients dying of AIDS in the Center for Human Caring, Denver, Colorado. Clients of this program attest to the value of humanistic caring in their progress through the process of their disease (Neil 1990).

Holistic models of nursing place client and nurse into an interaction that encompasses the health care system and the client-family. Often the client is within the hospital or nursing facility at the time of death. Some people choose to die at home, attended by special duty nurses or family. Other patients may die in nursing homes, which are organized to support patients and families at the time of death (Castle 1998). Regrettably some people die alone.

The moment of death is a powerful time in every model of health care that considers death at all. Erickson, Tomlin, and Swain (1983) agree that nurses involved in end of life care should allow clients and families to have control of the situation, that nurses care empathetically for them, and that the experience develops such that all have their spiritual needs fulfilled. Watson (1988) agrees that the spiritual side of grief and loss is an important occasion of caring in which the health professional fully participates as a member of the experience. Supporting the client and family in living the experience to a positive outcome allows the occasion of loss to become meaningful in the spiritual process for all individuals involved.

MULTIDISCIPLINARY MODELS AND THEORIES AND END OF LIFE CARE

Although physicians and nurses are likely to be in attendance at the time of death, other professionals are equipped to come to the aid of families during the dying experience as well. Family counselors, psychologists, social workers and clergy and pastoral care specialists all are available for counseling and grief care at that difficult time.

Elizabeth Kubler-Ross, a psychiatrist, interviewed very ill and dying patients in a large hospital and from this experience distilled a five-stage model of the patients' process of facing death and dying. This was an inductive theory; it was probably not the first attempt to theorize about death and dying, however it was grounded in scientific methods and was a breakthrough in the attempt to comprehend the world of those going through the process. Kubler-Ross (1969) found that initially patients who were very ill did not agree they were dying; they denied the possibility and seemed to build defenses to avoid the self-revelation of the seriousness of the problem. She also showed that patients were likely to retreat into denial even though they had entered a later stage in the process. Therefore, she indicated that patients often advanced and retreated into and out of denial, and might remain in denial to the end.

Kubler-Ross (1969, 50) found the second stage of the process to be anger. In this stage, she found the patients, who could no longer deny the seriousness of their condition, to be communicating "anger, rage, envy, and resentment. The logical next question in the process was 'why me?'" Kubler-Ross found that this stage was difficult for families and professionals to deal with since the anger was generalized to all who came in contact with the patient. She saw the avoidance that this stage led to and cautioned professionals to consider the state the patient was facing: This patient's life goals were being left unaccomplished, plans would never be fulfilled, and unpleasant treatments and tests had to be endured. Kubler-Ross begged that health care workers attend patients with respect and attention, giving the patient time to ventilate the frustrations of this stage. Meeting the needs of patients during the anger stage can have fruitful results for patient, family, and health care workers.

The third stage she called bargaining. In this stage, she found the patients offering some sacrifice for an extension of their lives or relief of pain or discomfort, even to attend an event which had been planned. Few of these patients kept the bargain, according to Kubler-Ross, and she stated it is a necessary stage for some to assuage their guilt over life events or omissions. She found it helpful with patients who were in the bargaining phase to have a multidisciplinary team to assist them in working through this stage.

Depression, the fourth stage of which Kubler-Ross (1969, 86) wrote, was viewed as being of two differing types. The first is the "reactive" type, seen when the losses mount up and the patient is confronted by the many problems posed by the disease. The second type of depression is a "preparatory" state, which patients go through as they view impending losses and prepare for the next stage. Kubler-Ross saw this stage as necessary preparation for the fifth stage: acceptance.

In the stage of acceptance, the patient had found some peace and was withdrawing into the self. The depression had been worked out and although the patient was weak and ever more tired, there was the impression of relief, as in a void. There was a detachment from those things that must be left unfinished and those loved ones who would remain behind. Kubler-Ross indicated that at this time the patient's loved ones probably needed more from the health care team than did the patient.

Although Kubler-Ross did not call this a theory of dying, nevertheless it has been extensively applied to the care of dying patients by nurses and other health care workers. Her stage model brings coherence to the otherwise chaotic process perceived by those who attend the dying. No doubt nurses and physicians who were sensitized to the needs of the dying by the work of Kubler-Ross, her students, and colleagues felt great relief to learn that there was a pattern to the final stage of life. Likely they were grateful for her insights on ways to attend the patients in this difficult time. Several writers have commented on and disputed Kubler-Ross's work, but its benefits as a heuristic for educating practitioners are important to recognize.

McClowry, Davies, May, Kulenkamp, and Martinson (1995, 149) identified the phenomenon of "the empty space" in a grounded theory research project in which they enrolled the same families who had been part of a two-year research project after the death of a child. The research took place seven to nine years after the death had occurred, and 49 of the original families took part. The theoretical structure that resulted indicated that three distinct patterns of response were expressed by the participants. The first pattern, getting over it, was seen as a matter-of-fact acceptance of the death which was not accompanied by intense or vivid memories of the deceased. The second pattern, filling the emptiness, was one of substituting activities to fill the void created by the death. Activities included such things as building a new home, divorce, adopting other children, creating altruistic works, or substituting food or drink for the lost child. The third pattern, keeping the connection, was described by those who did not get over the loss; rather, they cherished their recollections of the child, and these individuals "continue to reserve a small part of themselves for the loss of a special relationship which they view as irreplaceable (Martinson et al. 1986, 156). The phenomenon of the empty space assists the health care provider in comprehending those who still speak of and long for their loved one but have put their lives in order and are carrying on. This is in direct opposition to the theories of morbid grief (Mawson, Marks, Ramm, and Stern 1981). This model fills in the differences for the health care worker and enables the view that a person may still maintain an open place for the lost loved one without demonstrating emotional pathology.

Brabant's work (1996) is not touted as a theory, but it has the aspects of a model that can guide health care workers. Her vision of the period after death, the grieving period, is that of mending the torn fabric of a life changed by the death of a loved one. She writes of "places" (p. 10) "in which many people may spend time" (p. 16). In contrast to stage theories in which the person must complete the work of each stage in order to move along to the next, the person revisits the places intermittently, although in differing ways. Brabant redefines denial—which Kubler-Ross (1969) indicated was a walling off of consciousness from the loss—into a place of resting, a gift as the bereaved person gathers the self for the next place.

Anger is visualized by Brabant (1996) as total attention to the rage engendered by the loss, which leads to complete involvement in that place. She shows that the anger is value free and simply an emotion that is authentic and one of the places the bereaved person may spend time and may return to in similar or differing ways.

Brabant defines depression as a place that may require medical assistance to move out of, or as a place in which to release anger. She indicates that in either case, some outside assistance may be necessary lest the grieving person minimize the problem and the process of mending be halted.

Sadness to Brabant (1996, 20) is a place in which the grieving person can review the "fabric as it was before it was torn" and may be a place entered and reentered as needed to give emotional release. The crying engendered by sadness may even rid the body of chemicals manufactured during stress, she maintains.

Relief is a place to Brabant that, while sought out, may be problematic for some, since feeling relief over a death of a loved one may bring guilt. She shows that relief, like anger and denial, is an emotion that is acceptable and has its part in the mending process.

Brabant (1996) also defines fear and jealousy as places that the grieving person goes, each having its part in the mending.

Acceptance is the process of mending, rather than being a specific place, and one may go in and out of acceptance; each person will find this process in his or her own way (Brabant 1996).

Brabant gives two places to avoid—shame and guilt—indicating that climbing from these places may help the person avoid them in the future. Several paths may lead to the places persons who are mending should avoid. Cultural background may provide guidelines as to socially acceptable funerary practices and ways to grieve, but may also provide the seeds of shame and guilt. The person's history and the way other people define the bereaved person's loss may lead to shame and guilt. The pathway of the relationship with the person who died can end in shame and guilt. Brabant gives advice to the mending person on ways to avoid these problem places.

Needles and threads for the mending are defined, complicated mending is covered, and possibilities for assistance and support are given (Brabant 1996). She defines the mended fabric and indicates that although the fabric of the person's life is mended and can never be the same, it may be even more beautiful with the tears and the mends.

Although Brabant's mending the torn fabric model was not designed as a theory, it does frame the process of grieving and can be a guide to those who are grieving and to those who want to help them. While the largest proportion of people who will suffer the loss of a loved one are wives of elderly men (Beery et al. 1997), mending the torn fabric brings in the familiar to explain the difficult. This is one useful aspect of theory: It explains the abstract in terms of the real.

A CASE OF CARE AT THE END OF LIFE

A woman who had been with her mother at the time of death recounted the following situation. Even though the mother had reached the stage of acceptance of her death, the younger sister could not agree that her mother was dying. The younger sister insisted on life prolonging measures far after the signs of brain death had been diagnosed, prolonging the agony for the rest of the family. Finally, after long talks with her father, her eldest sister, and a nurse, the grieving woman allowed life support measures to be removed and the mother died quietly during the night. Just two years later, the father of the two women was diagnosed with a fast-growing cancer and lived just four months. He was given the best of care in a military hospital and died in the eldest sister's arms during the night. The younger sister resisted visiting her dying father until the very last day of his life. He became lucid, which he had not been for some days, in honor of her visit. She refused to believe that he was as ill as he actually was and flew home the next day. That night he died. She flew into a rage when she was called with the report of his death and charged her sister with many things. The elder sister took it in stride; as a nurse, she was familiar with the stages of death as Kubler-Ross has outlined, and this knowledge helped her to understand her sister. After the funeral, the sisters and a support team made up of other family members, pastoral care personnel from the hospital, and their own pastor worked to come to terms with the loss and the grief of each of them. The elder sister was comforted by the assistance, but the younger sister returned home still in a state of anger. Many years later, the sisters again spoke of the deaths of their mother and father. By this time, the younger sister had healed sufficiently to show acceptance and understanding. The accumulation of the loss of both her parents within a two-year period and the meanings that these sudden-seeming deaths had for the younger sister had overwhelmed her. She had not had the frame of reference that her elder sister had for comprehending the events, and she needed time with her grief.

SUMMARY

This chapter has been a description of several models and theories from nursing and other disciplines and their value in describing death and grieving. These theories are by no means the only theories that treat this realm of life. Watson's theory of transpersonal caring in nursing, Kubler-Ross's death and dying work, McLowry's spaces model, and Brabant's mending the torn fabric model all have the potential to assist health care workers in bringing care and relief to those suffering loss from death. The next chapter will assist in using some of the theoretical material in caring for persons who are experiencing dying and grieving.

REFERENCES

Alexander, J. F., De Meester, D. W., Laur, T., Tomer, A. M., Neal, S. E., & Williams, S. (1998). Virginia Henderson: Definition of nursing. In A. M. Tomey & M. R. Alligood (Eds.), *Nursing Theorists and Their Work* (pp. 99–111). St. Louis, MO: Mosby-Year Book, Inc.

Backer, B. A., Hannon, N., & Russell, N. A (1982) *Death and dying: Individuals and institutions*. New York: John Wiley & Sons.

Beery, L. C., Prigerson, H. G., Bierhals, A. J., Santucci, L. M., Newson, J. T., Maciejewski, P. K., Rapp, S. R., Fasiczka, A., & Reynolds, C. F. (1997). Traumatic grief, depression and caregiving in elderly spouses of the terminally ill. *Omega*, 35(3), 261–279.

Bowlby, J. (1961). Processes of mourning. *International Journal of Psychoanalysis*, 42, 317–340.

Brabant, S. (1996). *Mending the torn fabric*. Amityville, NY: Baywood Publishing Company Inc.

Castle, N. G. (1998). Innovations in dying in the nursing home: The impact of market characteristics. *Omega*, 36(3), 227–240.

Chinn, P. L., & Kramer, M. K. (1999). *Theory and nursing: Integrated knowledge development*. St. Louis, MO: Mosby, Inc.

DeVries, B. (1997). Kinship bereavement in later life: Understanding variations in cause, courses and consequences. *Omega*, 35(1), 141–157.

Dossey, B. M., Keegan, L., Kolkmeier, L. G., & Guzzetta, C. E. (1989). *Holistic health promotion: A guide for practice*. Rockville, MD: Aspen Publishers, Inc.

Erickson, H. C., Tomlin, E. M., & Swain, M. A. (1983). *Modeling and role modeling: A theory and paradigm for nursing*. Englewood Cliffs, NJ: Prentice Hall.

Fuller, S. S. (1978). Holistic man and the science and practice of nursing. *Nursing Outlook*, 26(11), 700–704.

Halterman, T. D., Dycus, D. K., McClure, E. A., Schmeiser, D. N., Taggart, F. M., & Yancey, R. (1998). Faye Glenn Abdellah: Twenty-one nursing problems. In A. M. Tomey & M. R. Alligood (Eds.), *Nursing Theorists and Their Work*. St. Louis, MO: Mosby-Year Book, Inc.

Henderson, V. (1966). *The nature of nursing: A definition and its implications for practice, research, and education*. New York: Macmillan.

Irish, D. P., Lundquist, K. F., & Nelsen, V. J. (1993). *Ethnic variations in dying, death, and grief*. Washington, DC: Taylor & Francis.

King, I. M. (1981). *A theory for nursing: Systems, concepts, process*. New York: John Wiley & Sons.

Kubler-Ross, E. (1969). *On death and dying*. New York: Macmillan Publishing Co, Inc.

Kubler-Ross, E. (1982). *Working it through*. New York: Macmillan.

Lindemann, E. (1944). Symptomatology and management of acute grief. *American Journal of Psychiatry*, 101, 141–148.

Martinson, I. M., Moldow, D. G., Armstrong, G. D., Henry, W. F., Nesbit, M. E., & Kersey, J. H. (1986). Home care for children dying of cancer. *Research in Nursing and Health*, 9, 11–16.

Mawson, D., Marks, I., Ramm, L., & Stern, R. (1981). Guided mourning for controlled grief. *The British Journal of Psychiatry*, 138, 185–193.

McClowry, S. G., Davies, E. B., May, K. A., Kulenkamp, E. J., & Martinson, I. M. (1995). The empty space phenomenon: The process of grief in the bereaved family. In K. J. Doka (Ed.), *Children Mourning Children*. (pp. 149–162) Washington, DC: Hospice Foundation of America.

McEvoy, M. D. (1990). The relationships among the experience of dying, the experience of paranormal events, and creativity in adults. In E. A. M. Barrett (Ed.), *Visions of Rogers' Science-Based Nursing* (pp. 209–228). New York: National League for Nursing Press.

Neil, R. (1990) Watson's theory of caring in nursing: The rainbow of and for people living with AIDS. In M. E. Parker (Ed.), *Nursing Theories in Practice* (pp. 289–301). New York: National League for Nursing.

Newman, M. (1994). *Health as expending consciousness* (2nd ed.). New York: National League for Nursing Press.

Nightingale, F. (1969). *Notes on nursing: What it is and what it is not.* New York: Dover Publications, Inc. (Original work published 1860).

Parse, R. R. (1987). *Nursing science: Major paradigms, theories and critiques.* Philadelphia, PA: W. B. Saunders.

Prigerson, H. G., Wolfson, L., Shear, M. K., Hall, M. Bierhals. A. J., Zonarich, D. L., Pilkonis, P. A, & Reynolds, C. F. (1997). Case histories of traumatic grief. *Omega*, 35(1), 9–24.

Rando, T. A. (1984). *Grief, dying and death: Clinical interventions for care givers.* Champagne IL: Research Press, Inc.

Rapheal, B. (1983). *The anatomy of bereavement.* New York: Basic Books.

Rhodes, C., & Vedder, C. B. (1983). *An introduction to thanatology: Death and dying in American society.* Springfield, IL: Charles C. Thomas, Publisher.

Rogers, M. E. (1970). *Introduction to the theoretical basis of nursing.* Philadelphia PA: F.A. Davis, Company.

Rogers, M. E. (1980). Nursing: a science of unitary man. In J. P. Riehl & C. Roy (Eds.), *Conceptual models for nursing practice* (2nd ed.) (pp. 329–337). New York: Appleton-Century-Crofts.

Rogers, M. E. (1990). Nursing: Science of unitary, irreducible, human beings: Update 1990. In E. A. M. Barrett (Ed), *Visions of Rogers' science-based nursing* (pp. 5–11). New York: National League for Nursing Press.

Schorr, J. A. (1983). Manifestations of consciousness and the developmental phenomenon of death. *Advances in Nursing Science,* 6 (1), 26–35.

Silva, M. C., & Rothbart, D. (1984). An analysis of changing trends in philosophies of science on nursing theory development and testing. *Advances in Nursing Science,* 6(2), 1–13.

Watson, J. (1988). *Nursing: Human science and human care. A theory of nursing.* New York: National League for Nursing Press.

APPLICATIONS OF THEORIES TO NURSING

Dr. Evelyn M. Wills

Theories that are based in practice, are tested in practice and research (Meleis 1997), and are of the prescriptive type (Dickoff, James, and Wiedenbach 1968) are probably the most useful at the end of life, especially for practitioners who are new to their discipline. Tested theories are not common, and therefore it is seldom that experienced nurses or other practitioners will label their care as corresponding to a particular theoretical perspective. Rather, the practitioner will work within a frame of reference (paradigm or philosophy) and use ideas and concepts from several theories and even from several disciplines. Nurses often combine theoretical materials from biology, psychology, sociology, and anthropology, as well as nursing and medicine to bring coherence to their work with the dying (Krisman-Scott 2000).

SOME THEORIES THAT ARE USEFUL IN END OF LIFE CARE

Brabant's (1996) work on "mending the torn fabric" has been used by her and others in assisting the grieving after a death has occurred. Brabant gives cases in her text showing outcomes of the grief work that has been done. This is a most useful model to help grieving families and significant others. Sarah Brabant, a sociologist, uses this work in counseling and in workshops. Her term *places* in the grieving process shows that there is some order in the grieving process without it being rigid; it considers that every person who is grieving will proceed differently to a healthy conclusion, although some may require assistance in leaving some toxic places.

Kubler-Ross's (1969, 1975) model of the stages of dying was a breakthrough for health care workers and made a difficult process open to study. She held extensive workshops and taught her perspective in five day long retreat-type settings and in shorter workshops and conferences. Her methods are still being studied and used and contribute to the completion of the grieving process.

A nursing theory that can guide nurses in the ways of caring for dying clients and grieving family members is Watson's theory of transpersonal caring. It is one of few in use in the nursing arena that deals with dying individuals. The components of this theory that help a nurse to integrate it into practice include the high regard for the whole person, protection of dignity, and the effort to gain insights into the patient's being-in-the-world through the "simple to complex human to human care process" (Watson, 1988, 63). The process takes time and concentration on the part of the nurse and may be too intense a relationship for the staff nurse working with many other extremely ill clients on a general service within a hospital. For nurses engaged in one-on-one care such as in a hospice or home care relationship, the holistic process of a reality-based perspective on the dying patient and the grieving family seems an excellent method.

INTERVENING AT THE END OF LIFE: A NURSING PERSPECTIVE

Disclosure of the impending terminal status of clients has not been a tradition in American health care. Krisman-Scott (2000) sees this as inappropriate because knowing about one's impending death allows the individual and loved ones to make appropriate plans, to prepare to manage the end of life, and to make choices about death. To nurses, disclosure of terminal status has typically been the prerogative of the physician. Although this is changing, nurses and professionals other than physicians typically do not inform the client of his or her terminal status. In order to fulfill Henderson's (1969) definition of nursing, that care contributes to a peaceful death when the ability to promote independence has faded, nurses or other professionals can perform in a consultant role to physicians who have difficulty disclosing terminal status to their patients. Knowledge of terminal status allows clients to grieve their imminent mortality and to make the necessary plans and decisions for the families. It is decried as deception by Kalisch (1971) when the patient is not told of the inevitability of death by the physician, yet to this day, many physicians still do not take this responsibility. Krisman-Scott states this is still an unclear area of practice in nursing and other disciplines. Nurses can be of service to other disciplines and to the physician through their careful and complete reporting of the events noted in their patient care that indicate a patient-family's readiness to deal with disclosure of impending death. Such events include patients claiming that they are "tired of being tired," "not long for this world," "looking forward to returning home," and other such verbalizations. Other clues to this readiness might be patients making lists of things to be given to certain family members, putting money and possessions into their successors hands, and asking to speak to family members who are at long distances away. According to several writers, patients have a knowledge that their death is near (Kalisch 1971, Kubler-Ross 1969) and will make plans to accommodate their last wishes. Nurses and other practitioners can help and support these plans by making telephone calls, telling family members what the patient would like, and, of course, notifying the physician of these findings.

Structuring End of Life Care Meaningfully Using a Holistic Model

This section is structured according to the process used by nurses almost universally and termed *the nursing process*. This is a logical problem-oriented method of structuring nursing care of patients and is outcome-based in that evaluation of the outcome is an integral part of the process. Each nursing theorist has constructed a process that coincides with the theory's concepts. Here a commonly used four-step process is given as a structure to insure that holistic care is provided.

Assessing the Client Family Holistically

Care planning using a holistic model means listening to client and family considering not only the biological and physical needs. To assess holistically means to consider the psychological, behavioral, and emotional situation of the client and family, which may be expressed differently, and to assess the cultural and spiritual needs of the client family (Irish, Lundquist, and Nelsen 1993). As much as possible the assessment should include cues to spiritual problems, such as negative verbalizations about God, so that the nurse can consult with other disciplines when needed. The patient's awareness of impending death should be assessed in the gentlest ways possible, recalling the information that many already suspect that they are terminal. The meaning of this particular death to the family is important, and this knowledge will allow the nurse to give more holistic care to the client and family (Watson 1988). It is important to note that there will be many meanings which will differ among the family members and that it may not be possible to learn of all of them. It is certain that the meaning will not be accessible to the nurse the first time an assessment is attempted. Watson indicates that only through union between client and nurse is holistic care possible. This bond or union can only be established through a developing relationship between client and nurse during frequent "caring occasions" (Watson 1988, 58).

Patients' desires about their care should be assessed and these desires communicated to other professionals and the family. Noting the attachment status of each family member to the dying client is important, determining those who are grieving but comfortable with the situation, those who are in other stages, and those who reject the idea that their family member will die. Since Kubler-Ross found that the families also traverse the continuum from denial to acceptance, care of each member wherever they stand is important in the care of the dying (Kubler-Ross, 1969, 1975).

Planning Care with the Client Family

The client and family must always be included in planning care at the end of life. The dying client should be assisted in having any desired control over the situation (Erickson, Tomlin, and Swain 1983, Krisman-Scott 2000). In the event that dying clients are unable to express their wishes, the selected next of kin should be consulted. Appropriate and complete physical care should be planned and dying clients never neglected, but interventions regarding nutrition and hydration, medication, and other therapies should be planned in consultation with client, family, nurse, and physician.

Clients and their families should be able to express their desires regarding the plans of the nurse and other professionals and have their wishes to provide aspects of the care seriously considered. Often family members experience great relief when allowed to provide some aspect of care to their loved ones; other family members may feel overwhelmed by this. Provisions should be made for respite for those who are grieving while caring for their dying loved ones. Nurses can assist in planning needed time away from the sick bed for a caregiver.

Intervening Holistically with the Client Family

It is important to provide for continuity of care, with the same nurses visiting over the course of the process. To fulfill the theories of holistic care of the dying, the nurses and other professionals rendering care need the contact that will give them the understanding of these particular clients to assess and intervene effectively. (Watson 1988; Erickson, Tomlin, and Swain 1983). Part-time personnel who do not know and understand the situation and are not properly oriented to the particular family's needs should never be sent to the home to give care. A cadre of nurses should assume a team responsibility for end of life care and carefully keep each member updated.

Pastoral care is usually a part of the hospital experience, but in the home care or hospice situation the nurse may feel impelled to call on the patient's spiritual advisor when confronted by situations that seem untenable. Many nurses may not feel competent to deal with spiritual problems with which they are unfamiliar.

Cultural care at the time of death and throughout the period of grief is important. People of every culture grieve differently, and the grief and mourning needs of each should be respected. Cultural diversity material may not be a part of the education of some levels of health care personnel and the differences in the client's culture from their own may be confusing. The agency that is providing holistic care is well advised to provide cultural information and sensitivity training to its practitioners to meet these needs of patients (Irish, Lundquist, and Nelsen 1993).

Evaluating Holistic Care Given to Clients and Family

Outcome of care is the standard by which health care is commonly evaluated (Kane 1998). The process of outcomes evaluation is a means of measuring the holistic nature of the care. Standardized self-report surveys, telephone surveys, and mailed questionnaires are possible methods of evaluation. Most often the information sought is simply a measure of acceptance of care and of satisfaction. According to Kane, these are subjective and of little value in determining actual quality of care. The Medical Outcomes Study (MOS) SF36 questionnaire is a standardized instrument which was developed using a holistic model, including the client's feeling of health (McHorney, Ware, Rogers, Raczek, and Lu 1992). It is less impacted by satisfaction with the care than many hospital marketing department-generated measures, but may best be used as a before–after measurement tool. The patient's satisfaction with nursing care is difficult to measure in hospitals because patient and family may have contact with many different, unidentifiable workers. But in home care and hospice care where an identifiable team of caregivers is present, measuring client-family satisfaction with the care is more reasonable. Measurement of care during the dying process is fraught with emotion, and many agencies, realizing this, forgo measuring outcomes to avoid further adding to the client-family grief. This may be legitimate, but clients and families should be able to have a feedback method to critique the quality of care received.

CARE AT THE END OF A LIFE: A CASE STUDY

Mrs. H., the wife of a prominent attorney in a medium-sized community was being treated for breast cancer. She was a socialite from a well-placed family whose life up to that time had gone as she had planned. She lived in a beautiful home, had two beautiful children, and the family appeared to be living a life suited to a spread in House Beautiful. *Mrs. H. rejected the idea of chemotherapeutic drugs and eventually began to lose ground to the ravages of the cancer. She denied that she would die of the cancer and consistently spoke of when she would be healed.*

She was being cared for by a home health agency in which a team of nurses were her caregivers. To relieve her pain, an intravenous medication device had been implanted into her upper chest through which she was being given constant infusions of a narcotic. She could also administer additional medication to herself using the equipment provided. The nurses visited on a regular schedule to care for her and the equipment. These excellent caregivers educated the family on when to call them and what needs would bring the nurse to the home at unscheduled times. The nurses reported faithfully to each other on the needs of Mrs. H and the family. Their work with Mrs. H. in coming to terms with her future mortality was stymied by her insistence that the problem would be resolved when she got her strength back and it would go away—an idea she held until the day she died.

On one weekend, a part-time nurse was given the assignment of going to the home and caring for and changing the intravenous equipment. Since there was an illness among the team of nurses, this substitute nurse did not get a complete report on the needs of the patient and family. When she arrived at the home, the client asked where "her nurses" were and the substitute nurse informed her that her usual nurse was ill. The substitute nurse attempted to do the care and was unsuccessful with the equipment for which she had been inadequately oriented to care. She called her backup nurse who came to the home and assisted in completing the care. Later the family called the agency complaining that the care by the substitute nurse was not satisfactory.

This family had come to expect a continuity of care that was not delivered. Their experience with the nursing team was one of concern, and the caring moments they were accustomed to were missing with the substitute nurse who was incompletely oriented to their needs. In the theory of transpersonal caring, the nurse would have been oriented to the ways the client family liked the care to be given, and the emotional and grief work that had gone before would have been brought to the nurse's attention. The nurse would have adjusted her care to the needs of the family and all would have had a more positive experience. If the nurse had been familiar with the transpersonal caring theory (Watson 1988), she would have paused initially to work with the client to create a caring occasion prior to trying to give the physical care. When she had equipment problems, they could have discussed it and resolved the fear that the nurse was not competent and helped the client come to realize that there was just an equipment problem. If these things had been done, the caring occasion would have had a more positive tone for both client and nurse, and the outcome would have been more satisfying.

SUMMARY

Holistic care at the end of life is an opportunity for the health care giver to bring comfort to the dying client and the grieving family and, if guided by realistic theoretical grounding, can bring lasting comfort to each member of the process. Theories abound in nursing and other disciplines, but few provide guidance for the care of the dying and grieving. In this unit the author has attempted to familiarize the reader with theoretical perspectives that can assist in providing complete and realistic care to dying clients and their families. Means to enact this care in concert with these theories have also been suggested. The care of the dying and the grieving family at the end of life is sometimes frightening and always meaning filled work.

REFERENCES

Brabant, S. (1996). *Mending the torn fabric.* Amityville, NY: Baywood Publishing Company, Inc.

Dickhoff, J., James, P., & Wiedenbach, E. (1968). Theory in a practice discipline, part I: Practice oriented theory. *Nursing Research, 17,* 415–435.

Erickson, H. C., Tomlin, E. M., & Swain, M. A. (1983). *Modeling and role modeling: A theory and paradigm for nursing.* Englewood Cliffs, NJ: Prentice Hall.

Henderson, V. (1969). *The nature of nursing: A definition and its implications for practice, research, and education.* New York: Macmillan.

Irish, D. P., Lundquist, K. F., & Nelsen, V. J. (1993). *Ethnic variations in dying, death, grief: Diversity in universality.* Bristol, PA: Taylor & Francis, Inc.

Kalisch, R. A. (1971). The onset of the dying process. In R. A. Kalisch (Ed.), *Death, dying, transcending* (pp. 5–17). Farmingdale, NY: Baywood Publishing Company, Inc.

Kane, R. L. (1998). *Understanding health care outcomes research.* Rockville, MD: Aspen Publishers, Inc.

Krisman-Scott, M. A. (2000). An historical analysis of disclosure of terminal status. *Journal of Nursing Scholarship, 32*(1), 47–52.

Kubler-Ross, E. (1969). *On death and dying.* New York: Macmillan.

Kubler-Ross, E. (1975). *Death: The final stage of growth.* Englewood Cliffs, NJ: Prentice Hall.

McHorney, D. A., Ware, J. E., Rogers, W., Raczek, A. E., & Lu, J. F. R. (1992). The validity and relative precision of MOS short- and long-form health status scales and Dartmouth COOP charts: Results from the Medical Outcomes Study. *Medical Care, 30* (5 supplement), MS253–MS265.

Meleis, A. I. (1997). *Theoretical nursing: Development & progress.* Philadelphia, PA: Lippincott-Raven Publishers.

Watson, J. (1988). *Nursing: Human science and human care. A theory of nursing.* New York: National League for Nursing Press.

UNIT II

THEORETICAL FOUNDATIONS

Critical Thinking Activities
1. Compare and contrast concepts of two nursing theories applied to end of life care
2. Apply Kubler-Ross's theory to a personal loss experience
3. Compare Watson's caring theory to Kubler-Ross's grief theory

Teaching-Learning Exercises
1. Choose a nursing theory and identify principles of palliative care
2. Write an annotated bibliography related to theories that apply to end of life care

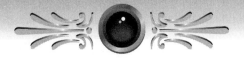

UNIT III

RESPONSES TO LOSS

Learning Objectives

1. Identify grief, bereavement, and mourning
2. Discuss factors affecting a loss reaction
3. Identify measures that facilitate the grieving process
4. Identify different cultural characteristics relative to death and dying
5. Discuss different stages and tasks of grief work
6. Discuss theories related to grieving
7. Define different types of grief

CHAPTER

LOSS, GRIEF, AND BEREAVEMENT

Pat Andrus

I am bowed down and brought very low. All day long I go about mourning. . .
Come quickly and help me, O Lord my Savior. (Psalm 38: 6,22)

INTRODUCTION

For thousands of years, grief has been recognized as a part of life. Extended families and neighborhoods helped the members cope with loss and grief. They shared in the ritualization of death and bereavement, and provided a sense of community and immediate, as well as lasting, support. Individuals and families turned to one another and to their religious leaders and institutions.

Changes in our world and the way we live have generated new needs and responses in times of crisis and grief. Decreased participation in formal religious activities, increased mobility of families, and a decreased sense of neighborhood unity have pointed people towards mental and physical health professionals for help with grief.

People turn to other people for help in handling their grief. Not everyone requires professional help to cope with his or her grief. Many, however, seek help outside the family. Nurses, as a result of their high level of interaction with a patient, often hear the stories, see the pain, and wipe the tears of the bereaved.

Bowlby (1980, 23) asserts, "Clinical experience and a reading of the evidence leave little doubt of the truth of the main proposition—that much psychiatric illness is an expression of pathological mourning—or that such illness includes many cases of anxiety state, depressive illness, and hysteria, and also more than one kind of character disorder." Nurses and other health care personnel need a core knowledge of grief and its related issues, conditions, behaviors, and effects.

Deepening our understanding of grief and the grief process requires building a foundation. We will define pertinent concepts, examine loss and normal grief reactions, highlight major theories about the process of grieving, and look at time as it interacts with the process. Throughout we will hear from the real experts in this field, the bereaved persons.

CONCEPTUALIZING GRIEF AND BEREAVEMENT

My years as a grief therapist working with a broad range of persons and losses have taught me much. I remind myself that I know much about grief and bereavement. I know little to nothing about this client's grief journey and grief experiences.

From early in our relationship, I begin to determine whether this bereaved person and I are talking from similar or vastly different life experiences. I outline for myself how this client understands the grief process. I seek to understand the cultural influences interfacing with this person's experience and to glean the definitions and frames of reference under which this person is operating.

One of the important pieces of my work is to create with the client a mutual understanding of the ways we choose to define loss, grief, bereavement, and other concepts while completing our course of grief counseling or therapy. This imbues a sense of rapport while eliminating some potential misunderstandings or misrepresentations. Thus, an educational component of the grief process is reflected in the treatment options I discuss with my clients.

Many persons will say they thought they understood grief. Most can and will tell about past events in their life or the life of a friend or relative to explain their knowledge and depth of the grief experience. This is indeed helpful in giving me insight into their conceptual framework. It does not mean they have ever taken time to define grief and loss. Words often elude them, and the challenge of having to find the right words may even seem overwhelming to some.

I offer clients, through a gentle discussion woven into a reflection of their own words and story, definitions that are easy to grasp. These definitions are simple and direct while applicable to many stories and losses. Brabant (1996) provides discussion of four such basic concepts:

- bereavement: a loss, any loss;
- grief: pain, the human response to loss;
- grief work: incorporating the loss into one's life so the loss no longer controls the person's life;
- mourning: what our culture, both "others" and "ourselves," tells us we should feel and do following a loss.

Grief, with its depth, intensity, and duration, surprises people. One woman explained to me, "These ideas are foreign to me. I feel like Alice in Wonderland, like I fell into the looking glass and no longer see things as they once were. My life was not supposed to be this way. I wasn't prepared to hold so much pain, so much grief. We laughed in our home. We were happy most of the time. This just isn't what I thought I would be doing at this time of my life."

Worden (1991) notes the increasing interest in issues related to death and dying as well as grief and bereavement. He claims people feeling stuck in their grieving seek mental health treatment. Most of my initial calls from clients come because the person fears he or she is "doing it wrong," that the process is not moving ahead or is taking too long, and that the painful grief and mourning will never come to an end. Often the caller sounds desperate, saying that he or she needs help to "get over it." Sometimes the person calls for an appointment because their physician, nurse practitioner, family member, or friend suggested that grief might be an underlying cause of their physical or mental condition.

Jon, a 46-year-old man, came to me after his family doctor explained that many of his physical symptoms were probably grief induced. Since shortly prior to his wife's death, Jon had suffered from headaches, shortness of breath, and feelings of being disconnected from what was going on around him. Medically, his tests were fine. In therapy, Jon began to recognize his fear of being left to finish rearing the teenage children and his need to begin separating from his dying wife. He shared his guilt about "going on" when she was "just going." With the passing of time, his yearning for her diminished. He began to see himself as a "forever loved and once-married man who has lost his first love."

Loss

A simple way of defining loss is "what we once had and no longer have." It could be an item, an event, an expectation, a belief, or a relationship. It might have been physical, intellectual, emotional, social, or spiritual in nature. The level of its importance can only be set by the person who lost it.

The observer or listener might be inclined to think the loss silly or unimportant while the person experiencing the loss may be devastated. The outer or physical manifestation of what was lost might seem simple, like a purse, piece of jewelry, photograph, or blanket. After all, these are only material things in life. The listener must determine the deeper, symbolic meaning of the item in order to better understand the depth of the loss.

Her grandmother's locket or favorite pie plate may serve as the symbolic tool which helps a woman connect with her ill or deceased grandparent, to what was or even to what might have been. Having the locket stolen or breaking the pie plate may open the grief of having "Grandma stolen from me" or reflect the "broken relationship" of death.

Rando (1993, 20) defines two general categories of loss as physical and psychosocial. She defines physical loss as "the loss of something tangible," i.e., items misplaced or stolen, or surgical removal of limbs. A psychosocial loss or symbolic loss is "the loss of something intangible, psychosocial in nature" such as divorce, retirement, diagnosis of chronic illness, or broken dreams. Physical losses are more often recognized and acknowledged by others than are psychosocial losses. A secondary loss is defined as "a physical or psychosocial loss that coincides with or develops as a consequence of the initial loss."

More than one widowed person has told me they thought they were doing fairly well after the death of their spouse. They were "doing okay" in handling the loss of their spouse (a physical loss) even in the aftermath of recently developing some chronic illness themselves (a psychosocial loss). They were dealing with the unfolding experiences of bereavement, mourning their losses by crying, and telling their story. They were better able to stay in the family home alone, even though they severely missed the spouses' presence (a secondary loss). The stumbling block came with a pileup of secondary losses: loss of personal safety in their home, having to move to another home, depleted income, or health care insurance issues.

Rando (1993, 20–21) explains:

> The mourner typically sustains much more than physical loss after a death. Loved ones play many roles in an individual's life. For instance, a spouse may be one's lover, best friend, helpmate, confidant, coparent, social partner, housemate, traveling companion, business associate, career supporter, auto repair person, housekeeper, and "other half," among myriad other roles. With the death, the mourner loses someone to fill these roles and to gratify the needs and sustain the feelings associated with them in the particular way the deceased did. In addition, the mourner loses a view of the world and the countless feelings, thoughts, behavior and interaction patterns, hopes, wishes, fantasies, dreams, assumptions, expectations, and beliefs that required the loved one's presence. The deprivation of the gratification the loved one once provided, the unfulfilled needs, the unreinforced behavior patterns, the unmet expectations, the emotional privation, the violated views of the world, the dashed hopes, the frustrated wishes, and the role relationships left empty are all examples of secondary psychosocial losses associated with the death.
>
> Each of these secondary losses initiates its own grief and mourning reactions, which ultimately may be greater or lesser in intensity and scope than those following the precipitating loss. At the proper time, each of these secondary losses must be identified and mourned just as the actual death precipitating it must be mourned.

We must never assume to know the full meaning of the loss for the client. Every physical loss gives rise to psychosocial loss. The intensity and value of the meaning may change over time and treatment. It is not a static process. Only the client can determine the definition of the loss in his or her life. Our professional role is to help the client or patient unfold the story, investigate the meaning of the physical, psychosocial, and secondary losses, and determine ways to live with these losses.

UNCOMPLICATED GRIEF RESPONSES

In 1942 E. Lindemann worked with the acutely bereaved family members of those killed in Boston's Coconut Grove nightclub fire. From this work evolved the broad group of characteristics widely recognized as normal or uncomplicated grief. He observed these six general categories of responses:

1. somatic or bodily distress of some type
2. preoccupation with the image of the deceased
3. guilt relating to the deceased or circumstances of the death
4. hostile reactions
5. the inability to function as one had before the loss
6. the development of traits of the deceased in their own behavior

Some attention has been paid to distinguishing between normal, uncomplicated grief and complicated grief. Worden (1991) generally denotes the normal grief process as one that shows a pattern of lessening intensity over time, while complicated grief reactions do not allow for movement in the direction of reduced intensity.

Rando (1993, 1996) indicates there are attempts to do two things in complicated mourning: 1) to deny, repress, or avoid aspects of the loss, its pain, and full realization of its implications for the mourner, and 2) to hold onto and avoid relinquishing the lost loved one. She put forth the premise that complicated mourning can be said to be present when, taking into consideration the amount of time since death, there is compromise, distortion, or failure of one or more of the six "R" processes of mourning. These are:

* Recognize the loss
* React to the separation
* Recollect and experience the deceased and the relationship
* Relinquish old attachments to the deceased and the old assumptive world
* Readjust to move adaptively into the new world without forgetting the old
* Reinvest

The list of normal grief behaviors is so extensive and varied that we could devote another chapter to it. Let it suffice to say the well-versed nurse will need to spend time studying the numerous psychological, behavioral, social, and physical responses of the bereaved. One of the best discussions of these can be found in Rando's *Treatment of Complicated Mourning*.

CURRENT THEORETICAL FRAMEWORKS

While still in its youth, the study of death and dying, grief and bereavement—known as the field of thanatology—is growing. Thanatology is drawing from sociology, psychology, nursing, medicine, family science, and social work as researchers build the literature. Each field interjects its own unique views and perspectives of death and dying as well as grief and mourning.

Universally some themes surface. While being bombarded by stage theories of dying and bereavement, most professionals agree that there are both commonalities and idiosyncratic occurrences in the human experience.

In studying human anatomy, plastic human body parts are used to demonstrate and explain structure and relationships. Yet, in working with cadavers, the student becomes aware that the plastic pieces were only meant as a guide. Each person has unique and individual features and idiosyncrasies. A person's grief will also be unique and individual even while fitting into some theoretical overviews and applications.

Studies of the psychological reaction to loss follow the work of Freud. In *Mourning and Melancholia*, published in 1917, Freud was the first to systematically analyze grief. He described mourning as the natural process of recognizing that the dead person would no longer be a source of satisfaction and thus be unable to fulfill another's needs. Freud first recognized grief as requiring "work"; thus comes the concept of the mourner doing "grief work."

Lindemann (1995) conducted early empirical research on acute grief which has become the basis for describing normal bereavement and complicated grief reactions. He studied 101 survivors and relatives of Boston's 1942 fire in the Coconut Grove nightclub. Nearly 500 people died in this fire. Lindemann's (1995, 185–186) observations about acute grief follow:

- Acute grief is a definite syndrome with psychological and somatic symptoms.
- The syndrome may appear immediately after a crisis or may be delayed, exaggerated, or apparently absent.
- In place of the typical syndrome, there may be distorted pictures, each of which represents one special aspect of the grief syndrome.
- Using appropriate techniques, distortions can be successfully transformed into a normal grief reaction with resolution.

Lindemann focused on initial grief responses, while later researchers began to examine the grief process as it develops over time. Kubler-Ross's stages of grief, Bowlby's attachment theory, Worden's four tasks of mourning, and Wolfelt's six tasks of mourning will be our focus in the chapter. These give the student a fairly well-defined historical perspective and current application of theory.

Most reading this text will be aware of Kubler-Ross's five stages of grief: denial and isolation, anger, bargaining, depression, and acceptance. Her research on "personal death" involved interviewing more than 200 terminally ill patients at a large university hospital. The data was summarized in *On Death and Dying* and served as a catalyst for thanatology as a field of study.

Unfortunately in some situations, her five-stage theory became the popular and overused explanation for what all bereaved individuals experience. Many persons interpreted their grief journey to follow these five stages in a linear, step design. There are numerous stories of people confused by their recurring feelings of anger and depression long after they believed they either were or should have been feeling acceptance. They found it difficult to understand the ebb and flow of their grief, certain they were at fault or not "doing grief the right way."

As Bertman reminds health care professionals in *Facing Death: Images, Insights, and Interventions*, "Cancers can be 'staged'; grief cannot. What is helpful about such theories is that they give us a sense of the emotional roller coaster experienced by persons who are grieving." (p. 198)

British psychiatrist Bowlby (1973, 1980) observed attachment behavior in young children placed in institutional settings away from their parents. His theory of mourning outlined three stages necessary for adaptation to separation: protest, despair, and detachment. From this he conceptualized mourning as a separation anxiety in the adult following the disruption of an attachment bond through loss. His phases of the mourning process are:

* numbing
* the urge to recover the lost object, evidenced by hopes and fantasies that the event had not really occurred and by action predicated on the continued outcomes of the lost object
* disorganization, characterized by disappointment and diminished hope of reunion
* reorganization, characterized by discrimination between behavior patterns that were no longer appropriate or productive and those that can be reasonably retained

Worden (1991, 7) contends: "Bowlby's attachment theory provides a way for us to conceptualize the tendency in human beings to make strong affectionate bonds with others and a way to understand the strong emotional reaction that occurs when these bonds are threatened or broken."

Worden developed his four tasks of mourning based upon Bowlby's attachment theory. His book, *Grief Counseling and Grief Therapy* grew out of a National Institutes of Health study called the Omega Project or the Harvard Bereavement Study. Initially an investigation of terminal illness and suicide, the expanded study investigated numerous areas within the general scope of life-threatening behavior. Worden's work included the families of the patients in the study. He theorized that all of human growth and development can be seen as influenced by various tasks. The same is true for mourning, which he defined as the adaptation to loss. He uses *mourning* to indicate the process that occurs after a loss and *grief* to indicate the personal experience of the loss.

Worden (1991, 10–18) contends that grieving persons must accomplish four tasks before mourning can be completed. An order is implied in the definitions of the tasks, and grief tasks which are incomplete may impair further growth and development. These tasks are:

1. to accept the reality of the loss (coming full face with the reality that the person is gone);
2. to experience the pain of grief (acknowledge and work through the emotional, physical, and behavioral pain associated with loss);
3. to adjust to an environment where the deceased is missing (adaptation of roles and behaviors associated with the deceased);
4. to emotionally relocate the deceased and move on with life (readjusting the relationship from one of physical presence to one of appropriate memory).

Wolfelt's six tasks of mourning contain some of the same elements as those of Worden, with the addition of developing a new self-identity and receiving ongoing support from others. These tasks are especially important in helping the bereaved person beyond the initial, acute phases of grief. Wolfelt's (1997, 2) tasks are:

1. acknowledging the reality of the death
2. embracing the pain of the loss
3. remembering the person who died
4. developing a new self-identity
5. searching for meaning
6. receiving ongoing support from others

Wolfelt denotes these six tasks as "yield signs" encountered during the grief process.

TIME AND GRIEF

Whether we discuss grief and bereavement from the stage, phase, or task conceptualization, the idea becomes evident of time passing and the process unfolding. Early on it was believed that a few weeks was adequate for adjustment. Now mourning is seen as a process requiring effort or work that changes over time. Each stage, phase, or task requires different approaches and shifts in beliefs and behaviors from the mourner. The process is fluid, often compared to the "ebb and flow of the tide" or a "roller coaster ride."

Although different words are chosen by different researchers and practitioners, most focus on the occurrence of sequential phases or time periods in the grief process. In normal bereavement, each schema indicates a positive growth movement or direction. The accepted philosophy is one of progression through difficult, yet potentially enriching, experiences and feelings, moving towards some sort of resolution of what happened.

Bertman (1991) uses (1) denial, shock, and protest; (2) disorganization, despair; and (3) reintegration, repatterning, transformation, or adaptation.

Rando (1993, 30) outlines her schema as (1) avoidance, (2) confrontation, and (3) accommodation. She contends the mourner, because these phases are not discrete, "probably will move back and forth among them depending upon

- the precise issue at hand (some issues are easier to cope with than others)
- how that issue stands with regard to other pertinent issues with which the mourner must contend
- where the individual is in the mourning process
- the interaction of factors circumscribing this particular loss for this specific mourner"

In other words, it depends on what the loss is, what else is happening in the bereaved person's life, how far into the grief process the person has traveled, and the personal twist the bereaved person gives to cultural and situational factors surrounding the loss. These, as well as the nature and meaning of the loss, characteristics of the mourner, characteristics of the death, social factors, and physiological factors, influence how the mourner moves in and out of avoiding or denying, acknowledging and working through the losses, while learning to accommodate the loss in their present and future lifestyle.

Most researchers now agree that grieving is an unfolding process, happening over time. The focus has shifted from time formulas based on specific categories of loss to viewing the duration of the grief process in the context of the uniqueness of each individual and each loss. More studies are indicating that grief does not follow a prescribed timetable, but rather has a variable course over time.

The adage "time heals" does hold truth, yet is not the whole picture. Bereaved persons must do their grief work as time moves forward. No one gets to just stay where they were when grief hit. Time continues forward. Whether the grieving person realizes it or likes it, the clock did not stop permanently when the death occurred.

Many have expressed anger similar to Marsha's: "When he died, my world ended. Time stopped. I just went numb and never wanted to admit to myself that I would have to go on. If I went on, it meant I did not care enough. If I never moved again, but just stayed still, sitting in our room, either he would come back . . . or I would just die, too. Why couldn't I die first? How dare he leave me in this world without him! I never wanted to go on without him. I still don't want to, even though I know I have to."

So, how long does it last? How long does it take for a person to adapt to a major loss like the death of someone close or important? How does one know when it is completed? Worden (1991) says it is finished when the tasks of mourning are accomplished. He uses the bereaved person's ability to think of the deceased without the wrenching pain and sadness it once held as one benchmark.

Some insist upon a timeframe in days, months, or years. If we look at the amount of time most corporations offer to employees who experience the death of an immediate family member, then three days is what it takes. The employee is expected to return to work at nearly full speed. A literature review would indicate a broad range of time limits from a few weeks to one or two years to forever.

While some might find it simplistic, a basic and honest answer is Brabant's (1996, 112), "How long will it take? As long as it takes."

I encourage clients to watch for a duality to exist. We slowly gain an overall sense of being able to embrace life's new roles with renewed interest, hope, and gratification while still recognizing that periods of sorrow can and will surface. We slowly turn towards the future even while looking over our shoulder at the past. This is not an easy task, nor a simple one.

Loving once and learning to grieve and fully mourn the loss of that love is a good indicator of being able to love again. We cannot just put that earlier love aside, though. It has played a significant role in us evolving into the person we are today. We tuck that love inside us, with all its teachings, and carry it tenderly as we turn to face what life is bringing on.

REFERENCES

Bertman, S. L. (1991). *Facing death: Images, insights, and interventions*. Bristol, PA: Taylor & Francis.

Bowlby, J. (1973). *Attachment and loss: Vol. 2*. New York: Basic Books.

Bowlby, J. (1980). *Attachment and loss: Vol. 3*. New York: Basic Books.

Brabant, S. (1996). *Mending the torn fabric*. Amityville, NY: Baywood Publishing Company, Inc.

Freud, S. (1957). Mourning and melancholia. In J. Strachey (ed. and trans.), *The standard edition of the complete works of Sigmund Freud* (Vol. 14, pp. 237–258). London: Hogarth Press. (Original work published 1917)

Kubler-Ross, E. (1969). *On death and dying*. New York: Macmillan.

Lindemann, E. (1995). Symptomatology and management of acute grief. In J. B. Williamson and E. S. Shneidman (eds.), *Death: Current perspectives* (pp. 185–195). Mountain View, CA: Mayfield Publishing Company. (Original work published 1944)

Rando, T. (1993). *Treatment of complicated mourning*. Champaign, IL: Research Press.

Rando, T. (1996). The increasing prevalence of complicated mourning: The onslaught is just beginning. In G. E. Dickinson, M. R. Leming, and A. C. Merman (eds.), *Dying, death and bereavement* (pp. 98–205). Guilford, CT: Dushkin Publishing Group.

Wolfelt, A. (1997). *The journey through grief: Reflections on healing*. Fort Collins, CO: Companion Press.

Worden, J. W. (1991). *Grief counseling and grief therapy: A handbook for the mental health practitioner*. New York: Springer Publishing Company.

CHAPTER

GRIEF AND BEREAVEMENT: YOURS AND MINE

Pat Andrus

> *Tears turned to ice do not flow.*
> *(Middle-aged woman whose father died when she was 12.)*

INTRODUCTION

When we begin speaking of grief, many will assume they understand what grief is. After all, most adult humans have had a personal loss experience. We tend to measure the experiences of others by our own experiences, just as we may judge our own experience against that of others. Our experiences might offer useful landmarks along the journey of grief. However, assuming another person's grief will be exactly like ours, or our grief like someone else's, is more harmful than helpful to the grieving person. In addition, we also miss out on a rich opportunity to learn more about ourselves and others.

When this happens, both parties are shortchanged in understanding what is being seen, heard, or experienced. The bereaved person loses the acknowledgment that his or her grief is important and the recognition that others are present for them during this time of their lives. We deny ourselves the chance to know "me" and "you" on a deeper level. We diminish awareness of their unique grief experiences intentionally or unintentionally. In doing so, we victimize them and us.

We will look at what happens when it is "my" grief and when it is "yours." Figure 6–1 offers helpful suggestions for working with bereaved persons.

- Be gentle with yourself, as you would with a wounded creature.
- Inventory your own losses—past, present, and future.
- Be vigilant in recognizing how your losses enrich and impede your healing.
- Make a plan for addressing unresolved grief and loss issues. Give yourself time, opportunity, and rewards for improvements.
- Hire your own therapist to debrief with you monthly.
- Treat yourself to a massage or other forms of healing body work.
- Take note of which you seem more connected to: earth, wind, fire, or water. Plant a garden, breathe deeply when the weather is changing, meditate with a lit candle, sit beside a lake, or install a recirculating rock and water garden.
- Enroll in ongoing professional development courses.
- Enroll in ongoing personal development programs.
- Attend a support group meeting.
- Sit quietly.
- Remind yourself of how far you have come.
- Decide what you want to learn to do. Take one step towards beginning.
- Write yourself a sympathy card.
- Start your own "kudo box" of favorite notes, cards, and memories.
- Create a personal ritual in memory of your special losses.
- Send yourself flowers.

Figure 6–1 Ways to Help Yourself Heal
© 2000. Reprinted with permission of Pat Andrus.

YOURS AND MINE

In regard to grief, we must learn to look at events and people through our personal kaleidoscopes. Grief is certainly one of the bumps and twists that can rearrange the color chips of life into new and unusual patterns.

When it is our kaleidoscope we may want others to see how different our life has become. At times, we may want to hold the changes close to our hearts, keeping it private and available only to our own examination. Sometimes we believe no one can see what is happening with us.

When it happens to someone else, they also may desire privacy in the midst of huge change. The more public the events surrounding the grief, the more the need for privacy and times of seclusion. Balancing what we offer or provide as professionals with the needs of the bereaved person or family is an awesome task. We are prone to do what seems appropriate based upon our own cultural training. Sometimes it will be well-received and sometimes not.

Having a loved one, or even perhaps a "not-so-loved" one die, is an intensely personal and painful experience for humans. It may be the most painful experience of a person's life.

Bearing witness to the pain, sorrow, and suffering of another person is both an honor and a burden. As health care professionals, we expect ourselves to be equipped to handle another person's pain, whether physical or emotional. Others expect us to be able to respond appropriately.

In the past, health care personnel and professionals were taught to not show any personal feelings, responses, or thoughts. Self-disclosure was looked upon as a sign of weakness or irresponsibility. Workers were terminated or chose to leave the profession because they "could not handle it." A "real professional" would not, or could not, show his or her own vulnerability. Thankfully this is changing.

A more well-balanced staff person is emerging—one who can deal with the stressful professional environment because he or she is better equipped to deal with personal losses. Nursing programs are including self-care components in coursework. Significant changes in employee assistance plans provide immediate and more encompassing services to help staff deal with high stress levels.

I have been invited to present in-service trainings, seminars, and workshops on de-stressing nursing personnel. Learning skills of appropriate self-disclosure, how to laugh and play to lower blood pressure and other symptoms, when to self-refer for therapy and support services, and quick yet effective tools for relaxation have helped audiences return to their demanding work with a lighter heart. Consider the following situations in which names have been changed for confidentiality.

May, an oncology wing nurse with decades of experience, once told me:

It's not that I don't want to care anymore. It's that it hurts too much to care anymore.

The only way I can continue doing what I do every day is to pull an imaginary cape around me before I go in each day. I can't remember when I first did it, but now I have to consciously do it every day. I know I am burned out. As a single mom, I have to count on my job to feed my three kids and buy their school things and keep my old car running. I cannot leave and yet it is getting harder and harder to stay.

If I allow myself to really see how many times I feel inadequate in caring for a patient, in keeping someone alive, or facing the family of the end of life patient—or, worse still, the family of one who dies— I'm not sure I could keep on. I am a really good nurse. I like what I do. I like who I am as a nurse. I don't like keeping myself so separated from my patients.

I have been told I can be insensitive and unfeeling. That is not the true state. I care too much and have to pull back from caring when I hurt so deeply. That way I can go in to perform whatever job has to be done.

A young nurse new in our area told me she did not know how I have done this work for so long. She admitted to me that she had already put in for another position. I won't leave my patients because I know I give them the best part of me, even though I sometimes don't seem compassionate.

I am tired, very tired. It seems so many are still dying, even though I know we have made huge strides in cancer research and treatment. I'm tired of saying good-bye to people I have come to like and care about.

May's story illustrates how complex the situation becomes for those in the helping professions. We work because we like what we do and we must have income to cover the expenses of life. We want to help others. We are skilled and experienced. Yet, we find ourselves caught in ambivalent emotions and thoughts.

We experience feelings of frustration, anger, and impotence, which make it painful to witness another person's suffering. We develop our personal defense mechanisms which help us deal with being vulnerable and afraid. As another nurse, Beth, said,

I must choose when and where I have the luxury of feeling what I feel. I go to the hospital chapel or sit on the toilet for an extra moment or cry in my car before going home to cook dinner. I schedule time to play racquetball because I pretend the ball is whatever illness that killed my patient that day. It helps a lot to slam that racquet, to hear the ball slap the wall, to really feel my anger working itself out of my body.

When my mom died a couple of years back, I nearly lost it. I couldn't stand going to work, having to deal with patients with the same kind of disease and diagnosis. Seeing them live and knowing my mom didn't was so hard for me.

I felt so guilty because I couldn't save her . . . and here I was a nurse and all. But I wasn't able to change what happened in the end. I wish I had been, but I wasn't. Now I have to make sure I handle things, like my emotions when a patient dies, as soon as I can. I won't allow the same mistakes I made then.

The difference between May and Beth is fairly obvious. Beth has learned ways which help her release her pent-up feelings. She makes time for herself. She recognizes healing herself as an important part of the total plan for helping others heal.

Health care professionals, specifically nurses for the purpose of our discussion here, are at risk for stress, burnout, and a fairly new concept called compassion fatigue and must take care to heal themselves. Staying close to burnout or in compassion fatigue decreases the person's ability to bounce back.

When chronically in burnout, the nurse risks escalating into compassion fatigue. Just one story that hits too close to home, that seems just a bit too possible in your own life, can flip you. Suddenly you might find yourself incapable of dealing with your patient. Feeling ill-equipped to deal with your own losses, experiencing a pileup of secondary losses or victimizations, having insufficient support systems, and facing multiple or sequential losses in a short period of time would be symptomatic.

Nurses are healers. They always have been. Somewhere along the way, as the field of medicine evolved, nurses became convinced that others, like doctors, did the healing and that the nurse supported the effort.

When nurses view themselves as powerful tools in a person's healing, the stage is set for success. When nurses practice what they teach, they allow themselves to experience a wide range of emotions, identify tools and techniques which help themselves heal, and recognize their own patterns of adapting to loss.

Just because we work well with other people in loss and transition experiences doesn't mean we work well with our own. It may seem like our personal losses are less important than the losses experienced by the patient and family facing death.

For example, the theft of your wallet may seem less important than the suffering you see in the family of the dying patient. You might be inclined to minimize your loss by comparing it to the death of this patient. Yet, the physical and psychological losses attached to that stolen wallet may hold deeper symbolic meaning. Losing the lock of baby hair tucked into the wallet's inner pocket after your now-estranged child's first haircut may open wounds. It may represent many losses, such as all the holiday meals eaten with that child's place at the table empty.

In addition, losing the wallet might serve as the proverbial "last straw" in a long list of events and losses. Ordinarily you could handle the theft of your wallet, even with all the inconveniences and sorrows it might bring. Your frustration and powerlessness in other parts of your life can spill over into how you respond to the theft. How you adapt to your own losses impacts how you work with others experiencing loss and transition.

Your losses are important. Your grief is important. Your bereavement process is important.

Your grief and my grief are not the same. Even if our stories were to match, our grief and our bereavement process would not be alike. Our histories and thus the ways we perceive losses are different. Even if we both experience the death of the same person, our grief and bereavement would not be the same.

Yours is yours; mine is mine. I cannot take yours away from you. You cannot take mine away from me. Each of us must experience it for ourselves and learn to live with our loss. We can facilitate each other's grieving process. We cannot do it for each other.

As Bertman (1991, 197) recommends: "Reflection on our own losses and how we coped with them is an excellent avenue to the empathetic sharing of other people's grief." This statement does not infer the ability or desirability of judging how another person handles loss.

It is often said that each person's grief is individual and unique. Because this is true, we can only come close to truly understanding what a person's loss means. To be equipped and prepared to enter the realm of another person's grief journey, we must first take care of our own grief and loss issues.

THE PROFESSIONAL'S GRIEF

The desire to help others is the core of our being in the so-called "helping professions." Nurses want to be able to help patients improve their life conditions. This premise holds true in grief counseling, except that the very experience of grief makes it difficult to be or feel helpful. The bereaved person does most of the grief work on his or her own, especially in normal or uncomplicated grief.

Worden (1991) discusses ways that our own grief can hinder our working with a bereaved patient. Even though Worden is addressing counselors and therapists, these also pertain to nurses. First, the nurse's need to be helpful may be challenged by feelings of frustration and anger associated with not being or feeling helpful to the bereaved. A nurse's excessive discomfort in witnessing the pain of the bereaved person, while not seeing herself or himself as successful in a helpful role, may result in the relationship being cut short.

Second, working with the bereaved may remind the nurse of his or her own losses, sometimes painfully so. Similarities between the bereaved person's and the nurse's losses can intensify this situation. A nurse who has adequately integrated the loss could be beneficial and useful to a bereaved person working through a similar loss. On the other hand, a nurse who has inadequately resolved a loss could impede or hinder the bereaved patient's movement towards appropriate grief resolution.

Third, the nurse may experience increased apprehension over feared or pending losses. Bringing our own anxieties about feared losses into consciousness and addressing the problem can help us deal more effectively with our own apprehension and with the bereaved patient.

Fourth, awareness of our own personal death and the existential anxiety attending this awareness can make a nurse more effective or less effective as a human being. We face the inevitability of death and our level of personal comfort or discomfort with the idea we will eventually die. "All of us are anxious to one degree or another about our own mortality, but it is possible to come to terms with this reality and not have it as a closet issue, making us uncomfortable and hindering our effectiveness" (Worden 1991, 134).

Learning to explore and address our own grief issues gives us a deeper, richer understanding of the grief process. My personal losses and grief experiences have helped me become more compassionate and patient in working with bereaved clients. I gained a valuable understanding of the strength required to face into the pain, to seek out coping methods, and to live in the grief even as I thought I was being remolded by it. Just about the time I naively believe I truly know about grief and the growth process it brings, life teaches me a new chapter and verse of the grief song.

Worden (1991) believes that exploring our personal history of losses also brings an opportunity to identify the kinds of resources available to the bereaved. We learn about coping styles, personal behaviors, and creative interventions. By recognizing what did and did not help us, we also recognize the value of different approaches to resolving grief. Figure 6–2 explains ways useful in helping others with grief.

- Just listen. . . and listen again and again.
- Hold back judgments of the person, and of their experience, and of their grief journey.
- Hear with all your senses—what they say with their words, expressions, behaviors, body language, and silences.
- Attend the funeral. Being present is an act of support often minimized yet seldom forgotten.
- Stay culturally aware and sensitive, even after a long or intimate relationship with the bereaved person.
- Be prepared for surprising behaviors or beliefs.
- Note on your calendar to call or send a simple note at regular intervals over the next year or so—in a week, month, quarterly, first anniversary date, at birthdays, or special anniversaries.
- Deliver a prepared dish, freezer wrapped with instructions for reheating. Use a nonreturn container. Or deliver a bag of paper goods, i.e. plates, cups, napkins, plastic forks, rolls of plastic wrap and foil, inexpensive storage containers.
- Women seldom have a nice handkerchief in today's world; tuck one into the widow's or daughter's hand with a note for her purse. Later she may not remember who brought it. Men also appreciate a fresh linen handkerchief.
- Care about the person and show it sensitively. Often the bereaved person is left to comfort the visitors more than to be comforted.
- Watch what you say. Listen to yourself before the words leave your tongue. Often-said statements like, "He or she is in a better place" are harmful and judgmental. Be thoughtful and considerate.
- Choose loving silence over well-intentioned words.
- Remember: Grief and mourning take many months and years, not days and weeks.
- Learn to say "I'm sorry" and mean it.

Figure 6–2 Ways to Help Others in Grief
© 2000. Reprinted with permission of Pat Andrus.

- Remember your own humanity. We make mistakes without intending to do so. Learn to forgive yourself for human inadequacies.
- Avoid gossiping about the situation, people, events, and possible outcomes. Change the subject or excuse yourself from others who wish to gossip.
- Be prepared for statements and behaviors that seem out of character to the bereaved person or family.
- Respect the mourner's anger with God, the expressions of that anger, and any questioning of God's will or plan. Assurances of God's plan may not bring comfort to the mourner at this time.
- Questions like "Why did this happen?" and "What will I do now?" do not require specific answers. Asking such questions is a part of the bereavement process.
- Use the name of the deceased. It is important to recognize the important role this person played in the mourner's life.
- Be patient with the griever repeating the story. Retelling his or her story helps the mourner adapt to a changed future.
- Use appropriate physical contact. A hug or touch on the shoulder or arm helps when words fail.
- Learn to be comfortable in shared silence. Chattering does not usually cheer a person.
- Occasionally sharing how you adapted to your own losses may be helpful to the mourner. Seek out your own therapist or friend to work on your own healing.

Figure 6–2 *Continued*

Out of this self-discovery, we can also identify any issues needing further grief work and resolution. Working with our own losses equips us to recognize our own limitations in working with other bereaved persons. We will be better prepared to know when to refer the patient, when to request reassignments, when to ask someone to share the support role, and when to seek professional help for ourselves.

Nurses, like counselors and therapists, fall prey to the notion that one is capable of handling all situations. Knowing our limitations is a valuable tool in working with bereaved populations. It is a sign of maturity when a nurse recognizes he or she would not be effective working with all patients.

In grief and bereavement work, my toughest cases usually share characteristics of my past losses or my most feared losses. I must remain vigilant to work on my own grief issues and to recognize my personal thresholds. I need to know where my support comes from and what I have to do in order to tap into it.

I participate in a weekly support group comprised of four bereavement professionals, as well as meeting weekly with a larger group of supportive professional women. Both groups regularly plan fun activities away from both our homes and jobs. I have access to case supervision discussions and have created a network of professional and personal friendships that allow me to debrief regularly.

I do not expect my husband or adult children to attend to my needs, even though I recognize their love and affection for me. It is my job to take care of me, to schedule massages and fun activities, not only work-related appointments. I have a cat and often find replenishment in the simple repetitive motion of stroking and petting him while I rest in my favorite chair. I keep a "kudo box" of my favorite cards and notes that brighten my spirits when I reread them. I pray and I meditate. I cook, crochet, and redecorate to be creative.

It sounds simple, perhaps. It has taken me years to identify the tools that work best for me.

REFERENCES

Bertman, S. L. (1991). *Facing death: Images, insights, and interventions.* Bristol, PA: Taylor & Francis.

Worden, J. W. (1991). *Grief counseling and grief therapy.* New York: Springer Publishing Co.

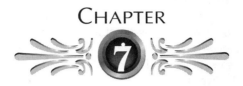

THE KALEIDOSCOPE OF CULTURE: ISSUES OF DEATH AND DYING, GRIEF AND BEREAVEMENT

Pat Andrus

"Death is one event that occurs in every society everywhere in the world, perhaps in the universe. And every society has a way of explaining death, each one believing that its way is the right way." (Kalish 1980, 2)

INTRODUCTION

Social relations take place within a cultural milieu. This coextensiveness shapes the family and the family forms the individual. From this, it may be reasoned that we as individuals think, live, and behave as we were taught as children from a specific family living in a specific culture and society. From babyhood we learn the language, norms, beliefs, attitudes, and values of our family who in turn had adopted those of the family's culture. As we age, we are afforded years of opportunities to see the world in which we live in new and diverse ways.

Culture helps us distinguish right from wrong, good from evil, acceptable from unacceptable. Culture provides the lens through which we see the world. As in photography and videography, the naked eye views the scenes of life through a series of lenses or filters which, when adjusted, clear or distort the images. For humans, cultural differences serve as the filters used to understand, interact, and deal with the world in which we live.

A person looking into a kaleidoscope sees colorful patterns which change with the slightest twist of the lens cap or bump of the hand holding the kaleidoscope. Some patterns are a delight to the eye; others are not nearly as attractive or appealing to the beholder. Similarly, as we become culturally sensitive, some of the patterns, behaviors, rituals, and beliefs we view in cultural scenes may be delightful. Others may seem morbid, ugly, wrong, crazy, ignorant, or otherwise undesirable.

Some incident, comment, or observation may twist or bump our cultural view of the world. Pieces of our experience resettle into new patterns. Sometimes there are parts never noticed before. Other patterns use the same chips in new and innovative ways.

We are often unaware any shift has occurred. Culture is such a part of who we are that we live within it without noticing much of what is happening. We take it for granted because we are comfortable with it and in it.

The old adage, "We see things not as they are but as we are" comes into play with culture. Prior generations handed us traditions and beliefs which serve as filters from our birth. We add our own life experiences and new lenses and filters begin to shape how we see and interact with our world.

We learn to live our daily lives in keeping with others around us, to meet the expectations of our culture. Too, we learn the socially acceptable and recognized ways to grieve and mourn our losses. Irish, Lundquist, and Nelson (1993, 187) conclude,

> Death and grief, though they are universal, natural, and predictable experiences that occur within a social milieu, are deeply embedded within each person's reality. When examining death and grief in a multi-cultural context, the myths, mysteries, and mores that characterize both the dominant and nondominant groups directly affect attitudes, beliefs, practices, and cross-cultural relationships.

RELIGIOUS EXPERIENCE

As a young married woman, I attended the South Louisiana funeral of my family's beloved African American housekeeper. I wore the same simple black dress I had worn just a few months earlier to the funeral of a family friend. Upon entering the small, rural church I felt somehow out of place, even though Lydia's family warmly welcomed me. I did not understand why her family members and friends were dressed mostly in white, not black as my Irish American heritage dictated.

I was uncertain where to sit in the small church. How close to the front altar and casket was "reserved" for the family members? Should I sit in one of the pews lining the sides of the church? I had never felt so "white" as I felt in that assemblage of African Americans. I felt out of place, out of step being the white woman wearing black in the sanctuary of black persons wearing white. For years I had been bathed and fed by this old black woman, yet I suddenly saw how much of her life and beliefs I did not know or understand. My set of lenses shifted, giving me a new image to discern and investigate.

As the funeral service unfolded, there was much singing and praising of the Lord accompanied by loud and forceful assurances that Lydia had arrived in a "better place" and was sitting beside the golden throne of the Savior. Having attended predominantly Presbyterian and Catholic prayer and funeral services all my life, this was surprising and awkward for me. I was unsure of when and exactly how to participate in ways appropriate to Lydia's culture while still honoring my own background and training. Even though her church was Catholic, it was not like the austere Catholic funerals I had attended in urban churches. It was as though all the same pieces had been shuffled and rearranged. I was seeing a very different picture of my life, its privileges and advantages in sharp relief against the images unfolding before me.

Brabant (1996, 29–30) describes mourning as

That part of our cultural background that has to do with loss, grief, and grief work. Mourning is a set of instructions you receive from your culture. . . . Whether or not to cry is only one of many mourning rules. In one culture it may be proper for the person who has died to be buried as quickly as possible. In another culture waiting several days or even a week or more is appropriate. . . . How and by whom the body is prepared and how and where the body is buried also differ widely across cultures. Whether or not there is a wake or a visitation before burial services, who is expected to come, and what that person is expected to do or not do are also mourning rules or customs and differ from culture to culture.

Now able to recognize the situation as one highlighting cultural diversity, I probably would choose to wear a lighter colored garment as a sign of respect for the culture of the deceased. I would be more comfortable with the style of service and music, being more relaxed and less anxious about what to do and not to do. I would be more accepting of the differences, more open to the beauty of the differences, and more honored to be included and welcomed. New lenses have been added over my years of life experience, which now give broader dimensions to how I view people, our backgrounds, and our perspectives of many life experiences and assumptions, including those about end of life and afterlife.

END OF LIFE ILLNESS AND LIFE EXPERIENCES

Decades later I recognize how being black in the 1970s in rural South Louisiana also dictated the kind and quality of care Lydia received as a cancer patient dying at home. Hospice care would enter our area several years later, after both Lydia and my sister had died at home of cancer, spending their last days being cared for by family and friends rather than lying in a hospital bed. Home health concepts would arrive even later. Although my understanding of the reasons was limited, I knew it was important to my family and to hers that both these women be allowed to die with dignity in their own bedrooms.

Today's terminally ill patient and the surrounding family face different attitudes and care models than several years ago. So do the nurses and other health care personnel attending these patients. Nursing students, as well as those in many other family and health care fields, must examine their own lens before addressing the care of patients. We must look through our own kaleidoscope. How we view the patient in front of us is deeply affected by our own cultural indoctrination and belief structure.

This is a lifelong examination which none of us dedicated to the care of others may ever really complete. There will inevitably be one more experience, another family, another situation which challenges the way we are thinking, the way we view that particular issue, the way we perform care for that family.

Societal issues drag us along, shifting our attitudes when we allow ourselves to be open to change and responsive to the needs of others around us. Seeing our children or friends choose mates from differing cultures or from belief structures in opposition to our own can cause personal stress which is, like it or not, transferred to our work. The care we provide is subtly restructured towards the patient with whom we differ. How we view the person always has and always will challenge the style and quality of care we give the patient.

An even greater challenge may occur when we become seriously ill, or when it is our own family, our own terminally ill loved one, or our own bereaved friend or family member. Our cultural kaleidoscope shifts with each new twist of our personal and professional experiences.

Personally being faced with decisions of care for a loved one is significantly different from those made professionally while dealing with relative strangers. Sometimes, when called to make end of life decisions with or for a loved one, a professional can hide within his or her role, assuming the persona of the nurse professional. After all, the art of depersonalizing and separating one's self from one's role is a refined skill, which allows nurses and other professionals to perform their work effectively and efficiently. Culture influences how stoic or demonstrative a person's visible reactions may seem. Having your own self or loved one in the sickbed may challenge long-held beliefs, customs, and rituals.

RELIGIOUS AND CULTURAL PRACTICES

Johnson and McGee (1986, 324) conclude from their editing *Encounters with Eternity; Religious Views of Death and Life After Death* that the 15 faiths presented shared some important views.

> Whether it be the Christian Gospel, the Law of Karma, the Book of Mormon, or the Baha'I Sacred Writings, the different faiths maintain that good thought or good behavior leads to happiness and/or heaven. On the other hand, evil thought or evil behavior leads to pain, torment, and/or hell. One attains salvation, or a place in heaven, or individual happiness through following religious teachings, engaging in good works done selflessly for the benefit of others, and/or having faith in prophets' teachings as sources to the door to eternal union with the

Creator. Hell, whether it be the literal, fiery state believed in by some branches of Islam or Christianity or the eight hot and cold hells of Buddhism, or the spiritual torment of being alienated from the Creator either in this lifetime or after, involves the tragic suffering of separation from God. Heaven, no matter what its description, time of occurrence, or location, exists when humans and Creator come together in a celebration of love and harmony.

They recognized that "faith and belief vary with each individual" and that it "is up to each of the rest of us to decide what we believe and how we interpret our faiths." Yet, their goal was to create a book which would "make available information about what a number of faiths believe about death and what happens after death. In the United States we are offered a supermarket of different beliefs" (p. 12). They encourage the reader to join them in searching for greater understanding of beliefs about death and what happens after death.

These authors recognized that persons claiming the same religious affiliation may hold a variety of beliefs and understandings about their faith structure. All Catholics are not the same, just as all Protestants are not the same. Members of any one church group may come from a spectrum of cultural backgrounds and hold unique interpretations of the religious structure of their church.

When viewed from a nursing perspective, respecting the faith and beliefs of a patient or the patient's family may cause conflict in our own lives. Being called upon to perform care tasks for a patient with a different faith structure can be satisfying or loathsome to a nurse. Being able to separate professional and personal beliefs may not be easy.

Continually finding a large, gregarious group of family and friends in the hospital room of the dying person may be frustrating for a nurse who believes the dying should be attended by only a few very close relatives. Having the elder Irish, Chinese, or Mexican women seen in the hospital room or hallway or even in the funeral home may be viewed as startling and inappropriate or welcome and reassuring.

RANKING IMPORTANCE OF A LOSS

In actuality, culture dictates how our losses are assigned importance. In America, the death of a spouse is generally more recognized as an important loss than is the divorce of a spouse, and the divorce of a spouse would carry more significance than the death of a fiance. This hierarchy disregards such factors as the level of commitment to daily living, the fact that the engaged couple cohabitated for many years, that the divorce was simply a final step after a long and mutually satisfying separation, or that the marriage was bitter and unhappy. It really disregards who each of the persons involved are, what they believe, and how they lived. The rules of the culture are applied to situations without consideration of their uniqueness or of the individuals involved.

Culture dictates that the death of the parents' child be more recognized than the death of a sibling. Thus, visitors to the bedside and later at the funeral may address their concerns with questions about how the parents are holding up or have taken the sad news of a daughter's or son's death. The adult sibling may never be asked how he or she is holding up or making sense of what has happened.

Losses such as the death of a dear friend or of a pet or the loss of precious possessions or a valued relationship are often viewed as socially unrecognized losses. Violent deaths, suicide, homicide, drug- or alcohol-related deaths, and abortions also become disenfranchised losses (Doka 1989). Culture sets the rules by which deaths and losses are viewed and measured.

Kalish (1980, iii) maintains

> Each society has developed roles, beliefs, values, ceremonies, and rituals to integrate death and the process of dying into the culture as a whole and to help individuals cope with the mysteries and fears of death. And each individual must adapt these folkways to his or her own needs, wants, personality, and situation. While aimed at being adaptive, these folkways can also have some harmful effects on certain members of the society.

Lesbian and homosexual couples face multiple issues in confronting illness and death. Long seen as a mental health problem and as a sexual deviance, being lesbian or gay is now viewed more as an identity and an all-encompassing lifestyle. In A *Cross-Cultural Look at Death, Dying, and Religion*, (p. 131), Evans and Carter refer to the population as an "invisible minority" and note the trend towards encouraging better understanding through higher visibility of lesbian and homosexual couples.

> Social workers, psychologists, and others in the helping professions are agreed that ethnic and minority group clients are entitled to competent professional services and that insensitivity to cultural differences in clients defeats the purposes of the helping professions.

With nursing at the forefront of helping professions, it fits that this comment be applied in health care settings. This change in perspective demands that health care organizations and personnel continue to make adjustments to the ways these individuals receive care.

Recently Laura, a highly respected nurse, stopped to visit, asking questions in preparation for prearranging her funeral. Her breast cancer had metastasized into her liver and sternum. Although her treatment plan was fairly optimistic, she lived with the threat of death from her cancer.

Several years after her first round with the breast cancer, Laura entered a committed relationship with another middle-aged woman, Betty. Their lives merged easily into a comfortable daily pattern of living. Recently, Laura's physician reviewed her latest tests, noting a new site of cancer and advising a rigorous treatment plan. With this new and more frightening occurrence, Laura has concerns about her ability to beat it, even using all the skills and the healthy lifestyle she has developed.

Because her brother is gay and lives openly with his partner, Laura felt secure in telling her parents and siblings about her choices. Her partner had been included in family gatherings for the last five years. Until recently Laura thought there would be no further problems with the ways her parents saw and accepted her lifestyle.

In the summer, there will be a large family reunion of Laura's father's family, all of whom live out-of-state. Laura was devastated when her parents tactfully but honestly requested Betty not attend the weekend functions. The kaleidoscope of culture twisted, giving Laura a new view of her family's belief structure.

Suddenly aware that their acceptance was contingent on other family members having no knowledge of Laura's "woman-friend," new questions have arisen. How will her family respond towards Betty when Laura dies? Will her family honor her pre-death wishes to include Betty as a very dear part of Laura's life? Will they ignore Betty, refuse her entrance to the funeral, thus denying the commitment she and their daughter shared? Will a durable power of attorney, designating Betty as Laura's decision maker should she become unable to make decisions or as her spokesperson if she becomes disabled, be enough to override the wishes of blood relatives? What stress and hurt will Betty have to bear in making funeral arrangements without the benefit of being a legal spouse?

Evans and Carter (1995, 143) suggest:

An assessment and intervention model appropriate for anyone facing terminal illness and coping with death must be based on the physical, emotional, spiritual, interpersonal, and legal-financial needs of the individual. In the case of lesbians, some additional factors that should be taken into account are level of visibility with which she is comfortable, her extended family and support groups, and her problems of confronting homophobia in herself, her therapist, and the health care system. We need to determine the strength of family ties and cultural bonds and how these impact on the lesbian relationship in times of crisis. We should find out what social support network the person has, and how this network will respond to terminal illness, death, and the needs of the surviving partner.

A surviving partner who has to deal with final arrangements while not being recognized as a legal spouse or family member faces stressful times. There may be conflict of values or plans for rituals, ceremonies, and final disposition between surviving partner and relatives of the deceased partner. The family of the surviving partner may be supportive or critical or denying of the importance of the relationship, and thus may create additional stress for the survivor.

Within months of his partner dying of AIDS, Roger's apartment complex was in the path of a tornado. It totally destroyed the bedroom where his partner, Joe, had spent a great deal of time, where Joe's belongings still resided, and where the treasured photos of their life together were displayed. The rest of the apartment showed serious structural damage, but the decorative pieces could be reclaimed. Shortly after Joe's death, Roger had closeted many of his personal items, tucked away in an attempt to compartmentalize some of his own pain and grief. He found it "simply too hard to see it all." The tornado sucked away many of these items, like a random hand fiercely and selectively stealing from Roger.

Roger's own health diminished severely in the weeks following the tornado. He confided to his hospice nurse that people had strongly advised him to be grateful it was *only* his partner's belongings and *not his own* that were destroyed. Further, they advised he just get rid of all that junk and start again. Caring persons had further harmed this gentle man by minimizing the importance of his partner's belongings, thus insinuating Roger and Joe's relationship and the rich life they shared was unimportant.

As his health wobbled, Roger struggled to make sense of what society was telling him and how he was to "start over" when he could barely climb out of bed each day. He was forced to move in with a sister, and he could only visit the site of their shared life and work in the cleanup of his apartment when a family member was available to drive him to the complex. His depression and isolation increased as his physical health decreased.

Finally he decided to be hospitalized rather than die in his sister's home. Surrounded by relatives, he no longer felt able to live openly as a gay man. His gay friends who had long been a part of his support system were unwelcome in his brother-in-law's home. His fatigue and grief left him "unable to keep on fighting against the tide."

IGNORANCE OF GOOD PEOPLE

Suarez worked as a US Army nurse in Vietnam. She refers to the "ignorance of good people" or the "arrogance of being good" in how we care for ill persons. Being well intentioned is valuable in nursing as in other social service and health care work. It is not enough! (Suarez, 2000)

Many times people say, do, or believe things because their own filters have prevented them from seeing the situation through the lens of another person. More often than not, no intent to harm was present; it was simply done out of ignorance or closed-mindedness. As nurses and others caring for the ill and the bereaved, we are mandated to open our hearts, hear what we say through the ears of the listener, and change our approaches. We must heal ourselves in order to help others heal.

PHYSICIAN-ASSISTED SUICIDE LEGALIZED IN OREGON

Oregon entered unchartered territory when it became the first place in the world to legalize physician-assisted suicide (PAS) in late 1997. Nurses have a recognized role in many end of life settings, such as hospice, long-term care, home care, and hospitals. How will this pioneering law ultimately affect other states? How will nurses feel and perform in situations where a terminally ill patient is legally able to end his or her life? More importantly, how will a nurse's cultural background and experiences affect how he or she views this choice made by a patient for whom he or she has been caring?

PAS and euthanasia are practiced openly in some parts of the world, such as the Netherlands. Technically PAS is performed illegally everywhere but in Oregon at this time. As in Oregon's law, the right of a nurse or other health care professional to conscientiously object to participation in PAS will possibly be written into laws adopted by other states. Religious beliefs create strong influences on how individuals view PAS and euthanasia. Agencies and health care professionals with religious affiliations often have set policies and procedures regarding these options. Attitudes and beliefs shape our perspective and interpretation of sensitive topics.

Miller (2000, 268) reviews Oregon's law and the implications for end of life care providers. The hospice philosophy supports patient control and autonomy, along with neither hastening nor postponing death.

> The right-to-die movement is alive and well in the United States, and some would say on a fast track. However, health care and technology also are on a fast track. Moving from the right to withhold or withdraw treatment to the federal Patient Self-Determination Act (PL 101-508) as part of the 1990 Omnibus Budget Reconciliation Act to double effect (pain medication potentially hastening death) to PAS happened in less than 10 years. Hospice was legitimized by Medicare only 18 years ago. . . . From a societal perspective, numerous polls and surveys indicate that a majority of U.S. citizens want PAS as an end of life option.

As the baby boomers become gerontology cases and the youth of Generation X mature into the workforce, nursing professionals will predictably contend with tough end of life issues having few clear answers. Nursing students may want to focus on direct care and avoid thinking about political issues such as those discussed in this chapter. Regardless of our efforts to avoid being drawn into thought-provoking and ethics-challenging situations, no one can fully avoid them.

A nurse's kaleidoscope of culture will twist throughout his or her career. The ever-changing pictures of life and its difficult decisions will pivot on nurses' beliefs brought forth from childhood and honed as adults.

Irish, Lundquist, and Nelson (1993, 187–188) drew four insights about death and grief from their project spanning 20 years.

First, although the topics of death and grief have taken on new life in re-cent decades, specific changes concerning those universal life experi-ences have been minimal when assessed within the parameters of multi-culturalism. Granted, countless books have been published on those topics, support groups abound in churches and hospitals, talk-show hosts focus on grief and loss, and individuals are less apt than formerly to speak euphemistically about death and dying. All those actions have had a posi-tive effect in reawakening society's awareness and acceptance of death and grief. Yet a concern exists that the processes of dying and grieving will be culturally stereotyped as a result of the tendency to generalize Euro-American theories about the stages of death across diverse cultures.

Second, death and grief engender different reactions from members of the dominant group when they occur among those groups that lie out-side the mainstream. Gang-related homicides, drug-related suicides, AIDS-related deaths, and the deaths of non-American combatants in war all tend to be depreciated. Indeed, because of the low status ascribed to members of "outside" groups, some representatives of the white, male, "Christian" mainstream seem to ignore, minimize, or give silent ac-quiescence to their sufferings and the grief of those who survive them.

Third, grief is a normal reaction to the death of a loved one, but indi-viduals from culturally diverse groups in our countries may be grieving for significant losses on a *chronic* basis. Such populations may be dealing simultaneously with the loss of their homeland, personal belongings, family members, economic status, professional identity, cultural tradi-tions, language, and sense of self. The chronic and deep-seated nature of such unresolved grief may complicate the bereavement process in terms of intensity and duration. Not only will culturally diverse popula-tions grieve differently over the death of a loved one but they may be grieving for other significant losses at the same time.

Fourth . . . lack of cultural understanding and sensitivity to cultural diversity in death and grief appear to have caused more problems than language barriers.

SUMMARY

When health care providers assume to understand the meaning of life's events for another person, we have significantly failed. We fail as profession-als, but more importantly, we fail as human beings.

We must remain alert to cues from the patient and the family, be willing to investigate new methods of communication, untangle miscommunications, gain more appreciation for cultures differing from our own, and value the family and friends of patients as resources for increased awareness and knowledge of customs and rituals.

It will always be easiest to support and assist others who share in our basic values and world views. However, no one is truly like us. The patients who teach us the most valued lessons of our careers are those who view the world through kaleidoscopes different from ours. It is from them that we gain the privilege of learning the meaning of death in their culture, the rituals surrounding death, and their ways of celebrating the life of the deceased. They are the bumps and twists which shift our kaleidoscope of culture into new patterns.

They are the ones who teach us the most about death and the most about living.

REFERENCES

Brabant, S. (1996). *Mending the torn fabric; For those who grieve and those who want to help them.* Amityville, NY: Baywood Publishing Co.

Doka, K.J. (Ed.). (1989). *Disenfranchised grief: Reorganizing hidden sorrow.* Lexington, Mass: D. C. Heath & Co.

Evans, I. M., & Carter, J. (1995). The lesbian perspective on death and dying. In J. K. Parry & A. S. Ryan (Eds.), *A cross-cultural look at death, dying, and religion* (pp. 131–144). Chicago: Nelson-Hall Publishers, Inc.

Irish, D. P., Lundquist, K. F., & Nelsen, V. J. (Eds.). (1993). *Ethnic variations in dying, death, and grief: Diversity in universality.* Washington, DC: Taylor & Francis.

Johnson, C. J., & McGee, M.G. (1986). *Encounters with eternity: Religious views of death and life after death.* New York: Philosophical Library.

Kalish, R. A. (Ed.). (1980). *Death and dying: Views from many cultures.* Farmingdale, NY: Baywood Publishing Co.

Mesler, M. A., & Miller, P. J. (1996). Incarnating heaven: Making the hospice philosophy mean business. *Journal of Sociology and Social Welfare, 23*(3), 31–49.

Miller, P. J. (2000). Life after death with dignity: The Oregon experience. *Social Work, 45*(3), 263–271.

Suarez, M. M., & McFeaters, S. J. (2000). Culture and class: The different worlds of children and adolescents. In K. J. Doka (Ed.), *Living with grief: Children, adolescents, and loss* (pp. 56–70). Washington, DC: Hospice Foundation of America.

Unit III

Responses to Loss

Critical Thinking Activities

1. Compare and contrast theoretical tasks of grief as presented by Kubler-Ross, Bowlby, Rando, and Worden
2. Compare cultural characteristics of own culture with that of a different culture
3. List 10 interventions to help support persons who are grieving
4. Discuss measures to assist with maladaptive grief responses

Teaching-Learning Exercises

1. Write own obituary
2. Have each student within a discussion group of five to six persons discuss a major loss that each has endured
3. Write a short paper regarding one's own loss experience, identifying perceptions of grief and cultural characteristics

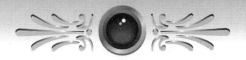

UNIT IV

ETHICAL AND LEGAL CONSIDERATIONS

Learning Objectives

1. Identify ethical principles in providing end of life care
2. Discuss importance of advance directives and health care proxy
3. Identify ethical and legal issues involving difficult and conflicting aspects of decision making in end of life care

CHAPTER

THE ETHICS OF END OF LIFE CARE

Dr. J. Brooke Hamilton III

END OF LIFE CARE IN THE UNITED STATES

Despite having access to the most technologically advanced medical system in the world, many patients under the care of physicians in the United States do not have good deaths. In November 1995, the Journal of the American Medical Association reported the results of the $28 million SUPPORT study funded by the Robert Wood Johnson Foundation, aimed at improving end of life decision making and reducing the frequency of mechanically supported, painful, and prolonged deaths. After a two-year observational phase, the study documented shortcomings in communication between doctors and patients and in the characteristics of hospital death: Only 47% of physicians knew when their patients preferred to avoid CPR, and 50% of conscious patients who died in the hospital endured moderate to severe pain at least half the time during their stay. A subsequent two-year intervention phase that provided information to the physician regarding the patient's wishes and condition failed to improve these outcomes. In 1997, an Institute of Medicine committee (Field and Cassel 1997) found that doctors and hospitals are poorly prepared to give appropriate care to the hopelessly ill. "Americans have come to fear that they will die alone and that they will die in distress or pain."

Perhaps in part as a reaction to these fears, 50% of Americans surveyed said that they favored physician-assisted suicide. Some patients availed themselves of Dr. Jack Kevorkian's help in ending their lives until he was put in prison. While the Supreme Court ruled in 1997 that people do not have a broadly defined constitutional right to a physician's assistance in ending their lives, the decision left the door way open for states to debate the issue. Oregon currently permits physician-assisted suicide under certain conditions. The results of these studies and the public's reaction are troubling for many health care professionals who see their role as helping patients to preserve life.

Whether patients receive aggressive medical care at the end of life, whether they die in a hospital or spend time in an ICU, and how much it costs for them to die are greatly influenced by the patient's zip code! A Dartmouth Medical School study (Wennberg and Cooper 1998) shows that hospital costs paid by Medicare in the last six months of a patient's life, adjusted for area cost differences, average $16,571 in Manhattan and $5,831 in several Oregon districts. Additional costs such as doctors' fees and out-of-pocket expenses would likely double the totals spent. In Newark, Medicare patients are likely to spend at least 20 days in a hospital during their last six months compared to 5.3 days in Salt Lake City. During their last six months, 46% of Medicare patients in Miami spend time in an intensive care unit, whereas in Sun City, Arizona, fewer than 9% utilize an ICU. In Newark 51.3% of Medicare deaths occur in a hospital compared to 22.2% in Portland, Oregon.

A number of factors could cause these wide variations in the cost and usage of hospitals and medical interventions. Patient and family preferences, the presence or lack of social support services to help patients die at home, the number of hospital beds per 1,000 population which correlates closely with the number of days of hospitalization, the attitudes of the medical community regarding medical interventions for the elderly, nursing home regulations that make nursing homes reluctant to have patients die there, and the presence of teaching hospitals and doctors in training who may be reluctant to let patients die are all factors that influence end of life care. Whatever the causes, this wide variation in the treatment of dying patients raises questions about what care is best. Are patients better off dying in a hospital surrounded by high-tech medicine or are they better off with fewer hospital days and less expensive treatment? Research has also suggested that critically ill children and their families may receive very different recommendations on appropriate medical care depending on the nurses and physicians involved in the case. Obviously our society has not settled on one best way to manage end of life care for adult or pediatric patients.

WHAT IS END OF LIFE CARE?

End of life care can be defined as medical and other supportive care given to a person during the final six months of life. But how do we know which are the final six months? When death will occur is clear with some diseases such as advanced stage cancers where physical manifestations are unambiguous and the progress of the disease well documented. The prognosis is much less clear in other conditions such as dementia, heart disease, stroke, lung disease, and liver and kidney disease. These are typically chronic conditions punctuated by acute episodes that the patient may or may not survive. Given the difficulty of predicting when and by what process death will come, end of life care can best be defined for purposes of ethics as that care which the health care team provides in what they think could be the final days, weeks, or months of the patient's life. If the patient is a conscious participant or the family is involved in the decision making, end of life care is also defined by the expectations of the patient and family as to the final period of the patient's life. Thus the boundaries of what constitutes end of life care are not definite. The reason to focus on the end of life period is that treatment chosen to deal with the aging or disease processes at this stage of life will have serious and even permanent consequences.

SHE JUST LOOKED AWAY

Mrs. T was a 65-year-old woman who presented with midsternal chest pain. She was a pack-a-day smoker who lived with her only daughter and fiercely guarded her independence. She was assessed by history and physical examination, determined to have an aortic aneurysm, and taken to surgery. Postoperatively, she had a little bit of respiratory difficulty, and after being transferred from postop to a telemetry unit, developed acute respiratory distress with arrest. No clear information was available as to how long she had been in arrest before CPR was initiated. She was placed on a respirator and was transferred to ICU, where she remained on the vent for two weeks. During this period, she had a collapsed left lung and had multiple problems with mucous plugs, for which she had three bronchoscopies. Right lower lung pneumonia was diagnosed, which had cultured as polymicrobial. It was uncertain whether her lung function would ever be restored to independent status, but removing her from the vent without a long weaning process would result in death. Her renal function had deteriorated. She was severely malnourished. The surgeon felt that each of her problems was potentially reversible and advocated aggressive treatment of each of them. Her family practice physician, given the multiple problems she faced, doubted that she would ever recover enough to leave the hospital. Her three adult children maintained that if she could not resume the independent life she had enjoyed before the surgery, she should be removed from the vent and allowed to die. They cited her many statements to them, at the time of her husband's death of lung cancer and later in her life, that she did not want to live in a dependent state and that she had not prolonged her husband's death needlessly. She did not have a living will or a health care proxy.

The patient's mental status was unclear. After being totally unresponsive for almost two weeks, her ICU nurses felt she was regaining her decision making capacity. She had begun to respond to simple commands such as "squeeze your right hand" and "squeeze your left hand." When the nurses explained to her that removing the vent would cause her death and asked if she wanted to have it removed, she seemed to look away. The nurses interpreted this response as a refusal to have treatment withdrawn.

At the end of the week, the patient would require a tracheostomy and a PEG tube in order to be maintained. The children saw this as a decision point after which their mother might be condemned to a life of dependency in a nursing care facility and asked for withdrawal of treatment other than comfort care. The physicians were unable to predict whether or not there would be improvement in physical or mental status, but the surgeon urged against withdrawal (Copyright 1997 by Julie Loup and J. Brooke Hamilton III. Reprinted by permission).

What treatment decision would you recommend? What diagnoses and prognoses are you basing your recommendation on? What values or ethical principles are you basing your recommendation on? Who should make the decision about the course of treatment? What institutional processes would you recommend to bring about a decision?

The Purpose of End of Life Care

One way to begin understanding the ethics of end of life care is to ask what is the purpose or goal of end of life care. What should the nurses, physicians, and other members of the team be trying to accomplish in providing end of life care? Knowing the purpose of end of life care will help establish what is right or wrong in providing that care. What accomplishes or contributes to the purpose is good. What takes away from the goal or frustrates the purpose is bad. Knowing the purpose will not give a final answer as to what is right or wrong. Some purposes for end of life care, such as suppressing respiration to hasten death and thereby gain quicker access to the patient's estate, would be unethical. Unethical means, such as turning off a patient's oxygen without her consent, can be used to gain ethical objectives, such as ending her pain. Looking at the purpose of end of life care, however, will give a starting point to deciding what is ethical.

Several possible objectives in providing end of life care are:

- To cure disease, halt the progress of disease, restore health or functioning, and thereby provide a longer life for the patient. The care team will provide the very best in aggressive medical treatment so that this patient and future patients may benefit by living longer.
- To maintain the patient in his current state until the nature of the disease processes can be understood and aggressive therapy or withdrawal of treatment can be decided upon.
- To withdraw aggressive medical interventions so that dying is not prolonged and pain and suffering are not increased. The care team will give comfort care and support to the dying patient so that pain and suffering are relieved to the degree possible and medical interventions are limited to those with clear benefits.

The first two objectives are aimed at a cure or at halting the progress of the life-threatening disease or aging process. These objectives are based on the value of life and seek to continue it even at the cost of pain and suffering and the utilization of expensive and sometimes scarce medical resources. The third objective is based on the value of relieving suffering and providing for a good death. This objective does not deny the value of life or the desirability of a longer life, but suggests that, in the face of great pain and suffering, a longer life may not be worth the price. If prospects for recovery are good and the quality of life the patient will return to is high, then the first objective is usually preferred. If the prospects for the patient are unclear, the second objective is usually preferred. If the prospects are bad or if the quality of life is poor, then the last objective may be chosen. Medical facts and value considerations must be weighed in deciding which objective to pursue.

If one of the first two alternatives is chosen, then the medical care team will play its usual role as the defender of the patient from death or disability. If the third objective is chosen, the medical care team will need to change its role of defender from death to the role of supporting the patient in dying a good death. With this change in roles will also come a change in the type of care provided. What would be acceptable therapy in an aggressive defense from death such as cardiopulmonary resuscitation (CPR), high-dose antibiotics, and intubation might be replaced in a comfort care plan with a Do Not Attempt Resuscitation (DNAR or DNR) order, high-dose pain relief which may suppress respiration, and withdrawal of a vent. Since there is not just one objective of end of life care and with the possible objectives being so different, there will not be a single standard for judging what is good care and what is not. The care team must remain flexible about adjusting its perception of what is right or wrong depending on the objective chosen.

In the case of Mrs. T, the objectives can be to return her to her prior state of independent living, to prevent her death and move her to a skilled nursing facility where her recovery will or will not progress, or to honor her previously stated wishes by removing her ventilator and allowing her to die with comfort care. The care that is appropriate for the first two objectives is not appropriate for the third objective.

The question then is whether all of these objectives are ethical. Is it ethical to withdraw aggressive therapies and allow patients to die when their life can be prolonged, at least for a while, by medical treatment? To answer this question, it is necessary to examine attitudes toward life and death in our society and the absolute value of human life.

ATTITUDES TOWARD LIFE AND DEATH

If end of life care can have serious and permanent consequences, death is certainly a serious consequence and a permanent state. Death is the end of life as we know it and the beginning of a new existence as a spirit or as a memory and presence in the lives of those who are still living. As the end of all a person's experiences and projects, death is an evil. It is an ending which is inevitable. All of us at some time will stop having new experiences and stop doing the things we want to do. Since it is inevitable and a necessary part of every life, death and the dying process that brings us to death need to be accepted, talked about, and planned for. In our society, however, we generally accept death, as long as it is not ours, not happening now, and not something we have to talk about.

Health care providers may project these attitudes toward death onto patients. It is not unreasonable to expect that patients want to avoid death and are willing to undergo pain and suffering to do so. If they were not, why would they consent to tortures by medical professionals that in any other circumstance would be cause for criminal prosecution?

Health care providers must recognize, however, that death is not always the greatest evil. With regard to life, longer is not necessarily better—just as with death, later is not always preferable to sooner. Patients who are experiencing intractable pain or who are suffering from a loss of dignity and sense of themselves may consider life a burden. Patients and families who see no hope for recovery and find no value in prolonging the dying process may see death as the restful end to a difficult struggle. Others in the same situation may see the process of dying as redemptive, to be prolonged because it is the last significant act of their lives and a time to bring their affairs to completion. Thus, just as there is as yet no consensus on the best way to manage the kind and cost of end of life care, there is no single best way to view death and the dying process which brings us to it.

Is Life an Absolute Value?

Some patients, families, and health care professionals may see life as an absolute value to be protected at all costs. They may believe that individuals are not allowed to choose to give up life. However true this position may seem, most individuals do not agree with it when they fully understand what it means. Nor do most societies or religious traditions uphold the absolute value of life.

All life, and especially human life, is valuable. We value our own lives. Because we see no real differences between our lives and those of other people, we value their lives also, whether they are young or old; rich or poor; of the same or different gender, ethnic group, religion, or nationality; are handicapped or not; are sick or well. After all, if we had been born them instead of ourselves, we would be in the same condition they are in and would want to be valued just as we want to be valued now.

Life, however, is not an absolute value for most of us, even if we think it is. Sometimes we value other things more than life, even more than our own life. We value our family and our country more than life because we would be willing to sacrifice our life to preserve them. We value our integrity and our freedom more than life since there are some circumstances in which we can imagine dying rather than lying or living under oppression. We value some exciting experiences more than life in that we raise the odds of losing it by climbing mountains, flying airplanes, and driving fast or even driving at all. In the same way, in medical settings life is not an absolute value or the only value. Life is a very important value but most people agree that sometimes it is ethical to choose goods other than life. In end of life care situations, when preserving the patient's life is the primary value, the decisions to be made are medical decisions about which course of treatment will best preserve life. These can be difficult decisions, requiring all of the art and science of the care team members to determine the facts and make accurate diagnoses and prognoses based on these facts. When other goods or values are in conflict with the value of life, the decisions are difficult from an ethical point of view. The medical decisions may be in doubt also and further complicate the picture. The decisions, however, about whether the management of pain, the relief of the patient's suffering, the preservation of the patient's sense of self, the medical professionals' commitment to best practices of medical care, or the society's concern for a just distribution of scarce medical resources are more important values in the situation than preserving the patient's life—these are ethical decisions.

The case of Mrs. T is a good example of how medical and ethical questions can combine in one situation. The physicians have not been able to determine with any certainty whether Mrs. T suffered permanent brain damage during her arrest. Her surgeon, looking at each of her other multiple medical problems separately, thinks that each is potentially solvable. Her family practice physician, looking at her as a whole person with multiple severe medical problems, doubts that she will recover to leave the hospital. It has not been determined whether she has recovered sufficiently to be capable of making her own medical decisions, though the ICU nurses contend that she has. These are all primarily medical questions, the answers to which are important for answering the ethical questions the case poses.

The primary ethical question is whether or not to withdraw treatment from Mrs. T, particularly the ventilator and antibiotics for her pneumonia, and allow her to die. Are her prior wishes as expressed, not in a legally recognized advance directive but to her family, grounds for allowing her to die at this point in her course of treatment? Should aggressive treatment of each of her problems, accompanied by a tracheostomy and PEG tube, be continued until the extent of her progress is better known? If the decision is made to allow her to die, should she be weaned from the respirator in order to maximize her chances for breathing on her own or should the machine simply be turned off? Is the possibility that she may recover only enough to leave the hospital but not enough to resume the life she thought worth living grounds for allowing her to die?

WHO DECIDES THE COURSE OF END OF LIFE TREATMENT ?

Who decides what care Mrs. T should receive? The medical questions are best answered by the combined resources of all the members of the care team. The physicians, and ultimately the physician in charge of the patient, must make the final determination of the most accurate diagnosis and prognosis; but nurses who care for the patient should contribute their expertise as well. Because of their training and their experience in caring for and observing patients over longer periods of time than physicians typically do, nurses have valuable information to offer the care team. This contribution of medical expertise is the first of the nurses' many roles in end of life care (Figure 8–1).

Who should decide the ethical issues in end of life care, such as those proposed in Mrs. T's case? Is it the patient, the family, the medical care team, the institution in which the patient is treated, or the society in which the patient lives? What values should guide that decision: the values of the patient, family, care team, institution, or society? The answer is that the primary decision maker is the patient, but others who have a role in the care of the patient must be considered also.

Medical care expert based on the special training and experience which a nurse has.

Translator of medical information into understandable language for the patient and family.

Values clarification counselor for the patient and family to help them become clear on what is really important to them in a stressful medical situation.

Guide to decision making by suggesting care options which are in accord with the patient's and family's values and goals, legal documents such as a living will and health care proxy, and institutional processes such as ethics committee consults which will aid end of life decision making.

Family mediator in discussions between patient and family members.

Patient advocate in making the patient's values and goals known to family and other care team members, and speaking out for the rights and best interests of the patient when no surrogate decision makers are available or when the family seeks to overrule the patient's advance directive.

Care team communicator insuring that members of the care team know the patient's wishes regarding end of life issues such as DNAR and confidentiality vis a vis her family, and that care team members have an ongoing discussion of appropriate end of life care based on a common knowledge of the facts and the prognosis in the case and a shared awareness of all of the appropriate value inputs from patient, family, medical professionals, institution, and society.

Figure 8–1 Nurses' Roles in End Of Life Care

Models for Health Care Decision Making

From the beginning of organized medicine until the 1960s, the primary decision maker for both medical and ethical issues was the physician (Figure 8–2). The physician, by possessing the specialized knowledge of medicine and being dedicated to the good of the patient, decided the course of medical care for the patient. The patient was "patient," waiting, sometimes for long hours in the waiting room at the doctor's office or in the hospital bed, and accepted directions from the physician. Nurses, other care team members and the hospitals ministered to the patient under the direction of the physician. The family and society also followed the physician's directions and paid the fees decided on by the physician.

This physician-directed model of medical care was severely criticized during the consumer revolution of the 1960s and 1970s as being paternalistic and

Hippocratic Tradition (Beginning of medicine until 1960s):

Primary Values:

Nonmaleficence—First do no harm.

Confidentiality is part of nonmaleficence.

Beneficence—medicine is acting in the interests of the patient.

Physician understands the means to promote the interests of the patient and society and so makes decisions about medical treatments. Paternalistic or authoritarian model.

Consumer Movement Changes (1960s & 1970s):

Primary Value: Autonomy—respect for individuals means patient makes decisions about medical care. Physician provides options available and patient makes choices.

Reaction against paternalistic model. Denies medical expertise of medical professions and responsibility of physician, hospital, and society to refuse inappropriate medical treatment.

Contractual/Community Model (1980s to the present):

Primary Values:

Autonomy

    Truth Telling

    Confidentiality

    Informed Consent

Beneficence

Nonmaleficence

Justice

Care team uses these principles as guides for ethical decision making. When principles conflict, must decide which is most important in this particular case. Understanding of the principles develops through application to cases. Decisions should reflect primarily the directions of the patient, conditioned by the professional values of physicians and nurses, the hospital or institution, and the community.

Figure 8–2 History of Medical Decision Making

authoritarian. Generalized suspicions of authority and charges that institutions were not being operated for the good of society led critics of medicine to suggest that the patient as customer should decide what medical care he or she wanted. Under this consumer model of medicine, the physician was to outline the options for care and the patient would decide which option best fit personal values and goals. The physician then provided the service ordered by the consumer.

The major shortcoming of this model was that it reduced the expertise of the medical professionals to medical knowledge and the skills. It denied that by virtue of using their knowledge and skills, they also gained ethical experience in what outcomes were or were not beneficial to their patients. The consumer model overlooked the values of the medical professionals—that they were dedicated to using their knowledge for the good of the patient and that they were unwilling to use their time and skills in futile or unworthy efforts. The model denied society's interests in insuring that important social institutions like medicine promote values which the society considers important, such as the use of pharmacological agents for pain relief but not for recreation. It also denied society's responsibility as the ultimate payor for medical services to decide what services and goods were worth paying for and what were not. Out of the need to balance the values of the patient, the medical professionals, and society grew a contractual/community model for medical decision making that recognized the legitimacy of many inputs into the ethical decisions in medical care (Figure 8–3).

PATIENT AUTONOMY

The most important factor in deciding what end of life care to provide is what the patient wants. The decision as to what care is appropriate is made by the patient in accordance with his or her values and goals in life. A patient who wishes to live as long as possible or who wishes to live long enough to mark an important birthday, holiday, or family event or to complete an unfinished task, such as reconciling with a relative, may choose aggressive therapy and pain in order to realize that goal. A patient who wishes to avoid pain or to avoid dependence on others may choose to forgo medical interventions and opt for pain control and comfort care or even, where it is legally available, assistance in ending his or her life. Pediatric patients, though not at the legal age of making their own decisions, do not arrive there suddenly at their 18th or 21st birthdays. They should be involved in the decision making to the extent that their reasoning abilities and emotional development approach that of an adult.

This recognition that the patient's wishes are primary is based on the importance given in our society to the value of autonomy. It is assumed that adults know best what they want. If everyone in the society is equal, then why should some be able to make decisions for others? The primacy of patient wishes can also be established in other ways. The 1990 Supreme Court case, In the Matter of Nancy Cruzan, pointed out that all U.S. citizens have a right to refuse medical care even if it is not perceived by others to be in their best interest to do so. Caregivers should also recognize that since they would like to be able to make their own decisions regarding medical care, they should not prevent patients from making those decisions for themselves.

Thus it is important that nurses on the care team do not impose their own values or society's values on a patient like Mrs. T if it can be avoided. It is also

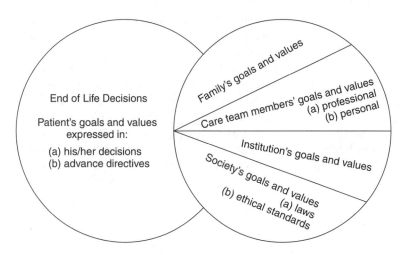

Figure 8–3 Contractual/Community Model
Who makes the decisions on end of life care?

important that the medical care team not assume that they know what the patient wants. Under the paternalistic model of medicine, the patient presented and the medical team decided appropriate care. The assumption was that the patient wanted to maintain health and live as long as possible and that the care team knew the best ways to realize these goals. The new contractual community model recognizes that the patient may have one of three possible goals in end of life care discussed above: aggressive treatment to extend life, temporary maintenance until more information is available, or comfort care until death.

Truth Telling

Truth telling is another important value which derives from autonomy. The need to tell the truth to patients regarding their condition and the expected outcomes is based on respect for autonomy of persons. Patients cannot make decisions if they do not have the relevant information. The level of truth telling, however, may be conditioned by the wishes of the individual patient and by the patient's cultural background. Some patients do not want to be told bad news, or they wish to have it in small installments so that they can deal with the emotional impact. Nurses learn to listen for clues as to whether a patient is ready to hear the facts or not and learn skills needed to deliver truth so that it is not harmful. Social work and pastoral care involvement can be helpful to support the patient who is receiving bad news.

In the absence of clues as to how much the patient wants to hear, the nurse can ask the patient how much he or she wants to know about the situation as it develops. Family members can also provide clues. Keep in mind that the suggestions of family members may be influenced by their own difficulties in facing the truth rather than the patient's desires. In some cultures the family acts as the filter for news or as the decision maker.

An additional benefit of truth telling is that truthful health care providers are seldom sued even when they make mistakes. Patients and their families can accept that members of the care team make mistakes much more easily than they can accept the fact that they are not told the truth about these mistakes. Truth telling in charting and reporting of mistakes to supervisors can also be very beneficial to the patients and the institution, since reports of a number of similar mistakes can allow the development of systems to avoid those mistakes in the future.

Following the Patient's Wishes— Respecting Autonomy

How can the care team know what the patient wants? The most direct way is to be told by the patient who has the capacity to understand the consequences of choosing among the various alternatives and has made a decision regarding an alternative. If there are doubts as to the capacity of the patient to consent and the consequences to the patient are significant, then a psychiatric or psychological consult should be requested.

Capacity versus Competency

In discussing the patient's ability to make decisions, it is important to distinguish between *capacity* and *competency*. *Competence* is a legal term indicating that a person is legally capable of making decisions regarding financial affairs or medical treatment. A competency determination is made by a court and can take several months. It requires the appointment of a lawyer to represent the patient and legal counsel to represent the family or institution seeking to have competency determined. Given the time required, these legal proceedings are not appropriate in medical decisions where the patient's status is changing quickly. The capacity to make medical care decisions depends on a patient's ability to understand the facts and consequences of various alternatives and to choose among them. Whether this capacity has been compromised by disease, dementia, unconsciousness, or delusions can be obvious or can require determination by trained medical personnel based on observation and a number of tests.

In Mrs. T's case, does the fact that she can respond to simple commands and squeeze the nurse's left or right hand indicate that she has the capacity to understand the consequences of removing the vent? When she looks away, is that an indication of refusal to have the vent removed, or is it a sign that the complex reasoning involved in making that decision is beyond her capacity? Both interpretations have some plausibility. The nurses involved in her care should be careful not to let their concern to have her improve influence their interpretation of which is the more plausible explanation. A consult to determine decision-making capacity would be in order here.

Nurse as Translator and Values Clarifier

Despite the fact that patients' wishes are primary in deciding end of life care, patients may not know what they want—what their values and goals are and how best to reach those given the limitations imposed by their medical condition and the medical resources available. Thus it is critical that nurses recognize the importance of their role as translator of medical information for the patient and values clarifier to help the patient understand what is really important at what may be the end of life (Figure 8-1). Ideally these discussions should be undertaken with a multidisciplinary team including the physician, the nurses assigned to the patient, social workers, and pastoral care.

Unfortunately, physicians are often not trained to conduct such discussions and are uncomfortable doing so. A skilled nurse will learn how to do the preliminary work of uncovering the patient's concerns and communicating these to the physician. The nurse should also create occasions for discussion to take place between physician, patient, and family by asking questions when the physician is seeing the patient and prompting the patient and family to voice their concerns. Sadly, research has shown that even when nurses were specifically assigned to inform the physician of the patient's end of life decisions and to enter a summary of these into the patient's medical record, more than half the physicians reported not seeing them (SUPPORT 1995).

A Patient Who Lacks Decision-Making Capacity

If the patient does not have the capacity to make decisions, then the procedure for deciding what routine medical care should be administered would be to consult the family members who are closest to the patient or responsible for the patient's care. State laws governing informed consent generally give classes of family members who can give proxy consent for the patient, beginning with the spouse not legally separated, the adult children, parents, siblings, and the patient's other ascendants and descendants. If the members of one class are not available, the care team is to consult the next class.

End of life care decisions are somewhat different. Because of the fear of patients in general that they would be subjected to end of life care that they did not want—to be put on a ventilator or have CPR attempted if their heart failed—and because of the concern of society that patients should not have their dying unduly extended by painful and expensive medical interventions that offer no change in the imminent outcome, states have passed one form or another of the Uniform Natural Death Act 1996 (www.choices.org). It allows patients to make an advance directive (the patient's directions given in advance) to govern what should happen to them if they lose the capacity to make their own decisions in the face of death. (Copies of advance directive documents for each state can be obtained from Choice in Dying at 1-800-989-9455.) Thus for end of life decisions, the first question to ask the family is not, "What should we do?" or "What would this patient have wanted?" but "Does the patient have an advance directive?" Fortunately federal law requires that patients be informed at admission that they have the right to make an advance directive, and most hospital and care facilities take this as an opportunity to urge patients to make their wishes known. The document(s) would then be included in the patient's chart.

Living Will

There are two types of advance directives, and the well-prepared patient will have executed both. The first document described in the Uniform Natural Death Act legislation is a living will. In the usual form of the living will, patients state that should they be dying and if medical interventions will not prevent death but only make it longer and more painful, and if they have lost decision-making capacity, then they wish to have medical interventions withheld or withdrawn and to receive only comfort care.

The patient is not limited to directing that care be withdrawn or withheld. The document can indicate that the patient wishes that all medically appropriate measures be done in the hope of recovery in spite of all odds to the contrary. Patients can even direct that "everything possible be done," though this wish may have to be reconciled with the professional values of the care team, the policies of the hospital, and the values of society.

In order for the living will to be put into effect, two physicians, one of whom is primarily responsible for the patient's care, must indicate in writing that the patient is in a terminal and irreversible condition. All of us are terminal in that we will die at some point. "Terminal and irreversible" under the Uniform Natural Death Act statutes means that the patient is in a continual profound comatose state with no reasonable chance of recovery or is in a condition caused by injury, disease, or illness which within reasonable medical judgment would produce death and for which the application of life-sustaining procedures would serve only to postpone the moment of death. Once the patient has been "qualified" as being in this condition by the two physicians, the care team is legally and ethically required to follow the wishes of the patient as stated in the living will in the same way that they would follow the directives of the patient if he or she were still able to make decisions and communicate them.

If a patient who has lost decision-making capacity can be qualified under the act but has not executed a living will, the act provides for a surrogate decision maker—someone who acts for the patient. Classes of surrogate decisions makers are listed in the act and are generally the same as those in the informed consent statutes. Unanimous agreement among all members of the class of surrogate decision makers is required by the act. If the patient has no spouse, for example, but has three adult children, then all three must agree to withdraw treatment; a majority of the children is not enough to direct the care. If all the members of the surrogate decision maker class do not agree, then standard of care medical treatment should continue.

Not only can the patient or proxy direct the end of life care even after the patient loses decision-making capacity, the legislation provides a safe harbor for the health care team. Caregivers cannot be sued for acting in accordance with the living will if the patient is "qualified" as terminal and irreversible under the terms of the act.

Inability to find surrogate decision makers or to get unanimous agreement does not mean that all possible care or all available care must continue. If standard of care medical treatment would be to withdraw therapies other than comfort care, the care team can make that decision but they will not have the safe harbor legal protection of the Uniform Natural Death Act. An ethics committee consult which confirms this decision will provide some legal protection. Some care teams may not consider an ethics consult sufficient protection from potential liability and may continue to administer futile and painful medical treatments. To do so is not really an ethical course of action since the patient is not benefiting from the treatments. Nurses on the care team should strongly consider advocating (Figure 8–1) for the patient's right to be free from unnecessary and burdensome treatments when the patient cannot advocate for himself.

Mrs. T did not have a living will. Even though she was in a severely compromised state, her physicians were not willing to declare her terminal and irreversible, so her children were not designated proxy decision makers under the Uniform Natural Death Act. Thus her care team did not have the safe harbor protection under the act if the children directed that care be withdrawn. The children did, however, have the right to refuse consent for the tracheostomy and the PEG tube. If the care team had decided to institute these therapies in the absence of the children's consent, they would have had to seek a court-appointed curator for the patient.

Models for Surrogate Decision Makers

There are several ways in which surrogate decision makers can make medical care decisions for a patient. The surrogate can decide based on advance directives received from the patient. The difficulty with this model is that the current circumstances may be different from what the patient envisioned. If the circumstances are similar, the patient's prior directives are a strong basis for a surrogate's decision. The surrogate can also use substituted judgment in which the decision made is based on what he thinks the patient would have wanted in this situation, given what is known about the patient. The difficulty with this model is that research has shown that surrogates often decide differently from what the patients report they would have decided. The surrogate can also decide based on what he thinks is in the best interests of the patient. This model is particularly useful when the surrogate has no prior directives to rely on. The care team should advise the surrogate based on their experience, but it is up to the surrogate to decide what the best interest is.

Under the directives model, Mrs. T's children reported that they had been told repeatedly by their mother that she did not wish to be kept alive in a diminished or dependent state and that if she could not live the way she had always lived, she would rather die. She had made decisions in keeping with that philosophy regarding the end of life treatment of her husband when he was dying of cancer, and she had used those decisions as an example of how she wanted to be treated. Under the substituted judgment model, the children, knowing their mother's feelings about end of life care, could have decided to withdraw treatment if the prognosis was for a life of dependency in a nursing care facility. If there seemed a good possibility that she would be able to return to her prior life of independence, then they would have decided to continue the treatments. The best interests standard would require a decision which represented the best interests of the patient. If she really hated the thought of being dependent and was unlikely to adjust to such a life, then her best interest would seem to be to discontinue treatment if dependence was the likely outcome.

When Family Wishes Conflict with the Patient's Advance Directive

Family wishes in conflict with the patient's advance directive create a difficult position for the care team. Hospital attorneys will often advise that dead patients do not sue but live families do. Thus, the legal wisdom suggests, it is better to follow the wishes of the family when they conflict with the patient's advance directive. This conflict usually occurs when the family wants everything done and the directive says no extraordinary measures. Failing to follow the patient's wishes as stated in an advance directive is clearly unethical. The directive is a legally binding document that speaks for the patients when they can no longer speak for themselves. The care team should honor these directions as if the patient were communicating with them verbally. When the family attempts to overrule the patient's clearly stated directive, the nurses on the care team should act as patient's advocate (Figure 8–1), using the arguments given above for the value of autonomy. If the family continues to press their demands and the care team gives an indication that they will go against the patient's directive, the nurses should call for an ethics committee meeting in order to gain additional support for honoring the patient's directive.

Health Care Proxy or Durable Power of Attorney for Health Care

A second type of advance directive, the health care proxy or durable power of attorney for health care, can provide additional protection for the patient who wishes to have end of life care directions honored. Living will forms will sometimes contain a health care proxy designation. In the health care proxy document, the patient designates an agent to make medical care decisions when that patient is unable to do so. The patient also designates alternate agents who can decide if the original agent is unable or unwilling to act as an agent. The agent is usually, but not always, a member of the patient's family, a spouse, child, or favorite niece for example. Only one agent is empowered to make decisions at any one time.

A health care proxy is different from a durable power of attorney, in which a patient designates an agent for legal and financial matters described in the document, such as signing checks or selling property. Some states require that a durable power of attorney explicitly state that making medical care decisions is one of the powers granted to the agent in order for the agent to act as a health care proxy agent or that a separate health care proxy document be signed. Care teams should verify that the power of attorney clearly includes medical decision making. Some attorneys maintain that health care proxy statements should be notarized in order to be self-validating, but this seems to be a difficult burden for persons being hospitalized for life-threatening conditions. Care teams and hospitals should accept health care proxy documents witnessed by two persons who are not related by blood or marriage and who do not stand to inherit from the patient. Nurses and other care team members should be willing to act as witnesses for hospitalized patients.

The agent's decisions are legally and ethically binding on the health care team. The agent can make decisions with the same rights as the adult patient, even deciding to refuse medical care which seems clearly in the best interests of the patient. The agent could refuse blood transfusions for a patient, for example, on the basis of that patient's religious convictions, even though that would hasten the patient's death. Since the agent will be making medical care decisions, it is important that the patient discuss values and life goals with the agent and what should be done in specific circumstances. Promises by the patient to return to haunt the agent who does not follow those wishes are sometimes effective, but trust in the integrity of the agent is the most effective guarantee.

One advantage of the health care proxy is its clear designation of one person who acts as the patient's agent. That person will consult with the care team and with family members but will be the one person whose decision the care team should honor when the patient is incapacitated. Family disagreement will not prevent the care team from acting. The health care proxy also covers a wider range of possibilities than does the living will. A stroke patient who is irreversibly incapacitated and lacks decision-making capacity but can be maintained successfully on a vent for a long period of time would not qualify for withdrawal of treatment under the safe harbor of his living will because the patient is not terminal in the sense of the law. Knowing the patient's wishes not to be maintained in such a state, the health care proxy agent could direct the care team to remove the vent and provide comfort care until death. Because of these advantages, nurses working in their role as guide to end of life care should urge patients to sign both a living will and a health care proxy (Figure 8–1).

Those Who Want All Possible Care

Some patients or families are unwilling to give up the most remote chance that the outcome will change and the patient will have a few more days, weeks, or even years of life. Society's faith in technological solutions and the wonder cures portrayed in emergency room hospital dramas on television strengthen their belief that a miracle could happen. These patients and families want to play the medical lottery no matter how long the odds of winning. If resources were not precious, if professionals did not object to working for futile ends, if society were not paying the price of the ticket, then all patients could receive all possible medical care for as long as they wanted. Professional values, standards of good medical practice (CPR, for example, is not good practice on end stage cancer patients with brittle bones), and justice (limited resources can better be used elsewhere) require sometimes that the medical system say no. Nurses can translate these considerations into language that the patient and family can understand and hopefully accept. Phrases such as, "We have reached the end of what medicine can do," or, "Medical care cannot provide any more benefits and will simply prolong dying," may be helpful in such discussions. Nurses can also help the patient and family understand their option of trying to obtain additional medical interventions from other care teams or other facilities.

Patients and families who are unwilling to give up any medical intervention in hopes of a divine miracle can be reminded that they do not need to put off dying in hopes of a miracle. Within the Christian faith, Jesus raised Lazarus even though he had been dead for three days.

Other End of Life Care Inputs Which Must Be Considered

Members of the end of life care team should not assume that the patient and the care team have the same goals for care, that the patient and the family want the same thing, nor that the patient and society want the same thing. To the extent possible, the patient's wishes should be given first priority. The patient, family, and care team members must realize that, under the contractual/community model (Figure 8–3), other values and goals come into the end of life decision-making process as well.

FAMILY WISHES

When a patient has family, the family is usually involved in end of life care decisions. These decisions impact the family as well as the patient, and their emotional and physical support are crucial. There are different traditions within families and within ethnic groups as to the level of involvement of the family. Despite the strong emphasis on the autonomy and rights of the individual, nurses should not assume that the family should be told everything about the patient's condition and care. This is particularly true with regard to the patient's HIV status. Thus nurses should discuss with the patient how much family is to be told and how much a part of the decision making family is to be. Confidentiality is an important value in medical care. Patients have a right to keep their medical information confidential, even from members of their family, though few will choose to do so. Some families are the translators for the patient. If a patient has agreed that the family is to play that role, then medical decisions should be discussed with the family first, and time and opportunity allowed for them to discuss the options with the patient. In other families the patient will want to be informed first and allowed to make a decision before telling the family what he or she wants to do. Having determined the patient's stance on confidentiality, the nurses should communicate these wishes to the other care team members (Figure 8–1).

While family members are usually the patient's most important supporters at the end of life, this is not always the case. Nurses should be alert to family members who have as their primary concern interests that are different than the patient's. This is not a problem as long as the patient's wishes are clearly known and the care team upholds the value of autonomy by following those wishes to the extent feasible. The difficulty arises, however, when the patient loses decision-making capacity and the family is called upon, in the absence of advance directives, to make decisions. If the nurse perceives that family members are acting contrary to the interests of the patient, this concern should be discussed with the physician and the nursing supervisor so that a decision regarding intervention on the patient's behalf can be considered. Nurses should also realize, however, that they may not be in a better position than the family to understand the wishes of the patient and to decide what is in the best interest. Nor can a nurse hope to change, in the course of a hospitalization, family dynamics developed over years of interaction.

PROFESSIONAL VALUES OF HEALTH CARE TEAM

While the directives of the patient are the most important in deciding what end of life care should be given, other values which must also be considered in the decision making process are those which guide the professional life of the care team members. To be a profession, a group of practitioners must be dedicated to service of others, must possess a specialized body of knowledge and direct the training and certification of those who utilize this knowledge, and the group must set the standards for using that knowledge for the good of society, with some input from the society that is being served. Two of the most important professional groups represented on the care team are the physicians and the nurses. Other groups also participate and their professional values are important, but the physicians and nurses have the central roles in providing care. Since the care team is usually directed by a physician, it is critical that the team understand not only the professional values of nurses but the values of the physicians as well (Figure 8–4).

Beauchamp and Childress (1998) suggest that clinical decision making is guided by a set of ethical principles, three of which—autonomy, truth telling, and confidentiality—have already been discussed in reference to protecting the patients' rights to make their own medical decisions. Autonomy can also

NONMALEFICENCE:

First do no harm.

Stronger duty than to do good for patient, based on acceptance of natural processes like disease and aging, which physician cannot prevent. Modified by principle of double effect: Harm is allowed if an unavoidable part of doing a good which is intended.

    Can conflict with: autonomy and beneficence.

TRUTH TELLING:

Based on respect for autonomy of persons. How can they make decisions if they do not have the relevant information? Level of truth telling may be conditioned by the culture. In some cultures the family acts as the filter for news or as the decision maker. Learn skills to deliver truth so that it is not harmful. Truthful providers are seldom sued even when they make mistakes.

    Can conflict with: nonmaleficence (when information will harm the patient) and beneficence (when withholding information will help)

CONFIDENTIALITY:

Based on autonomy. Control of information about ourselves. Strong element in Hippocratic tradition. More important as information has serious social consequences: HIV status and genetic coding.

    Can conflict with:

        nonmaleficence and beneficence (when telling others may be in patient's interest)

        justice (others who will be harmed by not knowing the information)

        truth telling (others may request confidential information)

AUTONOMY:

Based on respect for persons—being a person involves being able to choose what we think is important or valuable and to act on those choices. No one else can decide what is important to me as well as I can. If all persons are intrinsically equal, why should others be able to decide for me?

    Can conflict with:

        physician autonomy

        beneficence (paternalism: physician knows best)

    Can be diminished by illness—need for advance directives such as living will or health care proxy

    Competency requires ability to understand options and weigh consequences

    Can be very important to a patient in illness (ex. Texas burn patient, Dax Howard)

Figure 8–4 Ethical Principles for Clinical Decision Making

BENEFICENCE:

Doing good for the patient.

> Can conflict with:
>> autonomy (paternalism: do what is good for patient in spite of his or her choices)
>> truth telling (withholding information for the good of patient)
>> justice (concern only for the good of individual patient = hypocratic individualism)

JUSTICE:

Insuring that benefits and burdens are fairly distributed. Opposed to Hippocratic individualism—the concern for my patient only without regard for the needs of other patients, the health care system and society.

> Can conflict with:
>> nonmaleficence and beneficence (may not be able to do as much as possible for individual patient because of needs of others)

Figure 8–4 *Continued*

be expanded to include respect for the autonomous decision making and the professional values of the care team members. Two of the others—nonmaleficence (first do no harm) and beneficence (do good)—are physician-centered values because they govern the intent and effect of the physician's actions on the patient. These two are invoked by physicians to explain how their actions must be limited by concerns for benefit and harm and sometimes conflict with the directions of the patient or the family. Justice is a society-centered value in that it concerns the fair distribution of scarce medical resources including the care team's time and expertise, which the society has invested in creating, and the other medical resources, which ultimately the society as a whole provides.

These values can sometimes conflict with one another. Sometimes means can be found to resolve these conflicts through discussion which proposes further alternative courses of action, changes the way in which one of the parties sees his values being realized in an alternative, or gives the parties more time to consider. If no way can be found to resolve the conflict, then the care team and the patient or family must try to decide which values are most important in the situation. An ethics committee consult often can be helpful in resolving factual and value disagreements. There is also a rich literature on clinical ethics which can provide for practical, well-balanced guidance (Jonsen, Siegler, and Winsdale 1998).

Understanding what these values mean (Figure 8–4) and that these values can conflict with one another will help the nurse discuss ethical issues with physicians. Understanding that the physician-centered values of nonmaleficence and beneficence do not automatically trump the patient-centered values of autonomy, truth telling, and confidentiality, or the society-centered value of justice, will help the nurse advocate on behalf of the patient and society. A physician's statement that "I must first do no harm" when the patient requests palliative care that may hasten death is not the end of an ethical discussion, but only the statement of one value which must be considered.

It is also important to understand that these abstract ethical principles gain their meaning for medical practitioners through countless individual cases which they have experienced or which have been litigated in the courts and discussed in medical ethics literature. Nurses who wish to be effective in their discussions of clinical ethics with physicians and other care team members would do well to be familiar with the important cases in their area of specialization. For example, Jonsen (1998) provides a number of histories of important cases in the development of clinical ethics.

The Role of Personal Values

Nurses, physicians, and other members of the care team also have personal values that influence what they are willing to do or not do in giving end of life care. In the controversy that has arisen in the United States over physician-assisted suicide, for example, many health care professionals have indicated a willingness or an unwillingness to assist a terminally ill patient to end his own life if federal or state law allows it. Withdrawing medical treatment from severely deformed newborns is another topic on which equally ethical practitioners disagree. Their positions may be based on social or religious values or on interpretations of the purpose of professional medicine. These values or convictions may conflict with equally strongly held values of patients or families requesting their help. Based on the value of their own autonomy, it is ethically permissible for medical professionals to decline to provide services that they believe are wrong. Nurses who decline to provide a legally approved procedure have an obligation to help transfer the care of the patient to other care providers. This appeal to conscience may be limited, however, by being the only available provider of a legally approved procedure.

INSTITUTIONAL CONCERNS

Institutions such as hospitals, nursing homes, and home care services have a mission and have values and policies that flow from that mission. Many U.S. hospitals have religious traditions and values to uphold. Values such as "service to all in need" and "respect for the personal values of patients" and "in keeping with the Roman Catholic faith" may have important implications for end of life care decisions. These values are made specific through policies for patients' rights and responsibilities, DNAR orders, withholding and withdrawing life support, and ethics committee consults. Nurses should familiarize themselves with these policies so that they can advocate on behalf of patients and families and explain the limits on patients' and families' directions. Nurses should not assume that physicians will be familiar with the fine points of these policies since they may practice at a number of institutions with different policies. If the care requests of patients or families are contrary to the policies of the institution and no accommodation is possible, nurses should assist in finding alternative care facilities for the patient.

COMMUNITY AND SOCIETY'S CONCERNS

Society may also have certain values that it wishes to see upheld in end of life care decisions. Even though U.S. society is highly individualistic and upholds the importance of an individual's autonomous decision making, society as a whole does support medical education, research, and the funding of hospitals and other care facilities in which medicine is practiced. Thus society has a stake in insuring that those professions and institutions promote values which may limit the autonomy of individuals. The U.S. Supreme Court, in its recent decisions indicating that individuals do not have a constitutionally protected right to physician-supported suicide, pointed to the value of life as having been protected and promoted since the founding of the society. The judicial, legislative, and executive branches of government at both the federal and state levels have promoted other values, such as equal access and nondiscrimination and a just distribution of medical resources. Other social institutions, such as businesses, have also had an effect on the values promoted in medical care through their purchasing of health insurance for their workers. The move to managed care has been driven in large part by the desire of business to see medical resources used efficiently and in a cost-effective manner for the benefit of the workers and the employers who pay the premiums. Nurses who advocate for their individual patients against the limits on end of life care placed by private insurers or Medicare and Medicaid should realize the legitimacy of the values that place those limits while remaining free to disagree and work to bring about changes in the ways society has chosen to implement those values in health care policies. Being a contributing member of state and national nursing organizations that work to influence health policy is an important ethical obligation for members of the nursing profession.

WHAT PROCESSES CAN HELP WITH END OF LIFE DECISION MAKING?

Just knowing what is right in an end of life care situation is not enough. Nurses as members of an end of life care team are rarely able to make decisions and act alone. Care of an end of life patient is directed by one or several physicians and carried out by a number of nurses and other specialists. Thus it is essential that nurses be able to help in bringing about a consensus among the patient, family, and care team on what is appropriate care for each patient.

Ongoing Discussions Regarding End of Life Care

One method for reaching a consensus is to maintain an ongoing discussion with all those involved. This role as care team communicator (Figure 8–1) is discussed several times in this chapter. Nurses should also be willing to use the chain of command on the nursing staff and the institution's patient advocate to bolster their position on important issues of appropriate care. Fighting the battle alone or giving up are not the only options within a health care organization. An effective advocate for the patient looks for allies through both formal and informal networks.

An important effect of ongoing discussions to reach consensus on appropriate care is that a nurse's view of what is right or wrong may develop and even change. Being willing to listen to different points of view, especially from respected individuals, and remaining open to compromise and change is not a sign of ethical weakness or lack of integrity. Rather these characteristics show a commitment to the values of reasonable pluralism and democratic citizenship, which allow individuals to acknowledge the complexity of end of life issues, respect reasonable differences, and seek mutually respectful resolutions to reasonable disagreements (Benjamin 1990).

Ethics Committee Consults

Another important instrument for reaching consensus on complex end of life care decisions is an ethics committee consult. All hospitals are required by Joint Commission standards to have an in-house ethics committee or access to an ethics committee. An ethics consult is a valuable process for resolving disagreements or finding solutions to end of life dilemmas. Nurses should familiarize themselves with the procedures for calling for an ethics committee consult. Figure 8–5 presents a public teaching hospital's flowchart for calling an ethics consult. Some institutions also employ a clinical ethicist who consults on cases. In these institutions it is necessary to distinguish between an ethics consult and an ethics committee consult. Patients in nursing homes and home health care or under the treatment of a private physician usually do not have access to an ethics committee unless the facility or agency is willing to borrow one from a nearby hospital or a community-based ethics committee is available.

An ethics committee consult can be requested by a patient, a family member, or a member of the care team (Figure 8–6). The task of an ethics committee is not to determine what can be done but to conduct a discussion to determine what should be done. A patient may want to seek help from an ethics committee to clarify his or her values in order to be able to decide on a course of treatment consistent with those values. A medical professional may want

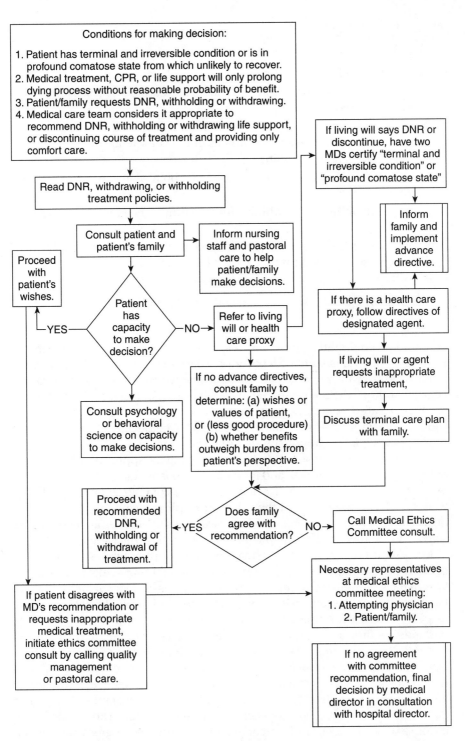

Figure 8–5 Decisions on DNR, Withholding and Withdrawing Treatment, and Ethics Committee Consultation Requests

Copyright 1997 by J. Brooke Hamilton III. Reprinted by permission.

An ethics consultation can be helpful if:

1. A patient is unsure of whether a course of treatment is consistent with his or her values.
2. A medical professional is unsure whether providing a course of treatment will be consistent with his or her conscience or professional responsibilities.
3. Family members are unsure or disagree about what should be done.
4. Family members differ with health care providers about what care is best.
5. Health care providers disagree with each other or with the family on the course of treatment that should be followed.

Figure 8–6 Who Needs an Ethics Committee Consult?

help in deciding whether providing a specific kind of treatment or withholding treatment is consistent with his or her conscience or professional values.

Most cases coming to ethics committees involve individuals or families deciding for others who are incapable of deciding for themselves. Should the patient be treated aggressively, maintained until further developments, or should care be limited to comfort measures? Are specific interventions appropriate, such as cardiopulmonary resuscitation, surgery, or the placing of a feeding tube? Is withdrawal or limitation of treatment appropriate? These are difficult questions to answer, and individuals and families are often conflicted over what is the best answer. Having access to a committee familiar with the values of the community and the ethics principles developed through legal decisions, academic research, and the discussions of other ethics committees across the country can be a help in arriving at the best decision.

Many ethics committee discussions consider whether the best course is to continue, withdraw, or withhold treatment. The meeting seeks to clarify the facts in the situation and determine the important issues and values involved. Figure 8–7 shows the Jonsen Box (Jonsen, Siegler, and Winsdale 1998), a widely respected format for ethics committee discussions, which divides the facts into medical indications, patient preferences, quality of life, and contextual features. Based on these facts and the value considerations of the patient, family, medical professionals, institution, and society, the committee will help the parties involved arrive at a consensus as to the best course of treatment. If disagreement persists, the committee will make a recommendation. The parties are free to act on or to reject the recommendation. The committee in its role as consultant enters its recommendation into the progress notes in the patient's medical record. All discussions and recommendations are held in the strictest confidence.

MEDICAL INDICATIONS

1. What is patient's medical problem? History? Diagnosis? Prognosis?
2. Is problem acute? Chronic? Critical? Emergent? Reversible?
3. What are goals of treatment?
4. What are probabilities of success?
5. What are plans in case of therapeutic failure?
6. In sum, how can this patient be benefited by medical and nursing care, and harm avoided?

PATIENT PREFERENCES

1. What has the patient expressed about preferences for treatment?
2. Has patient been informed of benefits and risks, understood, and given consent?
3. Is patient mentally capable and legally competent? What is evidence of incapacity?
4. Has patient expressed prior preferences, e.g. advance directives?
5. If incapacitated, who is appropriate surrogate? Is surrogate using appropriate standards?
6. Is patient unwilling or unable to cooperate with medical treatment? If so, why?
7. In sum, is patient's right to choose being respected to extent possible in ethics and law?

QUALITY OF LIFE

1. What are the prospects, with or without treatment, for a return to patient's normal life?
2. Are there biases that might prejudice provider's evaluation of patient's quality of life?
3. What physical, mental, and social deficits is patient likely to experience if treatment succeeds?
4. Is patient's present or future condition such that continued life might be judged undesirable by them?
5. Any plan and rationale to forgo treatment?
6. What plans for comfort and palliative care?

CONTEXTUAL FEATURES

1. Are there family issues that might influence treatment decisions?
2. Are there provider (physicians and nurses) issues that might influence treatment decisions?
3. Are there financial and economic factors?
4. Are there religious, cultural factors?
5. Is there any justification to breach confidentiality?
6. Are there problems of allocation of resources?
7. What are legal implications of treatment decisions?
8. Is clinical research or teaching involved?
9. Any provider or institutional conflict of interest?

Figure 8–7 Conducting an Ethics Discussion: The Jonsen Box from *Clinical Ethics* (4th Edition), Jonsen, Siegler and Winsdale, McGraw-Hill, 1998.

From Jonsen, Siegler, and Winsdale (1998), *Clinical Ethics* (4th ed.).

Two advantages to ethics committee consults is that they often provide the only time when all of the members of the care team and patient and family members are together in the same room at the same time to share information. Situations that seemed to present difficult dilemmas are often solved by this sharing of information. Ethics committee consults can also stand in as an honest broker for incapacitated patients who have no family members to act as decision makers. Having brought in these relatively disinterested parties to make a recommendation may prove to be helpful should family members surface at a later date with complaints about the care decided upon.

ETHICAL ISSUES THAT ARISE IN END OF LIFE CARE

In addition to the questions of who decides the course of end of life care and how can those decisions be made most effectively within an institutional setting, there are a number of specific ethical issues that care teams face when delivering end of life care.

DNR Orders and Withholding or Withdrawing Treatment

One such issue is who decides when to write a DNR order for a patient. As the discussion of who decides end of life care in general indicates, decisions to forgo attempts at resuscitation should be made primarily by the patient, with the advice of the care team. If the patient does not have decision-making capacity, then the decision can be made by the proxy decision maker designated in a health care proxy, by the patient's physician under the living will, or by members of the family designated in a state-informed consent statute. An ethics committee would be helpful if there is disagreement or if no one is available to represent the patient. The same decision-making procedure should be followed for decisions to withdraw or withhold life-sustaining treatment.

An interesting variant on the DNR decision is the status of DNR orders for patients admitted to surgery. Surgeons and anesthesiologists will sometimes maintain that DNR orders are automatically suspended when a patient is in surgery or immediate post-operative recovery. Anesthesiologists cite the difficulty of telling, when the vital signs are under their control, when a patient has truly arrested or is under the influence of the anesthetic. Surgeons cite the scarcity of their operating theater time and skill and are unwilling to use these resources for patients who are content to die. Patient advocates maintain that a DNR order is an agreement between the patient and the care team and that this agreement cannot be automatically suspended just because the patient comes under the care of another service. The literature suggests that there are some instances in which a dying patient would benefit from palliative surgery that is not designed to extend life and that in these instances the anesthesiologists, surgeon, and patient should discuss the status of the DNR order for surgery. An automatic suspension policy is not an ethical practice.

Pain Management

Another problem with end of life care that has an ethical dimension is the pain control for end of life patients. Both the SUPPORT study (1995) and the Institute of Medicine study (Field and Cassel 1997) reported an alarming incidence of inadequate pain control for dying patients. More than half of the patients who died in the SUPPORT study experienced moderate to severe pain during most of their final three days of life. Further studies have indicated that many nursing home patients who are dying of cancer are given inadequate pain medication.

Part of the problem with pain control is overcoming the false dilemma between psychotropic hedonism and pharmacological Calvinism. Hedonism is the belief that pleasure is good and, in fact, very good. Calvinism is the belief that suffering is good. Puritanism is the fear that somewhere, someone is happy. Nurses and other health care providers need to ask themselves what their attitude is toward pain and the use of psychotropic agents to control pain: Are you a hedonist who sees value in having your patient pain free, a Calvinist who feels that the patient's suffering is redemptive, or a Puritan worrying that your patient may be having too much fun when the pain is fully suppressed? It is often said that medicine should aim to relieve all unnecessary suffering. But what is the definition of necessary suffering?

Physician-Assisted Suicide and Patient Refusal of Hydration and Nutrition

Proponents of physician-assisted suicide (PAS) cite the values of patient autonomy and of fair treatment in support of legalizing the process. They maintain that even though society has an interest in protecting life in most instances, a patient should be able to choose death in limited circumstances. They also argue that society allows terminal vent-dependent patients to end their lives by directing that they be removed from life support, so why should non-vent-dependent patients be denied an equal right to end their lives? Opponents of PAS cite concerns that it is too easy a solution to society's problems with end of life care, that it robs patients of the chance to benefit from a good death, that it weakens society's efforts to protect life and show concern for vulnerable populations, that it runs contrary to the medical practice value of doing no harm, and that it weakens trust in the care given by medical professionals.

Is there a compromise in this dispute that would preserve the integrity of both sides? One compromise is that offered by the Supreme Court's decision to allow the practice in states such as Oregon while the discussion continues. Another compromise proposed by Martin Benjamin (1990) and others is to agree on patient refusal of hydration and nutrition (PRHN) as a way for patients in certain specified circumstances to end their own lives with medical support (Bernat, Gert, and Mogielnicki 1993; Eddy 1994; Quill, Lo, and Brock 1997). Proponents give up full measure of patient autonomy by forgoing the ability to demand quicker, more direct means of death; but they gain some measure of autonomy in that the patient does the action of ending life when he or she chooses to. Opponents give up their refusal to assist in dying since they will still be providing comfort care but do not have to provide the lethal agent.

Other Problems

There are a number of other ethical problems which arise in end of life care. Most of this chapter has concentrated on end of life care in a hospital setting. There are also problems specific to nursing homes and home health care. Some nursing homes refuse to allow patients to die in their facilities, in spite of the patient or family wishes. Any patient in distress is immediately transported to a hospital. Nursing homes have also been shown to administer inadequate pain control to cancer patients under their care. Are there also problems unique to home health care?

Another particularly difficult set of issues concerns the care of terminally ill children. Who decides when to withdraw or withhold care from very low birth weight or severely handicapped newborns? What factors should be weighed in these decisions? At what point and to what degree should teenagers and younger patients participate in decisions regarding their care? Nurses who plan to work in these areas should become familiar with the literature regarding these problems.

SHE JUST LOOKED AWAY: EPILOGUE

After a number of conversations between the family and the surgeon, the family and the family practice physician, and the family and the nurses, an ethics committee consult was requested by the family. The ethics committee met with the family and the members of the care team. The surgeon and the ICU nurses urged the family to continue treatment in the hopes of a complete recovery. The nurses maintained that whatever her earlier statements, Mrs. T was refusing to have treatment withdrawn by looking away. The hospital's ethicist disagreed, suggesting that the kind of thinking required for squeezing the right or left hand was not comparable to the complex reasoning that deciding to withdraw treatment required and that turning away could be interpreted as a sign that she did not understand what she was being asked. The hospital attorney insisted that the only way to fully withdraw treat-

ment in the absence of an advance directive was to have one of the children appointed by the court as a guardian and suggested that failure to provide nutrition would require notifying the Elderly and Protective Services to avoid possible prosecution under an elderly abuse statute. The ethicist questioned whether the medical prognosis suggested the kind of full recovery that the patient had always maintained she wanted as the outcome of continued treatment. He also disputed the hospital's responsibility to report withdrawal of medical treatment to Elderly and Protective Services. None of the children were willing to seek court appointment as guardian. Given the signs of improvements in Mrs. T's mental status, they agreed to put off the decision on withdrawing treatment until several psych consults could determine whether she had decision-making capacity or not. They also agreed to the tracheostomy and a PEG tube until her mental status could be determined. Aggressive antibiotic therapy brought Mrs. T's pneumonia under control and she was eventually transferred to the hospital's skilled nursing facility. She lived there for six months, never fully regaining her mental functions. Her daughter, who she was never able to recognize, stopped visiting her. The son who lived nearby continued to visit weekly but never felt that she understood where she was or what had happened to her. Mrs. T slowly declined and died in the nursing facility, never able to return to her home. (Copyright 1997 by Julie Loup and J. Brooke Hamilton, III. Reprinted by permission.)

REFERENCES

Beauchamp, T. & Childress, J. (1998). *Principles of biomedical ethics* (3rd ed.). New York: Oxford University Press.

Benjamin, M. (1990). *Splitting the difference: Compromise and integrity in ethics and politics.* Lawrence: University of Kansas Press.

Bernat, J., Gert, B., & Mogielnicki, R. P. (1993). Patient refusal of hydration and nutrition: An alternative to physician-assisted suicide and voluntary euthanasia. *Archives of Internal Medicine*, 153, 2723–2798.

Eddy, D. (1994). A Conversation with My Mother. *Journal of the American Medical Association*, 272, 179–181.

Field, M. & Cassel, C. (Eds.). (1997). *Approaching death: Improving care at the end of life.* Committee on Care at the End of Life, Institute of Medicine. Washington, DC: National Academy Press.

Jonsen, A. (1998). *The birth of bioethics.* New York: Oxford University Press.

Jonsen, A. R., Siegler, M., & Winsdale, W. J. (1998). *Clinical Ethics* (4th ed.). New York: McGraw-Hill.

Quill, T., Lo, B., & Brock, D. (1997). Palliative options of last resort. *Journal of the American Medical Association*, 278, 2099–2014.

Uniform Natural Death Act, www.choices.org

Wennberg, J. E., Cooper, M. M., Eds. (1998). *The Dartmouth Atlas of Health Care.* American Hospital Association Press, Chicago, Il. Chap. 4.

CHAPTER

LEGAL AND ETHICAL ISSUES AND ADVANCE DIRECTIVES

Tonia Dandry Aiken

INTRODUCTION

Mr. Alex Brett has terminal lung cancer. He has a living will and a do not resuscitate order on the chart that says he does not want to be coded if he has a respiratory or cardiac arrest. On the 11–7 shift, Mr. Brett turns to his wife and grabs his chest.

1. If the patient says at that time, "Do everything you can to save me," what should the nurses do? Has he revoked the do not resuscitate order?
2. Has the patient revoked his advance directive? Can he revoke his advance directive? If the answer is yes, then list the ways the patient can revoke a living will or health care agent in your state or facility.
3. If the wife tells the nurses, "No, just let him go in peace." Should you honor her request?
4. Assume Mr. Brett has a living will and a do not resuscitate order in place. He has a respiratory arrest and his wife, who is his health care agent, tells you to do everything you can to save him. Whose wishes do you follow?

THE PATIENT SELF-DETERMINATION ACT

Patient autonomy is a crucial factor that must be considered when making legal and ethical decisions in health care.

Senator Danforth sponsored and introduced the Patient Self-Determination Act of 1990 in an effort to ensure that patients' wishes about health care were upheld.

He stated in part:

Advance directives encourage people to discuss and document their views of life-sustaining treatment in advance. They uphold the right of people to make their own decisions. And they enhance communication between patients, their families, and doctors, easing the burden on families and providers when it comes time to decide whether or not to pursue all possible treatment options. . . .

Advance directives will not solve all problems related to end-of-life decision . . . they do not take the pain away from someone we love, but they do ensure that a person's voice continued to be heard, and they do ease the burden, pain, and guilt that families often feel when making decision(s) for their dying loved one.

Advance directives reduce the stress on family members who are forced to make end of life decisions for their loved ones. Also, the directives eliminate confusion or misunderstanding as to what the patient desires (Aiken 1994).

The Patient Self-Determination Act is a federal law that requires health care facilities that receive Medicare and Medicaid funding to provide specific information about advance directives to patients being admitted to the facility.

The law requires that

- the staff and community receive education about advance directives;
- information be provided to individuals about rights under state law about making decisions regarding accepting or rejecting advance directives;
- information be provided on the advance directives (living will and durable power of attorney for health care) and how to expedite them;
- policies and procedures on distributing information to patients be implemented and maintained, as well as information on how to implement advance directives;
- documentation in the medical records as to whether or not a patient has advance directives be maintained.

Right to Die Case Law

Quinlan Case.   In 1976, the New Jersey Supreme Court ruled that individuals have a constitutional right to refuse unwanted treatment.

Karen Quinlan stopped breathing unexpectedly for a short period of time on April 15, 1975. When she arrived at the hospital, she was unresponsive. Karen was diagnosed as being comatose and was placed on a respirator. She was in a chronic and persistent vegetative state; she wasn't brain dead, but her condition did not allow her to breathe on her own. Because doctors said her condition would not improve, Karen's father wanted to take her off life support, which caused a public outcry. He applied to be named her guardian, a move that would allow him to legally make any life and death decisions on her behalf. The court looked at issues involving patient, state, and federal rights. He was granted guardianship and thus permitted to do what he felt was best for his daughter: asserting her constitutional right to privacy under the New Jersey state and federal constitutions, which permitted termination of all extraordinary measures and treatment. Her death, then, would be brought about by "natural causes."

Conroy Case.   In a case involving progressive debilitation of an elderly woman, the nephew sought permission to remove a nasogastric feeding tube. Ms. Claire Conroy was in a semifetal position; she had decubitus ulcers on her hip, leg, and foot, along with gangrene of the left leg. She also had diabetes, hypertension, and cardiovascular disease. She was incontinent and unable to talk. However, she did interact and was not in a coma or persistent vegetative state.

The court held the case was significant because of the many legal and ethical issues discussed and the fact that it might influence patients to use living wills. The court made several findings. A basic societal philosophy was that a person had a right to control his own body and that right was protected by the patient's right to privacy. The court held that if the patient was competent she would have a choice to remove the nasogastric tube. The court also addressed what should be done if the person had not expressed her wishes in a living will or to anyone about life-sustaining treatment.

If there is some evidence that defines the patient's wishes and it is clear to the health care agent that the burdens of pain and suffering outweigh life in the form of physical, intellectual, and mental enjoyment, then life-sustaining treatment can be withdrawn. If there is lack of evidence, life-sustaining treatment can still be withheld or withdrawn if benefits are outweighed or the severe pain is intolerable. If a patient expresses that she wants everything done to stay alive, then health care providers must comply.

The court opined that there was no distinction between artificial feeding and hydration and other forms of life-sustaining treatment. The court stated artificial feedings were medical procedures. Ms. Conroy died before the matter was heard before the New Jersey Supreme Court.

Cruzan Case.   In January 1983, at age 25, Nancy Cruzan was in an automobile accident. She did not regain consciousness and was placed on life-sustaining treatment, including a gastrostomy tube. Nancy had no living will. In 1990, in the landmark case of *Cruzan v. Director, Missouri Department of Health*, the United States Supreme Court held that a person has a constitutional right to be free of unwanted medical treatment. For those patients who are incompetent, the court left the decision to the individual state.

The Missouri Supreme Court ruled absent "clear and convincing" evidence, Nancy's tube feeding had to continue indefinitely. No legal distinction was made between artificial nutrition and other life-sustaining interventions. After additional evidence about Nancy's wishes was provided, the parents' request to remove her from the feeding and hydration tubes was granted. She died within two weeks of removal of the tubes.

Advance Directives: The Process

The adult or emancipated minor (if allowed by state law) executes the living will. When the patient's medical condition is certified by at least one physician and documented in the medical record, the physician writes orders consistent with the instructions.

The legal document used to designate health care agents may be called any of the following, depending on state laws (Choices in Dying Inc. 1998):

- durable power of attorney for health care
- medical durable power of attorney
- medical power of attorney
- proxy appointment
- health care representative form
- health care surrogate form
- health care agent form

Table 9–1 identifies attributes of an advance directive.

TABLE 9–1   ATTRIBUTES OF AN ADVANCE DIRECTIVE

---

1. Living will: A legal document that defines what life-sustaining treatment the person accepts or refuses when the patient is no longer competent or able to make treatment decisions. State laws specify when the living will becomes effective—(e.g., when the patient's condition is terminal, irreversible; if the patient is in a continual, profound comatose state, or if the patient is in a persistent vegetative state.

2. Durable power of attorney for health care: Also known as the document to designate a health care proxy, health care surrogate, health care representative or health care agent.

The agent is designated by the patient to make health care decisions when the patient is unable to do so. If the patient regains capacity, the patient can then resume making decisions about his treatment.

It must be signed and witnessed and may have to be notarized. Some state laws allow for a second or successor agent. Many states do not allow health care providers to serve as agents or witnesses to advance directives if they are providing care to the patient in the facility. Laws also provide for oral and written communication changes in the document and immunity for health providers.

Enforcement

The Secretary of Health and Human Services and the Health Care Financing Administration (HCFA) have enforcement policies for the Patient Self-Determination Act that include:

- withdrawal of funding from the facility
- failure to renew a provider agreement
- on-site surveys

The facilities must have policies and procedures in place to ensure that the facility is in compliance (Table 9–2 and Table 9–3).

Do Not Resuscitate Orders (DNR)

Every health care provider must know the laws on DNR orders, along with the policies and procedures of the facility. Even if patients have stated in the living will that they do not want to be resuscitated and request a DNR order, there should be a DNR order on the chart. Many facilities also have DNR forms that are signed by the patient's health care provider or family and placed on the chart. Many facilities also designate DNR patients by using colored wristbands, or color-coding on the chart, over the patient's bed, or on the door (Table 9–4).

TABLE 9–2   The Nurses' Role in Promoting the Patient Self-Determination Act

1. Upon admission, ask the patient for a copy of the advance directive and place it on the chart.
2. Know specific state laws.
3. Determine if a health care agent has been designated.
4. Obtain the required physician orders.
5. Do not discriminate against the patients based on their decisions.

TABLE 9–3   Advance Directives

1. They must be in writing.
2. They must be signed by the patient.
3. They must be witnessed by individuals specified by law.
4. Some states require that they be notarized.
5. They can be revoked in various ways according to state statutes.
6. Most states offer health care providers immunity from civil, criminal, and disciplinary actions from licensing agencies (e.g., State Boards of Nursing) as long as they follow the patient's wishes as designated in the advance directives.

Source: From Brent, N., Nurses and the Law—A Guide to Principle and Applications. (Philadelphia: W. B. Saunders Co., 1997), 250–256.

TABLE 9–4   Do Not Resuscitate Order (DNR Order)

Definition: An order written by a physician instructing health care providers not to perform cardiopulmonary resuscitation in case of a cardiac or respiratory arrest.

Know the State Laws and Facility Policy Procedures:

1. When are DNR orders suspended? (Example: Surgery)
2. If there is no DNR order, must the health care provider resuscitate?
3. Must the DNR be reordered after a certain period of time?
4. Does the DNR order mean that the patient won't receive any treatment?

After a Decision is Made

When a patient makes a decision about the type of care desired at the end of life, treatments such as cardiopulmonary resuscitation (CPR), mechanical ventilation, hydration, artificial nutrition, and kidney dialysis should be discussed.

The patient must notify the health care provider, family, attorney, and physicians under what circumstances CPR is to be administered.

The physician should write do not resuscitate (DNR) orders on the chart if the patient is in the facility and the patient does not want to be resuscitated. Many facilities have policies and procedures regarding renewal of the DNR order.

It is important to stress to the patient that even if the advance directive states the patient does not want to be resuscitated, most facilities require that a DNR order be written as orders on the chart or else CPR will be performed if the patient suffers a respiratory or cardiac arrest.

Explain to the patient that a do not resuscitate order is not the same as a "do not treat" order. With a DNR order, the patient receives other types of treatment.

Also, list for the patient other medical treatments that should be discussed with the physician such as:

- intravenous lines (IVs)
- antibiotics
- chemotherapy
- radiation therapy
- blood transfusions
- diagnostic studies
- surgical procedures

This can avoid confusion, problems with the family, and potential litigation.

The patient must also be told that even though a medical treatment is started, it can be stopped. If a patient is competent to make decisions about health care issues, the health care provider must recognize and honor those wishes even if the patient refuses treatment that could be lifesaving. It is legally and ethically appropriate to discontinue medical treatment.

If there is a conflict based on personal values and beliefs, then discussions, conferences, and ethics committee meetings should be set up with the patient, patient's family members, health care providers, and physician.

DNR and Surgery

Hospitals may have an order rescinding all DNRs during surgical interventions. Others may determine whether a DNR will be upheld on a case-by-case decision. In most cases a DNR will be honored if an unexpected event occurs that can be corrected and is not related to surgical interventions. Health care providers and patients must discuss DNR orders when surgery is required.

EMS DNR

Many states also recognize nonhospital DNR orders that are known as EMS DNR (emergency medical services do not resuscitate orders). Such orders allow the patient's wishes to be carried out in the home or similar setting and do not require the EMS technicians to initiate CPR.

Legal and Ethical Dilemmas

Common dilemmas nurses face regarding DNR orders include some of the following:

- Lack of documentation in the medical records, especially the progress notes, indicating how the DNR decision was made. No DNR form on the chart.
- Interpreting DNR orders when a "no code" has been qualified as a "chemical code only," or "resuscitate but do not intubate."
- Performing a "slow code" or "show code" for the benefit of family members.
- Transfer of residents: Is a DNR order accompanying a resident transferred from one facility to another acceptable? Should a new one be obtained?
- Abandonment of care by health care personnel of patients designated as DNRs.

ARTIFICIAL NUTRITION AND HYDRATION

Through advance directives, every state law allows patients the right to refuse artificial nutrition and hydration. Some state laws treat artificial nutrition and hydration as a medical treatment in the advance directive, while others require the person to specify whether or not they want artificial nutrition and hydration. Some states also prohibit family members or agents from making decisions about stopping artificial nutrition and hydration unless they specifically know the person's wishes. A health care provider must know the state laws since they vary on this issue (Table 9–5).

Artificial nutrition and hydration is a form of life-sustaining treatment and is a chemically balanced mix of fluids and nutrients. It is given to the patient by placing a tube directly into a vein, intestine, or stomach.

Stopping this treatment is legally and ethically appropriate if there is no benefit to the patient or it is unwanted by the competent patient. Legal implications evolve when a patient's competency is put at issue. The courts may become involved to determine if the patient is capable and competent to make health care decisions.

TABLE 9–5   KNOW YOUR LAWS

Every health care provider and patient should know the laws about the following topics:

1. The patient self-determination act (PSDA)
2. Advance Directives
   a. Living Will
   b. Durable power of attorney for health care/health care proxy
3. The health care provider's obligation to comply with patient's wishes
4. Do not resuscitate (DNR) orders
5. Artificial nutrition and hydration
6. Physician-assisted suicide

Physician's Refusal to Honor Wishes

Various states passed laws that hold if the physician cannot honor the wishes of the patient, the physician must transfer the case to another physician who will honor them.

Some nursing homes and hospitals also have policies that prevent them from honoring patient's wishes on stopping artificial nutrition and hydration. If the facility has such policies, notify the patient and family so they can make an informed decision.

Suicide and Refusal of Artificial Nutrition and Hydration

It is not considered suicide to refuse artificial nutrition and hydration when the patient is refusing life-sustaining treatment at the end of life. Life insurance policies are not affected, because death is not by suicide when medical treatments are discontinued and the patient dies.

EUTHANASIA

Euthanasia or "good death" allows for making a death essentially pain free for the patient. There are several types of euthanasia:

- Voluntary means the individual has consented.
- Involuntary means that the person can't or has not consented, but there is a presumption he wants to die.
- Passive means that no interventions occur and nothing is done to hasten death.
- Active means that actions or steps are taken to cause death.

Physician-Assisted Suicide

In 1997, the Supreme Court ruled on the issue of physician-assisted suicide. *Washington v. Glubhebeg*, (an appeal from the United States Court of Appeals for the Ninth Circuit) focused on the due process clause of the Fourteenth Amendment of the U.S. Constitution. The court held that Washington state's prohibition of assisted suicide violated the due process clause of the Constitution. It denied competent terminally ill patients the right to hasten their death.

In *Vacco v. Quill*, the Equal Protection Clause of the Fourteenth Amendment was at issue. The United States Court of Appeals for the Second Circuit held that it was unconstitutional when the terminally ill were denied equal protection of the New York State's laws when the state prohibited assisted suicide.

The two issues in both cases were:

- Did a ban on assisted suicide violate terminally ill patients' constitutional rights under the due process clause of the Constitution?
- Are persons on life-sustaining treatments similarly situated to competent terminally ill adults not on life support but who wish to have a physician prescribe a lethal dose of medication to end life and hasten death?

The Supreme Court's Decision

Unanimously, the Supreme Court found that terminally ill patients do not have a fundamental right to physician-assisted suicide and, therefore, upheld the state bans on assisted suicide.

The Supreme Court's decision not to legalize physician-assisted suicide allows the states to make the decision as to whether or not they will legalize it.

In 1997, Oregon became the first state to legalize physician-assisted suicide by requesting a lethal prescription. A study done after the law became effective noted that individuals cited concerns over loss of bodily functions and autonomy versus pain control as the main reasons for requesting the lethal prescription.

Dr. Jack Kevorkian, a 79-year-old retired pathologist, was sought to assist a woman with early-stage Alzheimer's in committing her suicide. The case brought national attention to the issue of the right to assisted suicide and issues surrounding active, voluntary euthanasia. One of Dr. Kevorkian's stated goals was to push and test the limits of an individual's autonomy as a patient.

Dr. Kevorkian was convicted in March 1999 of second-degree murder for giving a fatal injection to a man with a terminal illness, amyotrophic lateral sclerosis (Lou Gehrig's disease). He claims that he has assisted more than 130 people in committing suicide. (Belluck, 1999.)

SUMMARY

Potential problems and conflicts arise when the person's wishes are not clearly known or a health care proxy has not been designated. Other conflicts arise when the health care provider believes it is never appropriate to discontinue or withhold life-sustaining treatment. In the future, laws passed to create national advance directives may eliminate problems faced by health care providers who care for patients in different parts of the country who have state-specific advance directives. A national registry for advance directives will aid health care providers who can obtain the patient's directives and honor their wishes.

The following internet sources are available for reference:

- www.jcano.org/index.htm-Joint Commission on Accreditation of Healthcare
- http:llwww.bioethics.gov-National Bioethics Advisory Commission
- http:llwww.healthlawyers.org-American Health Lawyers Association
- www.taana.org-The American Association of Nurse Attorneys

REFERENCES

Aiken, T. (1994). *Legal ethical and political issues in nursing.* Philadelphia: F. A. Davis Company.

Belluck, P. (March 27, 1999). "Dr. Kevorkian is a murderer, the jury finds." *The New York Times.* p. A2.

Brent, N. (1997). *Nurses and the Law: A guide to principles and applications.* Philadelphia, PA: W.B. Saunders, Co. pp. 250–256.

Choices in Dying. (1998). *Healthcare agents: Appointing one and being one.* New York: Author.

Unit IV

Ethical and Legal Considerations

Critical Thinking Activities

1. Compare ethical principles to principles of hospice and palliative care
2. Compare and contrast differences between advance directives and health care proxy
3. Discuss legal parameters in the provision of palliative care

Teaching-Learning Exercises

1. Divide class into groups of six persons each and give each group a topic to discuss and debate, such as withdrawal and withholding of food, water, and treatment; DNR orders; artificial hydration and nutrition; and physician-assisted suicide
2. Write own advance directive
3. Develop protocol for a community ethics committee
4. Create a list of Internet resources identifying laws in your state regarding consent to treatment and refusal of treatment

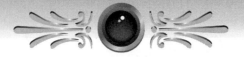

UNIT V

Patient Centered Care

Learning Objectives
1. Discuss the role of the nurse in palliative care
2. Discuss the importance of pain and symptom management
3. Discuss principles of pain management
4. Identify drugs commonly used for pain and symptom management at end of life
5. Identify assessment tools used to identify parameters of pain
6. Discuss special considerations in pain management for the young and elderly populations
7. Describe the WHO three-step analgesic ladder for pain management
8. Define hospice
9. Define suffering
10. Describe the importance of the therapeutic use of self in providing end of life care
11. Identify psychological responses of the dying patient
12. Discuss the role of religion in end of life care

CHAPTER 10

HOSPICE: TO MAKE THE PATH LESS LONELY

Michael Blanchard

INTRODUCTION: BARRIERS TO INFORMED CHOICE

In a 1992 Gallup Poll conducted on attitudes of Americans towards death and dying, 86% of those surveyed said that if they were terminally ill and had only six months to live, they would like to receive care and die in their own home or that of a family member. A similar number reported that they would be interested in a comprehensive program of care in which physicians, nurses, counselors, and other health professionals helped them remain comfortable at home (Baer 1994).

What respondents to that survey were describing—although many were unaware of it at the time—was a hospice program. It is no surprise that the hospice concept, even while it offers the kind of care seemingly preferred by a significant number, remains foreign to many people. For one thing, although hospice programs have proliferated rapidly and exist in every state, systematic programs of care for dying patients are a relatively recent phenomenon within health care. The first modern hospice was established in 1967. The first such program in the United States did not begin until 1974.

For another thing, death is for most an unpleasant topic, one which is avoided in conversation even with close friends or loved ones. A survey commissioned by the National Hospice Foundation (NHF) in 1999 showed that Americans are more likely to talk to their children about safe sex and drugs than to their terminally ill parents about choices in care as they near life's final stages. According to the study, one out of four Americans over the age of 45 say they would not bring up issues related to their parent's death—even if the parent had a terminal illness and less than six months to live (Stenrud & O'Connor 1999).

The NHF research also showed that Americans expect their loved ones to carry out their wishes about end of life care but have not made those wishes clearly known. One out of every two Americans said they would rely on family and friends to carry out their wishes, but 75% of Americans have never taken the time to clearly articulate how they wish to be cared for during life's final journey.

A third reason that the hospice choice is not readily apparent, despite the appropriateness of the patient's condition for admission, is the combination of knowledge deficit and misinformation about hospice services. Even in communities in which the local hospice organization is well-established and highly visible, lack of knowledge is a key barrier to informed choice. For instance, one Louisiana hospice commissioned its own public awareness survey in 1995. Despite having served the community for more than 10 years and having received considerable public recognition—including two presidential citations—the agency found a disturbingly low level of knowledge regarding specific services. Just over 80% of those surveyed responded that they recognized the name of the community's local hospice organization and had a favorable impression of the agency. However, only 50% had any appreciable awareness of exactly what services the hospice offered (Blanchard 1995).

Johnson and Slaninka (1999) conducted a similar study, using a broader sample. Most respondents to that survey could only describe their personal outlook on hospice rather than the services or care provided by a particular hospice organization. Misconceptions held by the respondents were that hospice was to be used only as a last resort, that hospice provided care only for cancer patients, and that admission to hospice care signified giving up on the patient.

In light of the many barriers to informed choice concerning admission to hospice care, this chapter proposes to serve as an introduction to the hospice movement, to its guiding philosophy and practices, and to the most commonly held misconceptions about hospice care. It is hoped that those who read this chapter will be better prepared to assist terminally ill patients and their families in making more informed choices concerning compassionate care at the end of life.

FOUNDER OF THE MODERN HOSPICE MOVEMENT

The word *hospice* may be used interchangeably to refer to an organization that provides compassionate care for patients with terminal illnesses and their families, to the place where such care is provided, or to the philosophy which guides caregivers in their efforts to comfort the dying.

The one person most often credited with articulating the philosophy of hospice care is Dame Cicely Saunders, a British physician. Born in London in

1918, Saunders attended St. Anne's College, Oxford University, where she studied political science, economics, and philosophy. At the outbreak of World War II, she left Oxford against her parents' wishes to pursue her long-held dream of nursing. She entered St. Thomas's Hospital Nightingale School in 1941 and completed her nursing training there in 1944. Forced to leave her nursing post due to chronic back problems, she returned to St. Anne's to earn a degree in public administration and was certified in medical social work in 1947.

That same year, Saunders met a patient who gave her life new direction. David Tasma was a refugee from Poland. He was 40 years old and dying. David suffered much pain and was often lonely and sad because he had no relatives. Saunders became very close to him. Together, they often talked about how hospitals could not provide more loving care than they did for dying patients. Patients who were dying were often left alone in constant pain, terrified of dying and worried about what would happen to their families. Saunders thought that such people should be cared for more lovingly and be allowed to die peacefully without pain and fear. An idea took shape in Saunders's mind. If she could build a special place for people who were terminally ill, with specially trained staff, then the patients could receive all the skilled treatment and loving care they needed and deserved.

After David's death, Saunders became a volunteer nurse at St. Luke's Hospital, one of the early "homes" for patients who were dying. There she learned how the nuns gave patients painkillers regularly, a practice that lessened both their physical pain and anxiety. One of the doctors at St. Luke's told her that if she wanted to help dying people, she had to change the attitude of physicians and that the best way to do that was to become a physician herself.

Heeding that advice, Saunders entered medical school in 1951 at the age of 33, while volunteering at St. Joseph's Hospice in London. After earning her medical degree in 1957, Saunders practiced at St. Joseph's, but her goal was to found a facility that would combine teaching and research with patient care. Her goal was achieved with the opening of St. Christopher's Hospice in South London in 1967, named for the Christian patron saint of travelers.

A deeply spiritual person, Saunders chose the name of her facility consciously. Derived from the Latin root word *hospes*—which means host or guest and which gives rise to our English words "hospital" and "hospitality"—the word *hospice* suggested to Saunders a place between a hospital and home, a place that would combine the medical competencies of one with the warmth, love, and openness of the other. Historically, the word was used in reference to places of rest and shelter for weary travelers. As early as the fourth century, monasteries ran hospices where pilgrims could stop and rest, be fed, and have wounds or illnesses treated before continuing on their journey. For Saunders, then, her hospice would be a place of rest and care for dying patients before they continued their journey to eternal life.

THE HOSPICE PHILOSOPHY

As envisioned by Saunders and as practiced today, hospice care is guided by the following basic concepts:

- Hospice care is patient-driven. Among the great fears witnessed by hospice caregivers is the patient's fear of losing control. Facing the end of one's life with equanimity indeed requires a gradual process of turning loose and of saying good-bye. One of the virtues of hospice care is that responsibility for making choices concerning care at the end of one's life rests with the patient. To the degree that it is possible, the patient remains in control of the decision-making process.

- The hospice philosophy is home-based. Another of the great fears witnessed by hospice caregivers is the patient's fear of dying alone and of dying in an alien environment. Hospices affirm the right of dying patients to spend their final weeks or months in peace and comfort, and to die with dignity in a place that affords warmth, freedom of movement, and openness to visitors. Following the model established by Cicely Saunders, many hospices today are residential facilities into which dying patients move, sometimes with family members. Many hospice programs, however, provide care directly in the homes of patients or of a close relative or friend. Still others participate in the treatment of patients within acute care settings, when hospital admission is necessary for the management of symptoms that cannot be managed in the home, and in long-term care facilities. Whether hospices visit the terminally ill at home or strive to create a homelike atmosphere, patients are not required to be bedridden or even homebound. In fact, the goal of most hospices is to allow patients to live as fully as possible. Achieving that goal often means encouraging patients to enjoy hobbies and other meaningful activities and making necessary accommodations for patients to do so. As one hospice nurse reportedly directed a patient, "You worry about living and enjoying life and let me worry about your illness."

- Hospice care is family-centered. Family members of patients are included in each step of the decision-making process. They are actively engaged as caregivers and receive training from hospice staff in comfort measures, including administration of medication, and in the signs and symptoms of approaching death. In addition, the entire family, not just the patient, is considered the unit of care. The terminal illness and impending death of a loved one is a crisis within a family that impacts its members physically, emotionally, financially, and spiritually. Hospices provide support to family members in coping with the crisis. Finally, most hospice programs include some form of bereavement support for families after the death of the patient. Typical bereavement services include individual counseling, support groups, memorial services, and the sharing of appropriate literature on the grief process.

- Hospice caregivers are privileged visitors in the lives of their patients. While patients are officially admitted to hospice programs, it is also true that hospice staff members are guests who have been admitted into the homes, lives, and families of patients at a time of dramatic significance. The dual meaning of the root word for *hospice* itself suggests that hospice employees and volunteers are both hosts and guests.

- The hospice philosophy stresses palliative care, as opposed to curative care. The World Health Organization (1990 pp. 11–12) has defined palliative care as "the active total care of patients whose disease is not responsive to curative treatment." Often, the decision to admit a patient to hospice care begins with the realization that aggressive measures to rid the patient of an illness are of no further benefit. This decision does not imply a passive acceptance of the patient's imminent death, however. Under the direction of physicians, hospices use sophisticated methods of pain and symptom control that enable the patient to live as fully and comfortably as possible. Often, relief from pain and discomforting symptoms is a necessary first step toward helping the dying patient achieve enhanced quality of life. As Saunders (1995, page 11) observed, "The greatest fear of the dying and their families is the fear of pain. Sadly, this fear has often been justified. Terminal pain is frequently treated ineptly and the public myth that death from cancer involves unremitting distress is perpetuated."

- Hospice programs promote quality rather than length of life. They affirm life and regard death as a normal process. Their goal is to enhance the patient's quality of life in his or her final months and weeks. Efforts of hospice caregivers neither hasten nor postpone death. Consistent with their respect for the patient's wishes, hospices believe in allowing a person to die when the time comes, rather than trying to keep him or her alive on machines or through resuscitation.

- Hospice care emphasizes a holistic approach and treats the whole person, not just the disease and its resulting physical complications. Saunders herself believed from experience that there are several ways of feeling pain, beyond the physical dimension. Patients often suffer the emotional pain of fear, anxiety, anger, depression, and helplessness. They suffer the pain of worry about burdening loved ones and the ache of uncertainty about their future lives. They suffer the pain of assessing their life's accomplishments and failures. Finally, they suffer the pain of uncertainty about life after death. The goal of hospice, as Saunders envisioned it and as it is practiced today, is to offer dying patients and their families a comprehensive program of medical care,

counseling, and spiritual direction that moves beyond physical pain to address all of the patient's fears and concerns.
- For that reason, hospice care is also team-oriented. Hospices assemble interdisciplinary teams comprised of professionals, support staff, and volunteers to address the medical, emotional, psychological, social, financial, and spiritual needs of the patient and family.

THE HOSPICE INTERDISCIPLINARY CARE TEAM

Typically, the hospice interdisciplinary care team includes the following members:

- The attending physician. Patients designate an attending physician to manage their care. It is usually the attending physician who makes the referral for hospice admission.
- The hospice medical director. The medical director oversees treatment by the hospice team, coordinates with the attending physician, and is available for consultation.
- The hospice nurse. Nurses coordinate the individualized plan of care for each patient, provide specialized palliative care services, and help educate family members on patient care.
- The social worker. Hospice social workers offer emotional support, counseling, and identification of available resources within the community.
- The hospice chaplain. Hospice chaplains provide spiritual direction and support, perform sacramental functions, and coordinate support with the patient's community of faith. They may also oversee a team of pastoral care volunteers.
- Home health aides. Hospice home health aides assist with personal care and perform light housekeeping duties.
- The hospice bereavement counselor. Bereavement counselors support the patient, family, and caregivers throughout the dying process and offer follow-up grief education and support.
- The hospice pharmacist. Pharmacists work with the hospice team to ensure the appropriate monitoring, supervision, and timeliness of pharmaceutical services.
- The hospice volunteer. Trained volunteers provide a variety of services, including companionship for patients, family, and caregivers.
- Other therapists and counselors. Dieticians counsel patients and families about nutritional issues. Physical, occupational, and speech therapists, as well as art, massage, and other allied therapists provide palliative care according to the patient's individualized plan of care.

WHEN TO DECIDE ON HOSPICE

Family discussions about the appropriateness of hospice care for a loved one may be guided by a knowledge of typical admissions criteria followed by most hospices:

- The patient has been diagnosed with a terminal illness of some type. While cancer is the most frequent diagnosis in most hospice programs, hospices care for patients with a variety of life-threatening illnesses, including end-stage heart disease, lung disease, liver or kidney failure, neuromuscular diseases, and AIDS.
- The patient has a life expectancy of six months or less. Often, this issue poses a challenge for family members. Bonham and Gochman (1988) observed that one of the most common barriers to accepting hospice care was the failure or refusal of family members to accept the patient's terminal condition. Admission to hospice care, however, does not insure that the patient will live only six months or that the patient will be automatically discharged from hospice if alive after six months.
- The attending physician, patient, and family agree that no further aggressive treatment will benefit the patient.
- The patient lives within the prescribed service area for the hospice in question.
- In the case of home-based programs, hospices may require that the patient has a primary caregiver (someone other than hospice staff) available within the home to help coordinate care with hospice staff.

COMMON MYTHS ABOUT HOSPICE CARE

As Johnson and Slaninka (1999) revealed, public misconceptions constitute a significant barrier to informed choice regarding appropriate care at the end of life. Figure 10–1 identifies and addresses the most common of the myths about hospice care.

MYTH	TRUTH
A patient loses Medicare benefits when he or she accepts hospice care.	One never loses his or her Medicare benefits. The hospice Medicare benefit is another form of Medicare coverage, and all services required for management of the terminal illness are provided by hospice.
A patient must be actively dying to receive hospice care.	A patient may be admitted to hospice at any time during the last six months of life. It is best when the patient is referred before death is imminent or there is a crisis situation. It is preferable to refer a patient early so that the hospice team can have adequate time to prepare the patient and family for the impending death.
Once a patient accepts hospice care, he or she can never be hospitalized. The patient must remain at home no matter what.	A hospice patient may be hospitalized to control symptoms that cannot be properly managed at home. Also, the patient may be admitted to a hospital to provide respite care for the family, if necessary.
Once a patient has been admitted to hospice, he or she can never get out of it, except by dying.	Hospice patients may choose to be discharged from hospice at any time or for any reason. It is also true that a patient may be involuntarily discharged alive from hospice if his or her condition improves to the point that he or she is no longer medically eligible for the program.
Hospice care is only for the elderly.	While the majority of hospice patients are elderly, hospice care is for all age groups. In fact, some hospices have special pediatric programs for children with terminal illnesses.
When a patient enters hospice, he or she must give up his or her regular physician.	A hospice patient is not required to change physicians. The patient's attending physician may continue to manage the patient's case, in consultation with the hospice medical director.
In order to be admitted to hospice, a patient must have cancer.	Hospice is for any end-stage or terminal illness, including heart disease and lung disease, among others.
Hospice care is only for those who cannot afford regular medical care.	Hospice care is reimbursed by Medicare and most commercial insurance plans.
Admission to hospice signifies a passive acceptance of the patient's impending death.	Hospices are very active and proactive in addressing the full range of medical, emotional, and spiritual concerns through the efforts of a comprehensive team of professionals, support staff, and volunteers.
Hospices advocate against advances in medical technology.	Hospices are supportive of advances in medical science and encourage patients to pursue any reasonable hope for cure. Hospice care is appropriate, however, for patients after it has been determined that curative measures are of no further benefit.

Figure 10–1 Some Common Myths Regarding Hospice Care

REFERENCES

Baer, K. (1994). A guide to hospice care. Boston, MA: Harvard Medical School Health Publications Group.

Beresford, L. (1993). The hospice handbook. New York: Little, Brown, and Company.

Blanchard, M. (1995). Findings of a survey: Public awareness and knowledge of hospice. Lafayette, LA: Hospice of Acadiana.

Bonham, G. S., & Gochman, D. S. (1988). Physicians and the hospice decision: awareness, discussion, reasons and satisfaction. The Hospice Journal 4, 35–53.

Byock, I. (1997). Dying well: Peace and possibilities at the end of life. New York: Riverhead Books.

Du Boulay, S. (1993). Changing the face of death: The story of Cicely Saunders. London: RMEP.

Johnson, C. B., & Slaninka, S. C. (1999). Barriers to accessing hospice services before a late terminal stage. Death Studies 23, 14–23.

Saunders, C., Baines, M. and Dunlap, R. (1995). Living with dying: A guide to palliative care, 3rd ed. New York: Oxford University Press.

Stenrud, C., & O'Connor, B. (1999, June). Baby boomers fear talking to parents about death. NHF Public Opinion Research. Retrieved May 10, 2000 from the World Wide Web: http://www.nho.org/porhtml.htm

World Health Organization. (1990). Cancer pain relief and palliative care. Geneva, Switzerland: WHO.

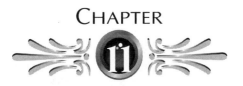

PALLIATIVE CARE:
THE ESSENCE OF NURSING

Julie Griffie

"It is very difficult to have to let go of all hope for life—one's own or that of a loved one. But when there was nothing more that could be done medically for my father, my sister and I gave him the only thing left that was important—we relieved his pain and held his hands. We are so grateful we had the opportunity for this."

Richard Stollberg

I believe there is no richer experience in nursing than to be allowed to walk with a patient who is at the end of life. When patients and family members have the opportunity to complete end of life work, heal relationships, and establish a plan for a dignified death, we are successful. The role of the nurse in assisting dying patients is multifaceted, at times complex, and very rewarding. Medical advances have not replaced the fact that we are not immortal beings. Each death is a momentous event with impact on a number of people. It requires caregivers to provide wisdom and have the ability to reassure, offer comfort, and understand who the dying person is (Bouwsma 1996). Assisting patients in recognizing and preparing for the end of life challenges the nurse to use a variety of nursing skills. Becoming more familiar with how we can assist our patients optimizes the goal of providing comfort and dignity at the end of life.

Palliative care is defined by the World Health Organization (WHO) as "the active total care of patients whose disease is not responsive to curative treatment. Control of pain, other symptoms, and of psychological, social, and spiritual problems is paramount. The goal of palliative care is achievement of the best possible quality of life for patients and their families. Many aspects of palliative care are also applicable earlier in the course of the illness, in conjunction with anticancer treatment" (World Health Organization 1990). Using this definition, palliative care activities should gradually intensify from the time of diagnosis of a life-threatening illness to the time of death. This is illustrated in Figure 11–1 (Griffie, Muchka, Nelson-Marten, & O'Mara 1999).

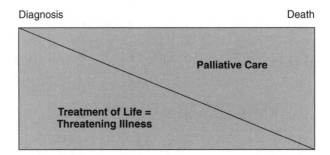

Figure 11–1 Continuum of Palliative Care

Palliative care is best accomplished using an interdisciplinary team approach. This assures a holistic approach to care and accessibility of expertise in all the caring domains. The nurse assumes the role of facilitator of a multidisciplinary plan of care. To accomplish this role well, our palliative care nursing skills need to be nurtured, honed, and refined by all nurses, in all settings. The following roles are essential aspects of everyday nursing practice:

- recognition of the patient in need of palliative care
- completion of the palliative care nursing assessment
- facilitation of the environment for care in the last days of life.

RECOGNITION OF PATIENTS IN NEED OF PALLIATIVE CARE

To provide palliative care, we must first recognize which patients are in need. In practice, we find that all patients with chronic, life-threatening illnesses have some fears or concerns about end of life. Considering this as a standard is perhaps the best way of identifying this broad population. Diabetes mellitus, cancer, heart disease, and Parkinson's disease are but a few examples of diagnoses that elicit thoughts or fear of death. The end of life may or may not be years away. To speak of it with someone who is willing to listen and assist in attending to tasks such as completing an advance directive or a living will or simply reaching out to mend a relationship are likely to be important to the patient. Nurses can play an important supportive role in facilitating these tasks. As functional status declines and complications increase in frequency and number, the need to address end of life issues intensifies and accelerates. Recognizing and validating disease progression is a critical competency we must develop. The nurse who is watching this progression needs to validate with the patient on an ongoing basis that personal needs are being met by the health care system and an acceptable quality of life is being achieved.

Criteria for identifying patients appropriate for intensive palliative care include the following: metastatic cancer, advanced dementia, nonreversible renal disease on dialysis, chronic illness with functional decline, and bedridden patients who have recurring infections. All care providers must assure that the patient's goals of care are clearly understood by the entire health care team. Because nurses may have the greatest amount of contact time with the patient, they may be the first to see cues of the patient's changing goals. Moreover, the patient may find it difficult to express or share changes in treatment wishes with the physician. The nurse may need to assist the patient in discussions of goals with the physician. Regular check-in points should be established with the patient to pose the question, "Is our care meeting your goals?"

THE PALLIATIVE CARE NURSING ASSESSMENT

The palliative care nursing assessment has been derived from a model suggested by Weissman (1997) for the palliative care consultation. Six key aspects are identified. A thorough physical assessment serves as a basis for the six aspects. The palliative care assessment begins with the traditional physical assessment and psychosocial assessment.

Assessment and Management of Physical Symptoms.   The foundation of palliative care is the relief of physical distress. The all-too-common absence of effective pain management has made pain the most frequently feared symptom at the end of life. Other common distressful symptoms are dyspnea, nausea and vomiting, constipation, diarrhea, and delirium. Additionally, patients may report distress from fatigue, bleeding, decreased mobility, anorexia, and edema. Multiple symptoms often exist simultaneously and can be overwhelming to the patient. To assist in goal setting, it is helpful to ask the patient, "What is the most important thing we can do to help you?" Patients may or may not respond with a physical symptom. Psychosocial issues may override the physical symptoms importance. All symptoms should be addressed. The starting point and goals should be mutually established by the patient and health care provider based upon the *patient's* identified priorities. For example, a patient who has just learned the diagnosis, is in physical pain, and is short of breath may tell you that the most important thing you can do for him or her is to help contact a particular person who will provide psychological support.

In an assessment of most physical symptoms, there are many common aspects such as: when did the symptom begin; intensity; quality; what makes it better; what makes it worse; what is its effect on activities of daily living; what does the patient think the cause is (meaning, of distress); and what are the patient's goals for management? Effective management of physical symptoms depends on an understanding of the physiological cause. Diagnostic workup of symptoms will gradually decrease in intensity as the patient approaches the end of life. Diagnostics should continue as long as the approach to symptom relief is dependent upon the information gained from the test results. In the last days of life, the value of doing diagnostic tests should be carefully evaluated. For example, the nurse may pose the question, "Will the results of the MRI (or other test) change what we are going to do?" or "Can we effectively manage the symptoms without the knowledge of the test results?" The burden of undergoing a diagnostic test or procedure must be carefully evaluated. For example, in the last days of life, anticoagulation may be managed based upon history rather than daily laboratory data.

Expertise in symptom management is an expected competency of hospice and palliative care nurses. The professional organization of this specialty group offers ongoing education and information on symptom management. Hospice nurses are excellent resources and can provide insights and suggestions for symptom management. Collaboration is always appropriate for assistance in managing difficult symptoms. Many successful interventions for symptom management are currently not well documented in the literature and are shared through the network of hospice and palliative care nurses. As this nursing specialty develops, increased research and documentation of innovative approaches is occurring.

Assisting Patients and/or Family Members to Identify Personal Goals. Quality of life is critical throughout the life span. As chronic illness intensifies, quality of life changes and may diminish. However, the definition of the quality of one's life comes only from one source: the patient. We must be careful not to impose our personal interpretation of quality of life.

At some point in the disease trajectory, it becomes appropriate to shift from life-prolonging care to maximizing the quality of the limited life expectancy. Focusing on intensive symptom management and the quality of life concerns identified by the patient and family will facilitate this shift. The nurse may help the patient to explore this point by questioning. For example, "Did the transfusion help relieve your fatigue and shortness of breath?" If the answer is no, continuing transfusions is inappropriate. Management of the dyspnea may shift to a focus on treating the symptom pharmacologically with opioids rather than treating the cause. It is appropriate to question patients about the burden of continuing to come to the clinic or repeated readmission to the hospital. Perhaps this time is better spent completing end of life tasks such as writing letters to children, spending time with family, or arranging for dispersion of cherished items to loved ones (Brody, Campbell, Faber-Landendoen, & Ogle 1997).

When this shift occurs, the health care team should address such issues as the continued value of cardiopulmonary resuscitation, tube feedings, non-oral hydration, continuing chemotherapy or radiation therapy, and the continued monitoring of pulse oximetry and blood pressure. If the goals of care can be clearly articulated, the decision to continue or not to continue treatments becomes much clearer. Stopping or withdrawing treatment may provoke psychological distress for the patient and family. The nurse must provide reassurance that discontinuing life-prolonging treatments even though quality of life is compromised is morally, legally, ethically, and spiritually acceptable. A family conference with the patient, all family members, the physician, and the patient's spiritual advisor may assist in providing support and understanding. Patients and family members need to be reassured that all efforts will be made to manage distressing symptoms when life-prolonging treatments stop.

The Assessment and Management of Psychological and Spiritual Needs. The assessment of physical symptoms overlaps with the assessment of psychological and spiritual needs. Gentle exploration of spiritual needs and concerns of the patient and family is part of our assessment. This is perhaps most challenging when we are caring for a patient at the end of life who, due to advanced illness, cannot speak. Careful assessment is critical to help us understand who this patient is and what the end of life represents to the family.

Fear of death, concerns about family being left behind, spiritual issues, and the need to "make peace" with loved ones may exacerbate physical symptom management and compromise quality of life. Perhaps one last goodbye needs to be said. Facilitating this aspect of care is the role of the nurse. Extenuating circumstances may require ingenuity and the support and assistance of the interdisciplinary team. Consider the patient who has an adult child who is incarcerated. How can we best assist in assuring the opportunity to say "goodbye," "I'm sorry," and "I love you" one last time (Byock 1997)?

Anxiety about death is common. There is no dress rehearsal for the experience. An open discussion of prognosis may assist in relieving anxiety. If possible, help make arrangements for the patient's return home, where he or she can have more personal control of the environment. Ask and allow patients to tell you how you can assist them to live well during this time.

Assessment of Support Systems.   Support systems for the patient may or may not be obvious. Family, friends, and community members may rally around the patient to offer support. Some patients may appear to have no support, and the complex needs brought on at the end of life may be particularly overwhelming. Assessment of support systems may begin with simple questions such as, "When you have been in a difficult situation in the past, who did you turn to? What did you do? What did you find helped you the most?" Understanding the patient's coping style and coping abilities will help us understand the patient's support systems. A patient with no biological family may or may not have developed strong skills of personal self support, which should be understood and respected. Based upon the responses to such questions, the interdisciplinary team may be able to develop interventions to support the patient. If no support systems exist, the interdisciplinary team of physician, nurse, social worker, chaplain, etc. becomes the patient's sole support system.

Assessment and Communication of Prognosis.   Clarification of prognosis is often the first step in goal setting and the shift to intensive palliative care.

Overall, it is a question most health care providers are uncomfortable addressing. Too often the response to the question of time has been dismissal, with a response similar to "only God knows." This is not a helpful response. We cannot say exactly when death will occur. A response of days, weeks, or years is much more helpful to the patient and family. Patients have a right to prognostic information to assist in goal setting. In the past, this has been considered a physician responsibility. With the growing awareness that all disciplines are responsible for enhancing end of life, it has become the responsibility of all disciplines, in particular nursing, to assure that prognosis questions are addressed. At a minimum, the natural course of the disease and common problems at the end of life should be discussed when patients request such information.

Patients may or may not want to know specifics of their prognosis. When asked, they may say they know time is short. Family members may need more specific information so that they can plan how to address care needs. The spouse who says "I need to see the doctor because I want to ask how much time my wife has left" in the presence of the wife who responds with "Don't ask that in front of me!" may simply want to know if it is time to arrange for a family leave of absence from work. The patient may be able to give the answer to this question, allowing the patient some control over the arrangements for care.

Functional status, nutritional status, and involvement of major organ systems are important components of making a prognosis. Functional ability is generally noted by Karnofsky scores (Table 11–1) (Ellison 1998). A patient's functional level is rated on a scale of 100–0, with 100 reflecting the healthy patient with no symptoms. Increments of 10 points are used to benchmark functional status. A score of 50 or lower is used for patients who are disabled. The rating continues to decline as patients approach death. Functional status is important to consider in long-term illnesses. Asking the patient or family member to give a history of functional ability over recent months will provide useful information for prognosis and allow the patient to reflect on the course of the disease. Questions such as, "What was life like for you a year ago? Six months ago? Last holiday?" provide an opportunity to discuss the speed of disease progression and open the discussion of goal setting.

The National Hospice Organization (NHO) has developed criteria for hospice admission of patients with nonmalignant diseases. This criteria defines when life expectancy is less than six months, thus making the patient eligible to utilize the Medicare Hospice Benefit (National Hospice Organization 1996). State health care programs for those in need of financial support generally have a benefit similar to the federal Medicare Hospice Benefit. The case manager should negotiate an end of life home care benefit for patients with private insurance plans that do not cover hospice. Most importantly though, hospice care should be thought of as a concept of care implemented when cure of the disease and prolongation of life is no longer the patient's goal.

TABLE 11–1   KARNOFSKY PERFORMANCE STATUS SCALE

100%	Normal, no complaints, no evidence of disease
90%	Able to carry on normal activity, minor signs of symptoms of disease
80%	Normal activity with effort; some signs or symptoms of disease
70%	Cares for self; unable to carry on normal activity or to do active work
60%	Requires occasional assistance, but is mostly able to care for self
50%	Requires considerable assistance and frequent medical care
40%	Disabled, requires special care and assistance
30%	Severely disabled, hospitalization indicated; death not imminent
20%	Very sick, hospitalization necessary, active supportive treatment necessary
10%	Moribund, fatal processes, progressing rapidly
0%	Dead

The decision to continue or discontinue hydration at the end of life is an emotionally charged issue for many patients and family members, and thus may require the full support of the interdisciplinary team. The patient who is not eating or drinking and is not being artificially supported cannot be expected to sustain life for greater than 14 days. Non-oral food and fluids may sustain life but may also prolong suffering as the disease progresses. Our focus must be to prevent suffering. At some point, as major organ systems shut down, non-oral hydration may cause symptoms of distress, such as edema, ascities, and respiratory distress. Zerwekh (1997) has identified seven questions that we should ask to guide the decision of continuing or discontinuing hydration:

- What do you expect the hydration to achieve?
- Are symptoms being relieved by hydration?
- Are symptoms being aggravated by hydration?
- Is hydration improving the patient's level of consciousness? Is this a goal?
- Is the infusion prolonging survival? Is this a goal?
- Are there psychosocial effects of the technology?
- Is the technology burden on the family justified by benefits?

We must help patients and families understand that the decrease or cessation of eating and drinking is a natural part of the dying process (Lindley-Davis 1991 and McCann 1999). Assuring that the patient and family members have a clear understanding of the disease status and prognosis will assist in allowing the establishment of clear goals. In turn, these goals will more clearly direct the decisions.

Treatment decisions concerning discontinuing non-oral fluids, blood transfusions, and life-prolonging treatments, such as dialysis and ventilator support, are difficult. Values of the nurse, patient, family, and other team members may conflict. The American Nurses Association (1991, 1992, and 1994) has issued a number of position statements that can assist us in defining our professional role as a nurse in end of life care issues. The recommendations of an ethics committee may assist in bringing consensus when there is uncertainty among the health care providers and patient and family members. Patients and family members need our support in the decision-making process. We can best assist by providing objective information about treatments and anticipated course of the disease.

Where will the Patient's Needs be Best Met at the End of Life?   What is the best environment for the patient at the end of life? The nurse must consider: where the patient desires to be, symptom management burden and the level of support necessary; caregiver support; and what type of reimbursement is available. Patients need to tell us where they desire to be at the end of life. Many patients desire to be at home, where they can more easily achieve control of the environment and have access to their family. By contrast, the young adult with young children at home may not be comfortable dying at home. Patients without caregivers may desire to remain independently in their homes for as long as they safely can, then later agree to other arrangements for care. Consider and negotiate the uniqueness of each individual's situation.

PROVIDING THE ENVIRONMENT FOR END OF LIFE CARE

Recognition of patients who are dying and assessment of their needs are critical roles for nurses. As this is accomplished, examination of the physical environment becomes our next focus. The physical environment for end of life care must be considered throughout the process of working with patients and family members, but perhaps is never more important than in the last days of life. Pierce relates three suggestions families have noted that address creation of a peaceful environment for the death experience in the acute care setting. Family members related that interactions between the dying patient and family should be facilitated; interactions between caregivers and patients/ families should be facilitated; and the environment or setting should be more conducive to these interactions. Family members want to be physically close to their loved one and to have their loved one's personhood acknowledged and respected (Pierce, et al. 1999). The environment does not need to be expensively furnished. Simple things—such as providing chairs for family members, space for them to gather to begin their grief work in private, and regular caring interactions with team members —are critical to support the family. A picture of the patient at the bedside that reflects who they are can help care providers more easily converse with the family about the personhood of the patient who no longer has a voice to speak. Reminiscing with family members about the life of the patient will help them begin the work of grieving. Asking a spouse "How did you meet your wife/husband?" generally assures a pleasant story in response. Simple interventions that reflect our care and concern are perhaps the most meaningful.

Palliative care helps patients to live well in the final days of life. Nurses have roles in recognizing that a patient is dying, successfully managing distressful symptoms, and providing an environment in the last days of life that acknowledges the personhood of the patient. These tasks are best accomplished by working with the interdisciplinary team. When patients are surrounded by love and support, their journey seems to become the natural conclusion of the cycle of life. To acknowledge that the patient has contributed in this life validates the meaning and purpose of life. Assisting patients in this process is indeed the essence of nursing.

MR. JONES: A CASE STUDY

Mr. Jones is a 62-year-old gentleman with pancreatic cancer. He has been receiving chemotherapy for the last six months. He is currently on his third chemotherapy regimen, having failed two others. He presents in the outpatient clinic with increased pain and fatigue, and states "I've run out of gas. I need a transfusion." A weight loss of 3 pounds in the last two weeks is noted.

Labs are done, blood is ordered, and Mr. Jones is settled in a clinic room for the transfusion. As you hang the blood, he asks, "What are we going to do about my pain?"

What critical pieces of the assessment would you focus on? Who is available to assist you? What would you communicate to the physician?

Response: You must address pain and fatigue during this clinic visit. Establish a plan for management before the patient leaves the clinic. If possible, clarify his understanding of the disease and the meaning of pain. Share this information with the physician and clarify treatment goals. It is appropriate to continue discussion with the patient via phone of the response to the new interventions. When pain is managed, do further assessment of the patient's understanding of the trajectory of the disease and discussion of goals as soon as possible. Based upon ongoing assessment, clearly communicate goals to the physician. Transitioning the patient to a more intensive palliative care approach is appropriate.

REFERENCES

American Nurses Association. (1994). *Position statement on active euthanasia.* Washington, DC.

American Nurses Association. (1994). *Position statement on assisted suicide.* Washington, DC.

American Nurses Association. (1992). *Position statement on foregoing nutrition and hydration.* Kansas City, Missouri.

American Nurses Association. (1991). *Position statement on promotion of comfort and relief of pain in dying patients*. Kansas City, Missouri.

Bouwsma, W. J. (1996). Conclusions: Retrospect and prospect. In H. M. Spiro, M. G. M. Curnen, & L. P. Wandel (Eds.), *Facing death: Where culture, religion, and medicine meet*, 189–198. New Haven, CT: Yale University Press.

Brody, H., Campbell, M., Faber-Landendoen, K, & Ogle, K. (1997). Withdrawing intensive life-sustaining treatment-recommendations for compassionate clinical management. *New England Journal of Medicine*, 336(9), 652–657.

Byock I. (1997). *Dying well*. New York: Riverhead Books.

Ellison, N. (1998). Palliative chemotherapy. In A. Berger, R. Portenoy, & D. Weissman, eds. *Principles and practice of supportive oncology*. Philadelphia, Lippincott-Raven.

Griffie, J., Muchka, S., Nelson-Marten, P., & O'Mara, A. (1991). Integrating palliative care into daily practice. *Journal of Palliative Medicine*, 2(1), 65–73.

Lindley-Davis, B. (1991). Process of dying defining characteristics. *Cancer Nursing*, 14(6): 328–333.

McCann, R. (1999). Lack of evidence about tube feeding-food for thought. JAMA, 282(14) 1380–1381.

National Hospice Organization. *Medical guidelines for determining prognosis in selected non-cancer diseases. 2nd Edition*. (1996), Washington, DC: Author.

Pierce, SF (1999). Improving end of life care: Gathering suggestions from family members. *Nursing Forum*, 34(2), 5–14.

Weissman, D. E. (1997). Consultation in palliative medicine. *Archives of Internal Medicine*, 157: 733–737.

World Health Organization. (1990). *Cancer pain relief and palliative care*. (Technical report series 804.) Geneva: Author.

Zerwekh, J. (1997, March). Do dying patients really need IV fluids? *American Journal of Nursing*, 97(3), 26–31.

CHAPTER

PAIN AND SYMPTOM MANAGEMENT

Tyla Ann Burger

PAIN MANAGEMENT

The management of pain and distressing symptoms is a major responsibility of the team caring for an individual with advanced disease. The fear of pain is a major concern for patients and families coping with terminal illness. Actual and potential pain are significant factors in the continuing debates about quality end of life care and choice in dying.

Our inability to directly measure pain and the attitudes and misconceptions of health care professionals has led to the institutionalization of the undertreatment of pain. Societal and cultural attitudes contribute further to the problem. The resulting impact is a greater incidence of untreated pain in women, the elderly, and minorities (Cleeland, et al. 1994). An increased understanding of the mechanism of pain, development of new treatments, and increasing efforts at pain management education should reverse the practice of chronic undertreatment. Recent guidelines on pain management have been issued by organizations such as the American Pain Society, the Joint Commission on Accreditation of Healthcare Organizations, the American Medical Directors Association, and the American Geriatrics Society. These guidelines should assist health care providers in improving the quality of life for patients and families.

The Joint Commission on Accreditation of Healthcare Organizations, American Pain Society, and the Veterans Administration, among others, have called for the assessment of pain as the "fifth vital sign." The concrete effect is to require that routine assessment of all patients include an evaluation of pain intensity (pain scales) along with pulse, respiration, blood pressure, and temperature. The more long-term goal is to change the mindset of the health care community to include pain management as integral to all aspects of practice.

Most professionals care for a series of patients who present with varying degrees of distressing symptoms. When providers do not have the knowledge or tools to address symptoms such as chronic pain, they often develop attitudes and strategies to cope with the distress in their patients and themselves. Health care providers often reinforce the myth that pain is something that "good" patients learn to deal with. Thus a patient in pain may receive admonitions such as "It's not really that bad," "Get a hold of yourself," and "You can get through this." Such statements devalue patient reporting. There is no objective method for directly measuring pain. Research also demonstrates significant variations in the degree to which individuals perceive and experience pain, including genetic factors (Uhl, Sora, and Wang 1999). Therefore, pain assessment and treatment must be guided by Margo McCaffery's (1968, 9) definition of pain: "Pain is whatever the experiencing person says it is, existing whenever the experiencing person says it does."

One misconception that both providers and patients may carry is that while pain may be an indicator of varying levels of disease or injury, the pain itself is not harmful. Further study has determined that the pain itself is detrimental to patients. Figure 12–1 identifies many of the effects of untreated pain (McCaffery and Pasero 1999). These include sleep and rest disturbance, decreased mobility, cognitive loss, and decreased immune response. Health care providers learn that the post-operative patient whose pain is not controlled is at risk for pneumonia and emboli due to unnecessary immobility. Elderly patients who take to their beds due to chronic unrecognized and untreated pain are at least as likely to develop a debilitating or fatal complication.

An attentive, timely response to reports of pain or discomfort can reduce anxiety about future symptoms and improve patient reporting. Appropriate treatment can improve quality of life for both patient and family. Well-managed symptoms reduce the overall costs: physical, emotional, social, and financial to families and society in general.

While this chapter addresses the assessment and treatment of physical pain and other symptoms, the provider cannot lose sight of the complete "picture of pain." In the model adapted from St. Christopher's Hospice in London,

---

- Loss of mobility, muscle tone, and joint function
- Decreased pulmonary function and capacity, leading to increased respiratory infections
- Confusion, loss of cognitive function
- Depression and anxiety
- Decreased bowel motility and urinary retention
- Alteration in metabolism, especially hyperglycemia
- Depressed immune response

Figure 12–1 Effects of Untreated Pain

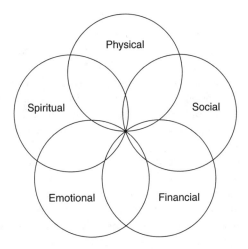

Figure 12–2 Adapted from St. Christopers Hospice, London

(Figure 12–2) physical, social, emotional, spiritual, and financial pain must be viewed as a whole entity in terms of their impact and treatment. Physical pain is often the most overwhelming concern. However, the patient with overwhelming emotional or spiritual pain will not have their physical pain successfully treated without appropriate intervention. The financial pain of advanced disease can as easily lead to consideration of suicide as can uncontrolled physical pain. Therefore pain management is an interdisciplinary team process. Medicine, nursing, social work, pastoral care, rehabilitation, and pharmacy are all disciplines that might be required to meet the pain management needs of patients and families.

CLASSIFICATION OF PAIN

Pain can, and should, be evaluated from a number of perspectives. There are several ways to define pain. This can be by classification, type (chronicity), and disease process (i.e. sickle cell pain). Determining the proper classification and type of a pain presentation is particularly important in determining the appropriate treatment plan. Identifying the underlying disease process will assist in determining the overall goal. The patient may require acute pain management while treatment is provided to address the causative disease or injury. Alternatively, in the presence of an unidentifiable or untreatable cause, long-term palliative pain management will be required.

The International Association for the Study of Pain issued standard guidelines for the classification of pain in 1994 (Merskey and Bogduk 1994). Classification is based on the mechanism of pain reception and transmission. The two major classifications are nociceptive and neuropathic pain. Nociceptive pain is further broken down into a number of subcategories. Nociceptive pain refers to pain experienced as a result of stimulation of nerve endings called nociceptors. Neuropathic pain results from injury or disease process affecting the nerve paths that transmit pain sensation to the brain.

Nociceptive pain occurs when nociceptors found in cutaneous, visceral, other soft tissue, and bone are stimulated. This classification is further divided by differences in pain sensation and response that are generally related to tissue type. Categories of nociceptive pain are somatic, bone, and visceral pain. In general, nociceptive pain is responsive to treatment with standard pain management therapies such as NSAIDs and opioids.

Somatic pain has also been called soft tissue or body pain. The pain results directly from stimulation of cutaneous nociceptors in skin, muscles, and other soft tissues. The sensation of pain is then transmitted through the normal nerve paths to the brain. The pain is generally localized to the area of injury. This localization may decrease if pain becomes chronic. The pain will be described in a wide variety of terms, depending on the source of injury and individual reporting. Somatic pain is generally highly responsive to anti-inflammatory, analgesic, and opioid medications.

Visceral pain is similar to somatic pain in that the pain results from stimulation of nociceptors. The actual presentation of pain produced by the activation of visceral nociceptors can be quite different from somatic pain. The descriptors used by patients to describe visceral pain are less often used for somatic pain. These may include cramping, irritation, pressure, wavelike, or "balled up" pain. Visceral pain also tends to be poorly localized and may be "referred" to a location away from the actual source of pain. While visceral pain tends to be quite responsive to anti-inflammatory, analgesic, and opioid medications, the provider needs to evaluate their use in terms of the likely underlying source of visceral pain. Many of these medications have properties that can exacerbate certain clinical situations. Using an opioid to treat pain related to impaction would need to be carefully considered in terms of the known opioid side effect of increased constipation.

Bone pain is also similar to somatic pain in that the pain sensation arises from stimulation of nociceptors that are found in bone and the periosteum. It differs however, in that prostaglandin activity is significantly higher in bone injury than in soft tissue injury. This results in an increased incidence of hyperalgesia and decreased response to mild analgesics and opioids. Effective treatment of significant bone pain will generally require use of an anti-inflammatory agent to address the issue of prostaglandin activity. NSAIDs are generally used first, though corticosteroids may be more useful in very aggressive disease. These agents may be used by themselves for mild pain or in combination with opioids for severe pain. A variety of non-pharmacologic interventions may be useful in bone pain including immobilization of acute injuries, thermal applications, and appropriate rehabilitation therapy.

Neuropathic pain is caused by abnormal processing of sensory input by the peripheral or central nervous system (McCaffery and Pasero 1999). It may result from injury or disease process. The most common sources of neuropathic pain are nerve compression, deafferentation pain, and peripheral neuropathies. Nerve compression occurs when tumors or other structures place sufficient pressure on a nerve to temporarily or permanently interrupt transmission of impulses along the nerve. Deafferentation pain results from traumatic injury to the peripheral or central nervous system. The most commonly cited example is phantom limb pain. Peripheral neuropathies are frequently described as burning, tingling, or numbness in extremities. HIV disease and diabetes are the most common causes of neuropathies. Some medications, including several antiviral agents can cause neuropathy.

Less common neuropathic conditions include central pain syndromes such as post-stroke syndrome and the complex regional pain syndromes. These conditions are also referred to as sympathetically maintained pain. Assessment and treatment of such syndromes is complex and detailed.

Neuropathic pain is rarely responsive to mild analgesics or opioids alone. Adjuvant analgesics are usually required. Tricyclic antidepressants, anticonvulsants, corticosteroids, and certain antiarrythmic medications are useful agents in addressing neuropathic pain. Once pain is controlled, rehabilitation therapy can be useful in restoring function and preventing some recurrent injuries. Consultation with appropriately trained physical therapists may be of benefit.

The potential for multiple pain issues should be considered. In a major study of 2,266 cancer patients, 4,542 separate pain syndromes were identified (Grond, et al. 1996). For example, a patient under hospice care identified two separate sensations of pain. The first, a tight, bandlike sensation in her chest which was thought to be related to tumor growth, responded well to opioid therapy. The second pain sensation, described as "a fuse box on fire" in her abdomen, did not respond at all to the opioids. This proved to be a neuropathic pain syndrome, possibly related to tumor invasion in her thoracic spine. It was first treated unsuccessfully with an anticonvulsant, then successfully with a tricyclic antidepressant.

TYPES OF PAIN

Most pain can be defined as one of three types: acute, cancer, or chronic nonmalignant pain (CNP). The line between these types is not always clear. Cancer pain is most likely to demonstrate overlapping characteristics as the disease process may create both chronic and acute symptoms.

Acute pain is short-term, related to injury or advancing disease and generally subsides with healing. The picture of acute pain is generally characterized by elevations in vital signs, expressions of discomfort, and active efforts to seek relief.

Chronic pain continues beyond the normally expected healing of the original injury. Chronic injury or disease may be present, not identifiable, or absent. The nervous system adapts to the presence of chronic pain. Vital signs are no longer elevated and the distressed expression is replaced by a flat or subdued affect. Prolonged chronic pain has progressive impact on function and lifestyle. Efforts to seek relief vary considerably with the personality and psychosocial resources of the individual.

Neuronal "windup" is a significant factor in chronic pain (McCaffery and Pasero 1999). With repeated stimulation of nociceptors, a state of hyperexcitability is created in the pathways that transmit pain. Thus chronic pain becomes progressively more centrally mediated. This causes increased sensitivity to stimuli in the forms of hyperalgesia or allodynia. Hyperalgesia is an abnormally increased pain response to a noxious stimulus. Allodynia is sensation of pain generated by a stimulus that is not normally painful (Merskey and Bogduk 1994). Both of these conditions can be illustrated by a person with significant sunburn. Exposure of the skin surface to heat, which might be minimally unpleasant in normal skin, will generally elicit noticeable pain in the already burned skin. This is hyperalgesia. Allodynia is presented in the form that even minimal touching of the burned skin will result in pain. Both of these conditions may be significant factors for patients experiencing chronic pain. There is also a decrease in localization. An original injury to a hand may result in a chronically painful arm.

Breakthrough pain is defined as a transient increase in pain of at least moderate intensity in a patient whose baseline pain is moderate or less (Foley 1998). Breakthrough pain is reported in about 65% of cancer patients (Bookbinder, et al. 1995). It is usually rapid in onset and brief in duration. The intensity of pain and frequency of occurrence is highly variable. Patients should have a fast-acting "breakthrough" medication available. Generally the fast-acting oral forms of morphine and oxycodone have been used. These generally have a 15–30 minute onset. Newer medications, such as fetanyl in a sucrose lozynge on a stick (Actig), are designed to have an even faster 5-minute onset.

Episodic, or incident, pain is a transient increase in pain that is caused by an identifiable activity or physical event. Movement, dressing changes, eating, and position changes can all cause episodic pain. Patients who regularly experience episodic pain should be premedicated with a fast-acting preparation. The medication should be administered early enough and at an appropriate dose to allow for the patient's comfort during the activity.

ADDRESSING MISCONCEPTIONS

Before providers can treat pain, they must determine what barriers exist to successful treatment. A significant obstacle to that success is the misconceptions about pain and its treatment held by patients, families, and other health care providers.

Provider Misconceptions

Many providers continue to have misconceptions about chronic pain. In repeated studies, nurses were more likely to devalue and underreport patients' assessments of pain if they did not appear uncomfortable (i.e. smiling instead of grimacing) (McCaffery and Ferrell 1997). A study of patients referred to a pain center demonstrated similar biases in physicians. The only significant factor differentiating patients who received opioid pain medication was observable pain behaviors (Turk and Olifiji 1997). Clearly, the basis of this problem is a lack of understanding of the differences between acute and chronic pain, including the adaptation of the nervous system. Control issues arise when providers are not educated to accept patients as the experts on their own pain. By transferring the responsibility for reporting on pain status to the patient, providers can avoid adversarial elements in the care relationship. Trust is a mutual process and necessary for successful outcomes.

Providers also demonstrate a significant bias to undertreatment when pain is not related to cancer or other terminal illness. The phrase "It's not going to kill you" demonstrates the effect of this bias. Even patients with cancer were less likely to receive adequate treatment if the pain they were reporting appeared unrelated to the cancer (Cleeland, et al. 1994). Patients with back pain and neuropathic pain syndromes have been particularly vulnerable to this misconception.

The need to identify a cause of pain can be a stumbling block for some providers. Some providers still label pain without an identifiable disease process or continuing injury as psychogenic or psychosomatic pain. This diagnosis has been removed from psychiatric manuals and does not appear in any recognized classification of pain. The true incidence of somatiform disorders is very rare within the population of patients with pain. Increased education about the role of central mediation in chronic pain might alleviate provider concerns.

Concerns about addiction and drug-seeking behavior can also limit provider's response to pain patients. The actual incidence of addiction in patients with pain has been studied repeatedly. These studies report signs of addiction in a dramatically small number, 7 out of 24,000 patients (Friedman 1990).

Providers who view opioid medications as "narcotics," a legal and criminalizing term, are less likely to adequately treat pain. This stems from both concerns about regulatory oversight and a lack of education about the proper use of these medications. The Federation of State Medical Boards (1998) has adopted new guidelines that should assist providers with concerns in this area. In 1999, a state medical board announced the first disciplinary action against a physician for regularly failing to provide adequate pain management.

Lack of communication between patients and providers has often been cited as a cause of undertreatment. The SUPPORT study (1995) significantly demonstrated that increased efforts to improve communication of patient and family wishes in end of life care were not effective in preventing undertreatment of pain. It appears that the underlying misconceptions of providers were of greater weight in determining outcome. The need for continuing education is readily demonstrated.

Patient and Family Misconceptions

Misconceptions about pain, its treatment, and the medications used to treat it are widespread in the general population. Significant areas of concern include addiction, safety of medications, running out of options for controlling pain, and multiple misconceptions about the nature and management of pain.

The misconception of addiction is even more widespread in the general population. News reports about addiction and the narcotics trade only reinforce these concerns. Education about the therapeutic use of opioids (not narcotics), and the clear evidence that addiction is not a factor in treatment of pain, is required to overcome these fears.

Concerns about safety of analgesic medications frequently lead to noncompliance with a treatment plan. Patients have reported the belief that even acetaminophen will significantly sedate them. Sedation, respiratory depression, GI effects, and "allergies" are all reported as preventing patients from taking medication. In light of these concerns, many patients adopt a "least amount necessary" approach. They take the medication intermittently and less than prescribed. Especially in the case of opioids, this can have a highly detrimental effect. The first problem encountered is clearly inadequate pain control. Secondarily, the very side effects they are trying to avoid are more likely to occur in the increasingly fluctuating blood levels created by intermittent dosing. Most side effects of opioids are transient and subside when steady blood levels are reached. Missing and unpredictable dosing will prevent steady state and prolong or increase side effects.

Many patients put off the use of needed pain medications because they worry about not having options when disease progresses and symptoms increase. The availability of a variety of medications and the lack of an upper dose limit for step III opioids prevents any real potential for running out of options for treating pain. An individualized combination of appropriate opioids and adjuvant therapies can be safely used as disease progresses to maintain pain control.

Patients and families require the same education about pain, its harmful effects, variations in pain sensitivity, and the concepts of chronic pain that providers require. Appropriate educational materials on pain, pain medication, and treatment are all necessary tools for any pain management practitioner.

A SYSTEMATIC APPROACH TO PAIN MANAGEMENT

Once the need for pain management has been identified a consistent approach is required. Response to previous treatment, educational needs, and resource issues (i.e. financial needs) all need to be considered in creating a treatment plan. All members of the team—providers, patient, family, and other caregivers—should be educated about the plan of care. All of these individuals have the potential to promote the success, or failure, of a pain management plan.

AIR

An overall approach to pain should be rooted in the concept that the need for comfort is very basic. Including pain management in care should be as simple as breathing. Thus the pneumonic AIR can represent the overall approach of assessment, intervention, and reassessment. The data collected by a complete assessment enables appropriate intervention. Routine reassessment allows for the evaluation of the effectiveness of the treatment plan.

Assessment

A complete assessment of pain requires development of a complete picture of the individual's symptoms, history, treatment, and response. The simple use of a pain scale documented in a note does not provide sufficient information to effectively treat pain. Good assessment technique includes appropriate environment, sufficient time, attentive listening, and proper training.

A significant factor in unnecessary pain and suffering experienced by individuals with advanced disease is the failure of health care professionals to properly assess pain and other symptoms (von Roenn, et. al. 1993). Factors that contribute to inadequate assessment include:

- use of inappropriate tools
- communication barriers
- inadequate training in assessment
- delayed assessment (i.e. awaiting verbal report of pain before assessing)
- minimal exploration of reported symptoms (making assumptions based on previous reports)

Assessment Tools
A wide variety of assessment tools have been developed. The choice of an appropriate tool requires awareness of the assessment goal, communication issues, and other issues related to the patient or population the provider needs to assess. One type of assessment tool may be suitable for use in an occupational health setting where most pain issues are derived from injuries in fairly ambulatory, verbally competent adults. It is unlikely that the same tool would be useful in a long-term care setting with disease-related pain and a significant number of nonverbal and dementia patients.

Types of pain assessment tools include trigger, comprehensive, and non-verbal assessments, brief pain inventories, and pain flowsheets. Any of these types of pain assessment can be incorporated into larger tools, such as admission and discharge assessments.

A trigger assessment is designed to screen a large population for pain or risk for pain. It is usually brief and completed as part of routine care, possibly on admission to a health care service. In order to be effective, a trigger assessment must be designed to the needs of the screened population and trigger systematic follow-up when a problem is identified. If the target population includes patients with impaired communication and cognitive abilities the assessment cannot be limited to verbal responses to a series of questions. Many trigger assessments create a numerical score based on responses to questions or observations of nonverbal indicators of discomfort or both. The level at which a positive "trigger" requires follow-up and what team members are involved is determined by the agency's procedures.

Comprehensive assessments are detailed tools designed to obtain a complete picture of the current symptoms, history, treatments, impact on quality of life, and resources or limitations for the patient and family. The assessment should be completed by a provider who has the proper training to effectively use such a tool. A comprehensive assessment provides a baseline for evaluation of treatment effectiveness and disease progression.

Brief pain inventories and pain flowsheets are used for fast, less detailed, evaluation of pain at the current moment. Brief pain inventories are often used by researchers to evaluate a specific aspect of pain and its treatment. Pain flowsheets are used by health care providers to monitor the ongoing status of a patient with pain. These must be updated consistently, even when the pain is well controlled.

Nonverbal assessments may be incorporated into any of these assessment tools. Providers who work with a large number of communication and cognitively impaired patients may develop separate assessments for this group. When a patient cannot respond to questions about their symptoms, other indicators must be used. Figure 12–3 includes behavioral indicators identified by geriatric pain management teams and groups such as Alzheimer's support groups to assist in evaluating pain and discomfort. It should be noted that the absence of normal behavior might be as significant as active behaviors, particularly in dementia patients.

Without an objective tool to directly measure pain, an alternative method is necessary for evaluating the degree and impact of symptoms on the individual. Pain intensity is best evaluated by the person who is experiencing the pain. The development of various pain scales was designed to provide a consistent method for evaluating pain intensity. The use of pain scales has been shown to be very successful when both patients and providers are properly trained in their use.

A variety of pain scales have been created. Some address the needs of particular groups (i.e., children). Others allow patients to choose those charac-

ACTIVE INDICATORS	ABSENCE INDICATORS
Rocking	Flat affect
Negative vocalization	Decreased interaction
Frown or grimacing	Inability to relax
Noisy breathing	Decreased intake
Irritability	Altered sleep pattern
Picking at objects	
Aggression	

Figure 12–3 Possible behavioral indicators of pain

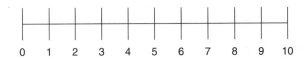

0 1 2 3 4 5 6 7 8 9 10

Figure 12–4 Numerical Rating Scale (NRS)—horizontal

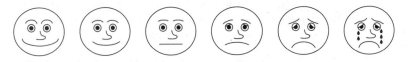

Figure 12–5 Wong-Baker Faces Scale

teristics that are easiest for them to use. Standard variations include visual analog scales (VAS), numerical rating scales (NRS) (Figure 12–4), descriptor scales, and picture-based scales, such as the Wong-Baker Faces Scale. All of these scales can be adapted and enhanced with color or other attributes to improve their effectiveness for a given population. The Wong-Baker Faces Scale (Figure 12–5) is frequently found to be most effective with children and the cognitively impaired. A vertical version of the NRS appears to be most easily understood by the general population. Most scales that include a numerical rating will be based on a 0–10 scale, with 10 representing the greatest possible intensity of pain.

Patients who are offered a choice of pain scales may be able to identify one that will be most effective for them. Children or the cognitively impaired should probably have an appropriate scale selected for them so they may concentrate on learning to use the scale. Once a scale has been chosen, all team members should use the same scale and document the results of its use in a consistent manner. Patients and families should be taught to use some form of a pain log, tracking frequency and intensity of pain, treatment, and its effectiveness. Such data is invaluable in reassessment and refinement of a pain control plan.

Several factors influence an individual's perception and experience with pain. Pain threshold is the level of stimulus that triggers the first perception of pain. This threshold and the individual's sensitivity to the intensity of pain will influence how a patient evaluates pain on the 0–10 scale. Pain tolerance is the level of pain that an individual is able to tolerate normally. For some patients, no pain sensation will be tolerable. For others a pain scale of 3–4 will be acceptable and allow fairly normal function. Thus simply knowing that a patient's pain is rated at 5 out of 10, without knowing if their tolerance is 0 or 2, is incomplete information. While the overall goal is elimination of pain, the patient's tolerance level may be a factor in difficult pain presentations or when comfort versus side effects is an issue.

Intervention

W.H.O. ladder

In the 1980s, the World Health Organization (WHO) identified cancer pain as a world health problem and proposed a systematic method of treating pain (WHO 1986). The method called for use of a three-step analgesic ladder (Figure 12–6). The WHO guidelines also call for using the following key concepts to ensure quality pain management (AHCPR 1994):

- Use the oral route as the simplest, least intrusive, and most dependable route of administration.
- Use regularly scheduled around-the-clock dosing to ensure steady levels and consistent pain control.
- Individualize the treatment plan to meet the needs of patient and caregivers.
- Give good attention to detail (such as full assessments, polypharmacy, potential side effects, etc.).

The WHO approach, particularly the analgesic ladder, has been carefully studied and documented to be 88% effective in providing good and effective pain control and maintaining that control over time (Zech, et al. 1995).

Step I—Mild pain. Step I calls for the use of mild analgesic and anti-inflammatory agents to treat mild to moderate pain. Pain that is consistently rated at up to 3 or 4 on a scale of 10 should be treated at this level. These drugs may be over-the-counter (OTC) or prescription medications. Step I medications include acetaminophen, nonsteroidal anti-inflammatory drugs (NSAIDs)—including aspirin—and corticosteroids.

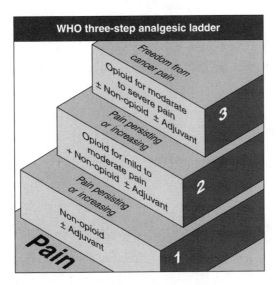

Figure 12–6 WHO Three-Step Ladder
Source: World Health Organization, 1980.

Acetaminophen is the most commonly used pain medication currently available. It comes in multiple forms and is highly effective for common pain. The drug has minimal to no anti-inflammatory properties. Pain that has a significant inflammatory source may benefit more from another choice of medication. It is generally well tolerated. Hepatotoxicity is a potential result from overdose, regular use with alcohol, and possibly with chronic high-dose use. The maximum daily dose is 4 gm, though some sources recommend staying below 3 gm for chronic use in the elderly. Since acetaminophen is an ingredient in many combination agents, both prescription and OTC, the potential for unintentionally exceeding recommended daily doses is significant.

NSAIDs actually consist of several groups of drugs, including salicylates, propionic acids, phenylacetic and acetic acids, and COX 2 inhibitors. Some of the more commonly used NSAIDs in palliative care include ibuprofen (Motrin, Advil), naproxen (Naprosyn, Aleve), choline magnesium trisalsalate (Trilisate), nabumetone (Relafen), ketprofen (Orudis), ketoralac (Toradol), and aspirin. All of these medications have significant anti-inflammatory effects and are particularly useful in bone and joint pain. They may be used alone as step I agents or as adjuvants to stronger medication at steps II or III.

The most notable adverse effects of NSAIDs include a wide variety of gastrointestinal (GI) symptoms related to damage to the GI mucosa. Gastritis, nausea, ulcers, and bleeding can all occur. The incidence of these adverse effects varies between groups of NSAIDs and between individual drugs. The new family of coacetyloxygenase 2 (COX 2) inhibitors, including celecoxib (Celebrex) and rofecoxib (Vioxx), has been developed with the intent of reducing the incidence of GI effects. While the incidence of such adverse effects has been very significantly reduced, GI bleeds have occurred in a very small number of cases. COX 2 inhibitors are quite new and costly. Nonacetylated salicylates, such as choline magnesium trisalsalate (Trilisate) and salsalate (Disalcid), have been overshadowed by newer agents. They have a somewhat lower incidence of GI effects in comparison to most other NSAIDs and are particularly easy to use. Trilisate comes in a liquid preparation, which may be beneficial to some patients and caregivers. Indomethicin (Indocin) has a particularly high incidence of GI effects and should be avoided, especially in the elderly. For patients with increased risk of ulcers, misoprostol (Cytotec) appears to be more effective than more commonly used agents, such as ranitidine (Zantac), in protecting the gastric mucosa from the effects of NSAIDs (Levy 1996).

Various NSAIDs have additional adverse effects including blood dyscrascias, hypersensitivity, and other effects. Providers should be familiar with the medications they use. Some agents will require monitoring of hepatic or renal function.

Corticosteroids (steroids) are strong anti-inflammatory agents. They also have a variety of multisystem effects that may lead to significant adverse reactions. Their use should be saved for specific conditions that require a high level of anti-inflammatory action or inflammatory pain issues that have not responded to less problematic drugs. Conditions where steroids should be considered include spinal cord or nerve compression, organ capsule pain, and some specific neuropathic syndromes.

Step II—Moderate pain.   When pain increases or persists after appropriate step I interventions, it should be treated at step II. If an initial pain assessment demonstrates pain consistently above 4 on a scale of 10, it should be treated starting at this step. Step II is defined as the use of opioids for mild to moderate pain. Traditionally this has meant the use of dose-limited opioids in combination agents with acetaminophen or aspirin, for their coanalgesic properties. Oxycodone in the form of the combination agent Percocet has also been frequently used. However, the use of combination agents has been found to contribute to issues of polypharmacy and incidental overdosing of acetaminophen. Many pain management experts recommend against the use of combination agents, while others continue to recommend them.

Dose-limited opioids are opioids that have an upper limit, or ceiling, to their use due to an increasing incidence of side effects related to dosage. The most commonly used dose-limited opioids are codeine (Tylenol with Codeine), hyrdrocodone (Lortabs, Vicodin), and propoxyphene (Darvocet). Propoxyphene is problematic and is addressed further in the section on inappropriate medications. Codeine is anecdotally reported by hospice staff to have a greater incidence of GI effects, especially constipation, than other opioids.

Several "no-ceiling" opioids are available at doses that deliver step II pain management. Oxycodone is available alone or in combination as Percocet.

Oxycodone	20 to 40 mg po. q12h (Percocet has 5 mg tablet for a max. of 60 mg day)
Morphine	15 to 30 mg. po q 12h
Hydromorphone	2 mg po q4h

Figure 12–7 Step II doses for no-ceiling opioids

Morphine and hydromorphone (Dilaudid) are also available at doses equivalent to the 5 mg. of oxycodone found in Percocet. An advantage to using the no-ceiling opioids at step II doses (Figure 12–7) is that if symptoms do progress, doses can be increased to step III levels. This saves patient and provider any difficulties that might arise from switching medications while increasing the relative dosage.

Tramadol (Ultram) is a unique step II agent with dual action properties. It is often mistaken for an NSAID, which it is not. The drug demonstrates weak opioid activity, at the analgesic level of other step II opioids such as codeine. It also acts on neurotransmitters involved in modulating pain in the spinal cord. The combined action appears to make the drug particularly effective for some patients. Anecdotally, there is also a small group of patients for whom the drug is completely ineffective, possibly because it is converted to its active metabolite via a pathway that may be absent in a small percentage of the population. Since the drug reaches steady state in two days of regular usage, 72 hours should be sufficient to indicate whether it will be effective. Adverse effects are considered to be at a level similar to other step II agents (i.e. codeine combinations), but with a comparatively decreased incidence of traditional opioid side effects such as sedation, respiratory depression, euphoria, and constipation.

Step III—Severe pain. When pain persists despite appropriate step II treatment or increases after previously effective treatment, it should be treated at step III. This step is defined as the use of opioids for moderate to severe pain. The increased dosages used at step III require the use of the no-ceiling opioids: morphine, oxycodone, hydromorphone, and fentanyl. Adjuvant medications should be considered when appropriate, especially in the presence of bone or neuropathic pain.

No-ceiling opioids do not demonstrate significant dose-limiting side effects. With proper titration, these medications can be increased over time to meet the pain relief needs of patients with advancing disease process. The maximum doses found in drug references are based on use of these medications in acute care. These guidelines are appropriate for opioid-naive patients receiving short-term therapy. No upper dose limits have been documented for opioid-experienced patients whose medication has been increased using appropriate titration. In a fairly small number of patients, symptoms of myoclonus or delirium may occur at higher doses. Switching to an equianalgesic (therapeutically equivalent) dose of another opioid will frequently alleviate such symptoms. It should be noted that oxycodone and hydromorphone seem to have a decreased incidence of these effects than morphine, though occurrence is rare overall.

Morphine is available in the widest variety of forms and dosages. Short- and long-acting preparations, oral tablets or capsules, liquids, suppositories, and a variety of parenteral formulations are all available. Long experience with morphine and therapeutic and its cost effectiveness make it the first line drug of choice for most patients. Proper and effective patient education will overcome most misconceptions and allow for effective use of morphine to control pain. However, patients or families who demonstrate a significant negative reaction to "morphine" should probably be started on another agent to prevent predictable treatment failure due to non-compliance with the treatment plan. Oxycodone is available in almost as many forms, but is not available in parenteral form in the United States. Elderly patients with an increased potential for cognitive impairment may benefit from the choice of oxycodone, which appears to have less incidence of confusion.

Usage of hydromorphone has been limited by the lack of a long-acting preparation. The drug seems better tolerated by patients who are particularly sensitive to opioid side effects. However, the every-4-hour dosing requirement places a significant burden on patients and caregivers. Several companies have long-acting preparations approaching approval. Addition of these formulations will significantly increase the options available for use of this medication.

One particular formulation of long-acting hydromorphone, currently pending approval, is designed with the ability to be given through feeding tubes or in small amounts of soft foods, such as applesauce, and still retain its long-acting properties. When approved this will provide an improved capacity for long-acting pain control in elderly, disabled, and actively dying patients who have difficulty swallowing. The only current option for long-acting preparations of morphine and oxycodone, which cannot be crushed, is rectal administration. While not documented in manufacturer's literature, safe and effective rectal use of oral preparations is well documented in case reports and anecdotal literature.

Occasionally both oral and rectal routes are either unavailable or ineffective in providing timely and effective pain control. Use of a CADD or other infusion pump may be necessary to deliver parenteral medication. Unless a long-term access is in place, subcutaneous infusion is preferred as the least invasive route. Morphine is the most commonly used medication. However, hydromorphone is more soluble than morphine in aqueous solution, so it provides more options for infusions at increased dosages.

Fentanyl is the step III opioid with the highest potency available. In comparison with the other available drugs, a very small amount is required to achieve the same therapeutic effect. Fentanyl is currently available in long-acting (72-hour) transdermal (Duragesic) or rapid-acting lozenge (Actig) forms. The transdermal patches are particularly useful for patients who have difficulty managing medications. Caregivers can change the patches every three days and maintain pain control. Duragesic is also useful for patients who have stable pain control and cannot take medication by mouth. The transdermal system generally provides very stable levels of medication. However, temperature directly affects the transdermal system and significant fevers can result in adverse effects related to overly rapid absorption. Transdermal patches should never be subjected to direct heat sources such as heat lamps or hot tubs. Titration is generally difficult using transdermal patches due to longer onset of effect and steady state. It should also be noted that the subcutaneous "reservoir" of drug created by the patches continues delivering medication for an extended period after the patches are removed. When Duragesic is discontinued, 17 hours or more are required for a 50% decrease in serum fentanyl concentrations (AHCPR 1994). This should be taken into account when converting to another medication or decreasing the drug.

The side effects most commonly associated with opioid therapy—sedation, GI distress, and confusion—are generally transient and will subside in three to five days of consistent dosage and frequency. Educating patients and caregivers will prevent treatment failure due to anxiety produced by predictable effects of the medication. Palliative care practitioners should be prepared to treat certain side effects, such as nausea, aggressively in the short-term after initiation of therapy or significant dosage increase. Stopping or decreasing dosages will generally result in uncontrolled pain and continuing side effects. Changing the medication should only be considered if side effects persist beyond three to five days or are unable to be controlled with appropriate treatment. Constipation is an opioid-induced effect that does not subside. All patients taking opioids on a regular schedule must have an appropriate bowel regimen. Many palliative care programs make this an indicator in their quality assurance programs. A wide variety of stool softeners, laxatives, and stimulants can be adapted to the individual treatment plan.

Respiratory depression has a very rare incidence of occurrence. When it does occur, it tends to be in opioid-naive patients receiving parenteral medication. Starting opioid-naive patients on the equivalent of step II dosages and titrating to necessary levels for appropriate pain control should prevent occurrence of this side effect. Respiratory depression occurs when both the frequency and depth of respiration decline sufficiently from the individual's baseline to cause some compromise. Far too often a patient who has had profound levels of pain controlled for the first time is found to be deeply asleep. An uneducated professional then evaluates the patient as being oversedated or in respiratory depression on the basis of an arbitrary rate, and administers a reversing agent such as naloxone (Narcan). The result is a wide-awake patient in unnecessary, severe pain. Proper usage, education, and—in the rare instance of actual compromise—respiratory support will usually address this concern. Patients who are actively dying may have respiratory depression related to either disease process or medications. The precipitating factor is irrelevant in comparison to the need to maintain comfort at this stage. It is inappropriate to reduce or withhold pain medication for an end-stage patient based on fear of respiratory depression or sedation.

ADJUVANT MEDICATIONS

Bone Pain

Increased prostaglandin activity is a major factor in the increased intensity and persistence of bone pain. In moderate to severe pain, it is likely that adjuvant medication will be required in order to provide acceptable pain control. NSAIDs will generally provide the necessary anti-prostaglandin effect. Anecdotal reports among hospice providers indicate that choline magnesium trisalsalate (Trilisate) seems to be particularly useful for bone pain.

Severe bone pain caused by malignant disease may respond well to radiation or chemotherapy. For some patients, pamidronate (Aredia), a biphosphonate, may be more therapeutic and cost effective for severe pain requiring large doses of opioids and NSAIDs. It is generally given every two to four weeks. Pathological fractures caused by invasive disease are generally treated with appropriate stabilization of the fracture and adequate pain control. The potential for healing varies considerably with the degree of disease and the individual.

Neuropathic Pain

Neuropathic pain nearly always requires the use of adjuvant medication since it is poorly responsive to most analgesics. Some experts recommend starting with anticonvulsant medications for sharp, lancinating pain usually associated with direct nerve injury. The underlying assumption is the need to decrease the threshold of excitation in the nerve pathway. Conversely, the burning, tingling, numbing pain associated with neuropathies and chronic pain syndromes may respond better to tricyclic antidepressants. Different medications within each of these categories act on different neurotransmitters. Neuropathic pain, and its modulation, can occur at different stages of pain transmission and be affected by different neurotransmitters. A process of trying several different medications, to a therapeutically effective dose, may be necessary before the one acting on the right pain pathway and neurotransmitters is discovered. Being appropriately informative about the complex nature of treating neuropathic pain may prevent an overly negative response to early treatment failure.

Side effect profiles can vary between these medications. While sedation, orthostatic hypotension, ataxia, and other side effects can occur with all tricyclics, the degree varies with each drug. Many providers use amitriptylline

(Elavil) as the first line tricyclic. It is well known and low in cost. However, desipramine (Norpramin) and nortriptyline (Pamelor) both have better side effect profiles, especially for the elderly or cognitively impaired. Most tricyclics should be given at bedtime due to sedative effects. Some of the newer anticonvulsant medications, such as gabapentin (Neurontin) and lamotrigine (Lamictal) (McCleane 2000), seem to be more effective for neuropathic pain, with better side effect profiles.

In certain types of complex or persistent pain syndromes, nonpharmacologic or more invasive treatments might be beneficial. TENS, acupuncture, and surgical or chemical nerve blockade should all be possible options for comprehensive pain management.

EMOTIONAL DISTRESS

In general, emotional distress will improve or resolve with the achievement of good consistent pain control. Thus providers should not rush to place patients in pain on anxiolytic or antidepressant therapy. Emotional pain should be addressed by the interdisciplinary team. A small number of patients will experience anxiety, fear, or depression significant enough to affect quality of life and interfere with pain control. Such patients should receive complete assessments and a competent evaluation of the appropriate short- or long-term use of medication to treat these symptoms. Medications with a shorter half-life and appropriate side effect profiles should be used.

DOSAGE AND ADMINISTRATION OF OPIOIDS

A lack of provider education is responsible for a significant degree of poor outcomes associated with opioid therapy. An improved understanding of the properties and proper usage of these medications will enable greater treatment success and improved education for patients and families.

Short- versus Long-Acting Preparation

Opioid analgesics are generally short acting with effects that last no more than four hours. Long-acting preparations do not change the properties of the drug. Instead they are designed to release the drug into the system incrementally over an extended period of time. This is the reason why most long-acting preparations cannot be crushed.

Short-acting preparations are easy to titrate for initial therapy and increasing disease. Breakthrough and episodic pain is most effectively treated with short-acting medications. Long-term treatment of baseline pain with short-acting drugs places an unnecessary medication burden on patients and families. The more significant fluctuations in medication levels with more frequent dosing may also exacerbate the potential for side effects.

Long-acting medications are a little more difficult to titrate rapidly for initial or increasing symptoms. However, the decreased burdens associated with fewer scheduled doses and steadier blood levels are important for long-term pain management. Therefore most patients require a combination of long-acting medication for control of baseline pain, with an available short-acting agent for breakthrough and titration with progressing symptoms. It is generally best when the short- and long-acting agents are different forms of the same drug. This eliminates the often-difficult question of "which drug?" when adverse or unexpected responses are obtained. Figure 12–8 lists some of the more commonly used forms of the step III opioids.

Drug	Long acting	Short acting
Morphine	MS Contin, Oramorph SR	Morphine sulfate, MSIR, Roxanol
Oxycodone	OxyContin	Ozycodone, OxyFast, OxyIR, Roxicodone
Fentanyl	Duragesic	Acting
Hydromorphone	Several pending FDA approval	Dilaudid

Figure 12–8 Commonly used short- and long-acting opioids

Titration

Titration is the management of opioid medication to maintain optimum pain control in the presence of advanced disease. It presumes a framework of continuing reassessment for adequacy of pain control and indications of new or recurrent symptoms.

The frequency of adjustment of a pain regimen should be based on the severity of active symptoms and the properties of the medications being used. A medication with a fairly short duration of effect, such as four hours, can be titrated fairly frequently, every 12 to 24 hours. A 12-hour controlled release medication requires a little more time between dosage increases, 24 to 48 hours. The time between dose increases is necessary to allow the medication level to approach a steady state at the new dosage. The effectiveness of a new level of medication cannot be assessed based on the response to the first dose. This does not mean that a patient should be left in pain while the baseline medication is adjusted. Breakthrough medication should be available to control pain until the new dosage becomes effective or can be increased again. Parenteral infusions can be titrated quite frequently, every 30 to 60 minutes, since absorption is not an issue and steady levels are quickly reached.

The amount of dosage increase can be calculated using two methods (McCaffery and Pasero 1999). The most common is fairly simple and dependent on the degree of continuing symptoms.

- If pain is mostly controlled, but a small increase is needed, increase the baseline dose by 25%.
- If there is a need for a moderate improvement in effect, increase the dose by 50%.
- If pain is severe and a significant effect is needed, increase the dose by 100%.

If the provider is uncertain about how much of an increase is necessary, reviewing the amount of breakthrough medication being used will provide the information necessary to use the alternative method. First confirm that the patient is taking all doses of the scheduled baseline medication. Baseline pain medication should not be increased because of failure to comply with dosage schedules. Calculate the amount of breakthrough medication the patient has taken in 24 hours. A variety of pain logs and flowsheets has been developed to assist patients and families in tracking this information. Add the amount of breakthrough medication used to the total daily dose provided by the scheduled baseline medication. Divide the new total by the frequency for the baseline medication to arrive at the new dosage. A maximum increase of 100% of the previous dose should be used at each titration.

For example, a patient with lung cancer is taking OxyContin 80 mg q12h. On reassessment, the pain logs show that for the last two days he has scaled his pain at 3–6 out of 10. He has also taken an average of 60 mg of OxyIR for breakthrough each day. The provider can simply increase his baseline pain control to OxyContin 120 mg q12h based on the pain scales indicating a moderate amount of continuing pain, and therefore the need for a 50% increase. Alternatively, the 60 mg of breakthrough medication can be added to the 160 mg total daily dose of OxyContin to achieve a new total of 220 mg/day. When divided into two 12-hour doses, a new baseline dose of 110 mg q12h is indicated. Since the medication comes in 20, 40, 80, and 160 mg tablets, the closest appropriate order would be 120 mg q12h.

If the new dose is still insufficient, breakthrough medication will continue to be available until the medication can be titrated again. If the pain remains severe, pain may need to be controlled using a method that can be quickly titrated, such as continuous infusion. The patient can be switched back to oral medication once control is achieved.

Breakthrough and Episodic Pain

Short-acting medications with rapid onset should be used to treat breakthrough or episodic pain. Several formulas have been developed for calculating breakthrough, or rescue, doses for patients on opioid therapy. The most current formula is 1/10 to 1/6 (10% to 15%) of the total daily dose (McCaffery and Pasero 1999). Rescue doses can be given as often as q2–4h., in severe pain q1–2h is acceptable. If a patient requires frequent rescue doses in order to be comfortable, the baseline pain control is probably inadequate. More than three to four rescue doses for several days should trigger a reassessment of the long-acting dosage. When the baseline pain control is increased, the rescue doses should be increased accordingly.

Since episodic or incident pain is predictable, it should be pretreated in order to prevent unnecessary pain. The usual dose is the same as the breakthrough or rescue dose. The medication should be administered at a time appropriate to provide relief when the care or activity is going to occur. This should generally be between the onset of action and the peak effect of the medication. For example, if short-acting morphine has a 15-minute onset of action and 1-hour peak effect, it should be given 30 to 45 minutes prior to the anticipated dressing change or activity.

Stopping or Decreasing Opioids

Opioid pain management should only be reduced or discontinued if the underlying cause of the pain has been effectively treated or if clinically significant adverse effects continue after appropriate time for adjustment and treatment. Patients who have been on step III therapy for greater than three days must have the medication tapered down to prevent occurrence of physical withdrawal. Physical dependence, not addiction, is the basis for this requirement. This situation is similar to the need to taper corticosteroids after sustained therapy. Opioid regimens at step III will need to be reduced at a rate of 25% to 50% per day (Levy 1996). Step II level use does not require tapering.

For example, a patient with end-stage AIDS had been taking 560 mg of OxyContin q12h for several months, resulting in very stable pain control and fairly good quality of life. The disease took a sudden and severe decline, and he became completely unresponsive in a relatively short period of time. Since he was unable to swallow and showed no indication of discomfort, the nurses simply withheld his OxyContin. The hospice nurse who visited him 36 hours later observed that while he remained unresponsive, he was also diaphoretic and tremulous. The patient was experiencing physical withdrawal. After consultation with the physician, a tapered regimen of rectal OxyContin was administered for the remaining 48 hours of his life. The symptoms subsided quickly after restarting the medication.

INAPPROPRIATE MEDICATIONS

Medications used to control pain in advanced and chronic illness should be the most effective drug with the least potential for untoward effects. A number of drugs that have been, or currently are, being used for pain management have known properties that should exclude them from general use.

Perhaps the most problematic of these medications, because of its wide use in long-term care, is propoxyphene. As a combination agent in Darvocet and other preparations, propoxyphene has been widely used as a step II pain reliever. This drug has a long half-life and a toxic metabolite, norpropoxyphene. The side effect profile of this drug includes sedation, confusion, and dystonia, making it particularly inappropriate for use in the elderly. The drug can precipitate seizures and biliary spasm. It also carries a warning against use in addiction prone patients.

Meperidine (Demerol) is also a poor candidate for ongoing pain control. The buildup of the CNS toxic metabolite normeperidine, short duration of action, and extremely poor oral bioavailability are all well documented. These properties create a high potential for side effects combined with a less-effective therapeutic performance in comparison to other opioids. Additionally, meperidine has an increased occurrence of GI side effects, compared with other available opioids. This may have contributed to a higher expectation of GI side effects from both providers and patients, when using opioids in general.

Methadone can be a very effective pain management medication. Some pain management providers use it regularly with excellent outcomes. It has a long half-life and a number of active metabolites. This can lead to very complex titration and management of the regimen. In general, only providers who are familiar with the complex pharmacokinetics of methadone should use this drug for routine pain management. Patients who are receiving methadone as treatment for addictive disease should be maintained on that treatment at the normal dose (McCaffery and Pasero 1999) and have their pain management provided using the medications and doses used for any other patient.

Opioid agonist-antagonist agents, simultaneously promote analgesia at some opioid receptors while reversing that effect at other sites. These drugs, such as nalbuphine (Nubain) and butorphanol (Stadol), were widely used in acute care in the 1970s and 1980s in a misguided effort to address beliefs about addiction and opioid pain management. These drugs have no place in current pain management practice.

REASSESSMENT

Reassessment is a continuous process. Algorithms that have been written for controlling pain in chronic and advanced disease never have an ending point. When pain is controlled or a symptom is successfully treated, the provider does not stop providing pain and symptom control; reassessment continues. Palliative care patients will always have the potential for new, recurrent or increasing symptoms.

Efforts to specify timeframes for reassessment of pain in institutional policy are limited in success. The frequency and depth of reassessment is a professional judgment, based on the severity and frequency of an individual's symptoms. Patients with active symptoms should be assessed with greater frequency. When pain control is achieved, reassessment can decrease in frequency, but not stop.

Team members cannot assume that today's "pain" is the same pain as previously reported without doing a complete assessment. Providers have overlooked acute illness and advancing disease that unnecessarily led to premature loss of quality of life and death by failing to properly evaluate new and continuing symptoms. At intervals, a complete comprehensive reassessment of the entire patient and family should be undertaken. This can identify changes in pain presentation, tolerance, support systems, coping strategies, and a variety of other factors.

Pain Management in the Elderly

The basic principles of pain management do not change when working with elderly patients. However, certain factors in developing a safe, effective treatment plan deserve greater consideration when treating older individuals. The presence of and potential for additional disease process and related medications can complicate care. Actual and potential cognitive impairment can create medication problems and an increased sensitivity to certain side effects. Age-related changes in the body's processing of some drugs require consideration when adjusting pain medication.

Particularly in the older elderly (above 75), renal and hepatic function may decline, even without the presence of significant end-organ disease. This will influence the metabolism and elimination of many medications. Decreases in lean body mass may influence medications differently. If the medication is lipid-soluble (fentanyl), it may have a slightly delayed onset and increased potential for accumulation. If it is water-soluble (hydromorphone, morphine), the opposite might occur. Decreased gastric motility seems to delay absorption of NSAIDs and may add to the GI side effects of those drugs.

In general, the best observation for pain management in the elderly is, "start low and go slow." In choosing between a range of options, take the more conservative choice. To titrate controlled release opioids, increase doses every 48 hours, instead of 24. Start medications at the lowest appropriate dose for the medication and step. If calculation of an increased dosage is between two available strengths, choose the lower dose.

When choosing between different medications in a category, consider side effect profiles in terms of the increased potential for detrimental effects on the elderly. Confusion, sedation, ataxia, hypotension, and anorexia should all be minimized to prevent adverse outcomes.

With appropriate education and support, older adults can fully participate in development and implementation of a pain management plan. Caregivers, both institutional and family, sometimes demonstrate a tendency to disempower the elderly by taking the "burden" of decision-making out of their hands. The provider has an obligation to ascertain the patient's goals and information needs to the extent appropriate for that person.

PAIN MANAGEMENT IN CHILDREN

Children are not simply small adults. Using appropriate medications and dosages requires training and guided experience. Involving children in their treatment plan requires an ability to assess developmental abilities while creating a trusting relationship. Parents and other caregivers will need support and thoughtful education while coping with advanced disease in their children. Palliative care of infants and children should be undertaken with care and appropriate training and resources.

At the same time, children are the subjects of additional misconceptions that create barriers to pain control. Belief that infants have a decreased sensitivity to pain and assumptions that they will not remember the pain experience have been thoroughly refuted (Taddio, et al. 1997). Pediatric practitioners have as much need for improved education in pain management as any other provider.

Children with advanced disease should have access to appropriately trained providers. Either palliative care specialists with training and experience in working with children, or pediatric providers with additional training in pain management and palliative care can be useful. Hospice or palliative care teams that admit and care for children have the responsibility to provide adequate clinical resources and training to all staff members.

SYMPTOM MANAGEMENT

The appropriate management of symptoms is dependent upon a complete assessment. Symptoms that arise as side effects of medications or treatment will likely be treated differently from those that arise from the disease process. Symptoms that result from advancing disease may have multiple etiologies and therefore different responses. Shortness of breath, experienced by a person with advanced lung cancer, may result from tumor invasion, pleural effusion, or excessive respiratory secretions. The response of the practitioner might be different in each of these situations.

Additional medical and psychosocial history should be considered. A history of difficulty with urination, due to prostate or other disease, should caution the provider to consider carefully the use of anticholinergic agents. Clear indication of fear of morphine or opioids in general will require a significant educational intervention or a different plan of care. A proper assessment of the entire patient-family unit is crucial in developing an appropriate plan of care.

Many hospices place "emergency kits" in patient's homes at some point in care. These kits contain the most commonly used medications that the hospice and its physicians use for emerging and urgent symptoms (Figure 12–9). They generally contain only a few doses of a particular drug. When symptoms are likely to reoccur, an appropriate assessment, continuing orders, and additional supplies are obtained. Use of these kits, along with procedures for standing or emergency orders, vary from state to state. Providers using this type of anticipatory supply must make certain they are in compliance with all legal and regulatory requirements.

The common use of a medication by a palliative care program does not excuse the provider from making a complete assessment of its appropriateness in a given situation. A lung cancer patient may experience dyspnea due to tumor or other obstruction, without excess secretions. Use of hyoscyamine (Levsin) for dyspnea under these circumstances is unlikely to improve the

Medication	Uses
Morphine—oral, sublingual, or suppository	Pain
	Dyspnea
(Oxycodone less common)	
Lorazepam (Ativan)—oral, sublingual, or suppository	Seizures
	Anxiety
(Valium much less common)	Muscle spasm
	Agitation
Hysocyamine (Levsin)—oral, sublingual or	Excess secretions
	Dyspnea
Scopolamine—TD patch or gel	Secondary use for nausea and vomiting when GI obstruction is possible
Haloperidol—oral, suppository	Agitation
	Nausea and vomiting
ABHR—suppository or troche	Nausea and vomiting
(Compounded Ativan, Benedryl, Haldol, and Reglan)	
Prochlorperazine (Compazine)	Nausea and vomiting
Phenytoin (Dilantin)	Seizures

Figure 12–9 Medications frequently found in "emergency kits"

symptoms and may create new ones. Oral or nebulized morphine is more likely to control the immediate symptom while a long-term approach is considered. In another case, profound dyspnea in the presence of significant secretions is unlikely to improve with the use of bronchodilators alone. Hyoscyamine (Levsin) or another agent will be needed to address the excess secretions.

In general, the approach to symptom control should be summarized as: Use the lowest effective level of treatment, via the least invasive method, while minimizing the potential for creating additional problems. Such an outcome is, of course, ideal and sometimes not possible. The entire team must focus on providing effective treatment without adding unnecessarily to the burdens of advanced disease.

RESPIRATORY SYMPTOMS

Dyspnea

This is perhaps the most distressing symptom regularly experienced by patients and caregivers. Its prevalence is estimated at 25% to 70% (Billings 1985). It has a wide-ranging and somewhat subjective definition. Profound shortness of breath, air hunger, and "an uncomfortable awareness of breathing" (Bruera, et al. 1993) have all been used to describe this condition. The need for air is so basic that the experience, or even anticipation, of dyspnea is likely to have a significant impact on the physical and emotional resources of patient and family.

Anticipation of and readiness for the occurrence of dyspnea is important in providing care to patients at risk. The associated fear and anxiety can exacerbate the symptoms if they are not controlled early. Figure 12–10 summarizes various causes of dyspnea in advanced disease (Ahmedzai 1998). The most likely presentation at assessment and most commonly used treatment strategies differ somewhat for each etiology. As with pain, the potential for multiple causative factors or, conversely, the inability to identify a cause is a reality of treating dyspnea. Relief of the symptom is the primary responsibility of the provider. In the presence of acute symptoms or the inability to identify a specific cause, morphine is an appropriate first-line treatment.

Oral versus nebulized morphine remains an area of contention in palliative care. While review of the literature shows increasing use and perceived benefits of nebulized morphine (Fancombe, Chater, and Gillin 1994), there are several areas of continuing discussion. Some experts report that oral morphine is sufficiently effective to make nebulized administration with its additional equipment and teaching needs unnecessary. Others report a greater effect on respiratory symptoms, with decreased systemic effects, when the medication is provided in nebulized form. In light of the significant impact of anxiety and emotional distress on the presentation and resolution of dyspnea, the most successful treatment is likely to be the one that meets the patient's perception of ease of use, availability, and effectiveness.

	Assessment	Treatment
Tumor or other obstruction	Breathlessness Areas of decreased areation on ascultation. May have localized rhonchi if fluid or secretions are trapped by obstruction Cough (+/−)	Oral or nebulized morphine Nebulized bronchodilators or steroids Positioning If advancing tumor is suspected, radiation or chemotherapy may be appropriate
Excess secretions	Congested sensation Audible secretions in upper airway and bronchii on ascultation. Productive cough	Positioning: side-lying with elevated head of bed or semi-prone Anticholinergic such as: Scopolamine (Scop TD) Hyosciamine (Levsin) Atropine
Cardiac failure	Progressive dyspnea Rales on ascultation Jugular vein distension (+/−)	Diuretics Morphine Intropic agents Activity and diet considerations as appropriate for quality of life
Chronic obstructive pulmonary disease (COPD)	Wheezing, rhonchi on ascultation Persistent cough Chronic shortness of breath	Nebulized bronchodilators Steroids Morphine
Pleural effusion	Distant or absent breath sounds in lower fields, most often unilateral Progressive shortness of breath	Positioning: elevate head of bed Morphine Thoracentesis, with or without sclerosing therapy if appropriate for quality of life
Pneumonia	Fever Productive cough Rhonchi or consolidation on ascultation	Acetaminophen or ibuprofen for fever Positioning and anticholinergics to control secretions Antibiotic therapy if desired for quality of life
Superior vena cava (SVC) syndrome	Acute shortness of breath Jugular vein distension Swelling of neck and face	Emergency radiation therapy High dose steroids Morphine
Treatment related pneumonitis	Increasing chronic shortness of breath Cough	Morphine Nebulized bronchodilators Steroids

Figure 12–10 Causes and treatment of dyspnea

Nebulized morphine should be started at 2.5 to 5 mg in 3 cc of normal saline q4h. The dose can be titrated up in 5 mg increments until 4 hours of relief is provided. Fast-acting morphine can be given orally for dyspnea. If the patient is not on opioids for pain, a starting dose of 5–10 mg q3–4h should be tried. If the patient is already taking opioids, the usual breakthrough dose should be given, followed by a 25% to 50% increase in baseline medication if effective for controlling dyspnea.

Bronchodilatora and steroids have known side effects. The patient's ability to tolerate the most common effects should be considered before these medications are started. Anxiolytics may also be useful.

The use of oxygen for treatment of dyspnea is controversial for some providers. Some question its therapeutic value without documentation of decreased saturation. Others provide oxygen to all patients with respiratory symptoms based on some combination of therapeutic and emotional effect. Generally, if oxygen is readily available and the patient reports the perception of increased comfort as a result of using it, it should be offered when symptoms are active. The least obtrusive delivery method is via nasal cannula. If the patient is reliant on the availability of oxygen for comfort, efforts must be made to ensure that a supply remains available. An empty tank or nonworking concentrator can cause serious anxiety and severely exacerbated symptoms.

Excess Secretions

As patients approach the final terminal stage, commonly referred to as active dying, they may develop excess secretions in upper airways, trachea, and bronchi. Conditions that will increase the risk of this symptom include lung or head and neck tumors, pneumonia, heart failure, renal failure, and the presence of intravenous hydration.

Patients generally experience a decreasing ability to clear such secretions independently. This symptom may appear in a variety of presentations ranging from a persistent cough to noisy respirations accompanied by some degree of dyspnea. Excess secretions are also responsible for the phenomenon known as the death rattle. This is a particularly unpleasant sound caused by trapped secretions in the upper airway.

The initial response to this symptom is to reposition the patient. Repositioning should be done in a calm and reasonable manner, considering patient and family issues. Side-lying with the head elevated and the semi-prone "coma" position are most likely to reduce the immediate effects of excess secretions. Reduction of the secretions can then be addressed, usually with an anticholinergic agent. Hyoscyamine (Levsin) is frequently used because of its ease of administration (sublingual tablets and liquid), effectiveness, and low cost. Transdermal scopolamine is also used, though it is more costly. The increased sedative effect of scopolamine, in comparison to hyoscyamine, needs to be considered. Sedation may be a desirable effect in some cases and a major issue in others. Atropine injections, which have been used in some settings, are not recommended since the availability of the previously noted medications should make repeated injections unnecessary. If the patient is receiving intravenous hydration, it should be significantly decreased or discontinued in the presence of this symptom.

Use of anticholinergic agents will frequently lead to dry mouth. Regular mouth care will readily overcome any discomfort from this symptom. Constipation and difficulty with urination may also occur. Hyoscyamine can sometimes cause CNS excitation, especially in the elderly. This can be addressed by switching to scopolamine.

Cough

Persistent uncomfortable cough may be caused by respiratory distress, increased secretions, or respiratory infection. Treatment of these underlying conditions is discussed above. Cough may also be caused by allergies, smoking, medications, bronchitis, or an irritable diaphragm. Generic treatment of such cough can be provided with the expectorant guaifenessin, either alone in high dose form (Humibid LA) or with codeine for suppression (Robitussin AC). Phenergan in various combinations or benzonatate (Tessalon) may also be useful.

Hiccough

Intractable or persistent intermittent hiccoughs are generally caused by irritation of the diaphragm due to gastrointestinal disease, nerve damage, or other neurologic disorders. The drug of choice is chlorpromazine (Thorazine). If this drug is ineffective or too sedating, metoclopramide (Reglan), prednisone, and various benzodiazepines are all possible alternatives.

Altered Respiratory Patterns

Altered respiratory patterns generally occur when patients are actively dying. The most common altered patterns are Cheyne-Stokes respirations and apnea. Cheyne-Stokes respiration is characterized by a pattern of fast, then slowing respirations, usually ending in a pause or apneic period. The cycle then repeats. These patterns have a large degree of variability. Apnea may present with or without Cheyne-Stokes respirations.

These symptoms are far more likely to cause distress to caregivers, family, and friends than to the patient. In general, these symptoms occur when the respiratory centers of the brain become insensitive to changes in CO_2. This "insensitivity" creates a condition in which the patient rarely has any awareness of the respiratory changes, but the surrounding family may become acutely uncomfortable. Education and emotional support is the most effective response to family concerns. Direct intervention is only needed when other symptoms, such as acute dyspnea or excess secretions, occur in combination with these altered patterns.

GASTROINTESTINAL SYMPTOMS

Nausea and Vomiting

The potential sources for nausea in a patient with advanced disease are almost unlimited. Medications, end-organ failure, pain, emotional distress, decreased GI motility, bowel obstruction, tumor, metabolic disorders, diet, and increased intracranial pressure can all precipitate nausea and vomiting. After certain specific concerns have been addressed, general treatment of nausea is a matter of identifying the most effective antiemetic agent.

If medication side effects are suspected, a determination of the importance of the possibly offending medication needs to be made. The drug should be discontinued if it is optional or an alternative is available. If it is necessary for maintaining comfort, a decrease in dosage may be attempted. An antiemetic should only be added to medication regimen if no alteration in the use of the suspected medication is possible. The burden of multiple medications and potential effects of polypharmacy should be avoided when possible. Nausea and vomiting that is caused by chemotherapy is best treated with agents, such as ondansetron (Zofran), that were specifically intended for this purpose.

Partial or complete bowel obstruction may be caused by tumor or other factors. Delay in treatment will usually result in symptoms advancing to a severe degree. Reducing the pressure in the bowel is very important for controlling immediate symptoms. A combination of restricting intake and anticholinergic agents, to decrease motility and reduce secretions, may be effective. Decompression using a nasogastric tube may be necessary to achieve comfort. Surgical correction of a confirmed obstruction should be considered if life expectancy and quality of life are sufficient to justify the invasive nature of major surgery and its follow-up.

The most commonly used first line antiemetic is chlorpromazine (Compazine). It is available in oral, suppository, and injectable forms and is generally effective. Other commonly used antiemetics include trimethobenzamide (Tigan) and haloperidol (Haldol).

Many palliative care programs have developed their own recipes for compounded combinations to treat nausea and vomiting. These combinations are compounded as suppositories, troches, or other preparations. Most of these recipes include two to four of the following medications. Traditionally these combinations have been referred to by the first letters of their trade names.

- (A) Lorazepam (Ativan)—anxiolytic, muscle relaxant
- (B) Diphenhydramine (Benadryl)—antihistamine
- (H) Haloperidol (Haldol)—antiemetic
- (R) Metoclopramide (Reglan)—cholinergic agent (increases GI motility)
- (D) Dexamethasone (Decadron)—steroid

The different combinations may be created for specific situations or simply provider preference. Metoclopramide should be removed from any combination when increasing GI motility is likely to exacerbate symptoms (i.e. possible obstruction). Dexamethasone usually replaces metoclopramide under these circumstances.

The concept of bowel rest is not easy for families focused on nurturing (feeding) a patient with advanced disease. However, even a few hours of restricted intake can allow for significantly better response to efforts to control nausea and vomiting.

Constipation

Constipation is a frequent issue for patients with end-stage disease. The largest cause of this by far is opioid or other medication-induced symptoms. Tumors, neurologic abnormalities, and alteration in food and fluid intake can also cause constipation. Treatment is done by either increasing bowel motility (laxatives or stimulants), softening the stool to facilitate its movement through the bowel, or both.

Most palliative care programs develop "stepped" bowel regimens to be used routinely. These usually start with a combination medication such as Senokot S for daily use. If regular bowel movements do not result, this medication may be increased or the bowel regimen can step up to stronger agents such bisacodyl (Ducolax), lactulose (Chronulac), milk of magnesia, or magnesium citrate. Fleets or other enemas, glycerin suppositories, and manual disimpaction may be necessary to remove hardened stool. Untreated constipation can advance through impaction to bowel obstruction.

Anorexia

Anorexia or loss of appetite can have a variety of causes in end-stage disease. Dysphagia, fatigue, stomatitis, tumor, AIDS wasting syndrome, and medication effects may all be relevant issues. Efforts should first be made to address factors such as fatigue or mobility issues. Identifying community resources to assist with shopping and meal preparation will occasionally address this symptom. Identifying changing diet preferences, offering smaller and more frequent meals, and reducing the focus on eating may also be beneficial.

Treating stomatitis, dysphagia, and other mechanical issues should be addressed if these conditions are identified. The generic treatment of anorexia starts with megestrol acetate (Megace), which has been found to be effective for both cancer and HIV disease. Alternative therapies include prednisone and dronabinol (Marinol).

Diarrhea

Diarrhea can result from medication effects, food intolerance, impaction, and disease process. Kaopectate or loperamide (Immodium) given after each loose stool will generally control most incidents of diarrhea. More persistent cases may require diphenoxylate/atropine (Lomotil). Profound diarrhea related to the disease process, such as HIV-related infections, may require the use of injectable octreotide (Somatostatin).

NEUROLOGICAL SYMPTOMS

Seizures
The most common causes of seizures in advanced disease are brain tumor, metabolic abnormalities, and medication-related effects (Waller and Caroline 1996). Less common causes include fever or sepsis, hypoglycemia, and hypoxemia. Since the incidence of seizures is very small, prophylaxis is not indicated. However, many hospices choose to have appropriate medications available for treatment of potential seizures in patients with brain tumors or seizure histories.

Seizures are very distressing to families, and anticipation of seizures can cause emotional distress for the patient. Assurance that the needed medication is available, clearly understandable instructions, and dependable team response will enable caregivers to successfully cope with a difficult situation.

Actively occurring seizures should be treated with fast-acting medications, usually rectal or injectable lorazepam (Ativan). If the seizure ends before administration, do not give the medication. If the seizures persist, additional benzodiazapine doses may be necessary. Continuous seizures—status epilepticus—should be treated with midazolam (Versed) or phenobarbital infusion. If the cause of the seizures cannot be identified and corrected reliably, phenytoin (Dilantin) or other anticonvulsant medication should be started for prophylaxis.

Restlessness and Agitation
Restlessness and agitation are different degrees of a spectrum of ill-defined behaviors that indicate distress or discomfort. The possible sources of this distress are myriad. Terminal agitation is associated with the last stages of life. Both cause and an effective treatment that does not completely sedate the individual may be very difficult to identify.

Medication-related effects should be considered and adjusted. Possible metabolic abnormalities can be assessed and treated. If the patient is able to communicate, issues of emotional and spiritual distress should be explored. The possibility of uncommunicated physical pain should never be overlooked.

If a cause cannot be identified, agitation should be treated empirically. Medications with a shorter half-life are preferred. Therefore lorazepam (Ativan) is usually the first-line drug. Some patients may be more responsive to Haloperidol (Haldol). Dosage and frequency can generally be increased to control the symptoms. Occasionally, the presence of severe nonresponsive agitation may require sedation with a continuous infusion of one or more agents. Palliative sedation should be fully discussed with the involved family members and supervised by an experienced practitioner.

SEDATION

Sedation may be opioid induced, or caused by other medications or by disease process. The most common factor is disease process. However, most families will focus on medication issues rather than assume advancing disease. Opioid-related sedation is transient and will generally subside after three to five days of regular scheduled use. Occasionally if sedation persists, reducing the opioid dose by 25% may be effective. Sometimes the opioid dose cannot be decreased because of pain control needs or because the causative factor is disease process. Under those circumstances, and if sedation is interfering with quality of life, a trial of methylphenidate (Ritalin) may demonstrate some improvement. If effective, the medication can be continued.

The palliative care team must be prepared to support patients and families coping with sedation due to end-stage disease or medication required to treat otherwise overwhelming symptoms.

FATIGUE

Anemia, medication, decreased intake, emotional distress, infection, and disease process can all contribute to the experience of profound fatigue, which significantly interferes with function and quality of life. Anemia should be treated by correcting the cause and the use of erythropoietin. Medication that can cause fatigue should be reevaluated for alternative agents and benefit-burden analysis.

Teaching energy conservation strategies and identification of available resources are interventions that can be utilized by team members. Infection, sleep problems, and emotional concerns should be explored. The patient and family may require assistance in adapting to the persistent fatigue associated with some disease entities, such as end-stage AIDS.

SKIN INTEGRITY

Creating a treatment plan for maintaining skin integrity and treating wounds in the framework of palliative care requires an evaluation of goals for the individual patient. Decreased nutritional intake, decreased mobility, loss of body mass, medication effects, and a wide variety of additional issues all contribute to the potential for loss of skin integrity and decreased potential for healing. The occurrence of bed sores may be emotionally distressing to some patients and families. The degree to which a patient may be willing to tolerate aggressive wound care, repositioning, and nutritional support will be heavily related to perceived quality of life.

Cachexia or wasting syndromes can result in significant discomfort even without any breakdown. Appropriate pressure relief and positioning devices should be available simply for patient comfort. When a pressure area or wound develops, discomfort and distress is likely to increase. A treatment plan should be initiated with the intent of preventing additional breakdown and relieving discomfort related to loss of skin integrity. Discomfort can be relieved by treating wound-related pain, choosing wound treatments that require less frequent dressing changes, and gentle positioning as tolerated. Treatment with the long-term intent to heal wounds should continue. The level of aggressiveness of such treatments should be guided by the patient's desires and condition.

REFERENCES

Agency for Health Care Policy and Research (AHCPR). (1994). *Clinical practice guidelines: Management of cancer pain.* (DHHS Publication No. AHCPR 94-0592). Rockville, MD. Agency for Health Care Policy and Research, U.S. Department of Health and Human Services, Public Health Service.

Ahmedzai, S. (1998). Palliation of respiratory symptoms. In D. Doyle, G. W. C. Hanks, & N. MacDonald (Eds.), *Textbook of palliative medicine* (2nd ed., pages 586–602.) New York: Oxford University Press.

Billings, J. A. (1985). *The management of common symptoms, outpatient management of advanced cancer.* New York: Lippincott.

Bookbinder, M., Coyle, N., Kiss, M., Goldstein, M. L., Holritz, K., Thaler, H., Gianella, A., Derby, S., Brown, M., Racolin, A., Ho, M. N., & Portenoy, R. K. (1996). Implementing national standards for cancer pain management: Program model and evaluation. *Journal of Pain and Symptom Management, 12,* 334–347.

Bruera E., MacEachern, T., Ripamonti, C., & Hansen, J. (1993). Subcutaneous morphine for dyspnea in cancer patients. *Annals of Internal Medicine,* 119: 906–907.

Cleeland, C. S., Gonin, R., Hatfield, A., Edmonson, J. H., Blum, R. H., Stewart, J. A., & Pandya K. J. (1994). Pain and its treatment in outpatients with metastatic cancer. *New England Journal of Medicine,* 330: 592–596.

Fancombe, M., Chater, S., & Gillin, A. (1994). The use of nebulized opioids for breathlessness: A chart review. *Palliative Medicine,* 8: 306–312.

Federation of State Medical Boards (1998, May). *Model guidelines for the use of controlled substances for the treatment of pain.* A policy document.

Foley, K. (1998). Pain assessment and cancer pain syndromes. In D. Doyle, G. W. C. Hanks, N. MacDonald (Eds), *Oxford textbook of palliative medicine* (2nd ed. page 313.) New York: Oxford University Press.

Friedman, D. P. (1990). Perspectives on the medical use of drugs of abuse. *Journal of Pain and Symptom Management*, S2–S5.

Grond, S., Zech, D., Diefenbach, C., Ralbruch, L., & Lehmann, K. (1996). Assessment of cancer pain: A prospective evaluation of 2,256 cancer patients referred to a pain service. *Pain*, 64: 107–114.

Levy, M. H. (1996). Pharmacologic treatment of cancer pain. *New England Journal of Medicine*, 335: 1124–1132.

McCaffery, M. (1968). *Nursing practice theories related to cognition, bodily pain and man-environment interactions.* Los Angeles: UCLA.

McCaffery, M., & Ferrell, B. R. (1997). Nurses knowledge of pain assessment and management: How much progress have we made? *Journal of Pain and Symptom Management*, 14: 175–188.

McCaffery, M., & Pasero, C. (1999). *Pain: Clinical manual* (2nd Edition). St. Louis, MO: Mosby, Inc.

McCleane, G. J. (2000). The symptoms of complex regional pain syndrome; Type 1 alleviated with lamtrigine: A report of 8 cases. *Journal of Pain*, 1: 171–173.

Merskey, E. V., & Bogduk, N. (Eds.). (1994). *Classification of chronic pain: Descriptions of chronic pain syndromes and definitions.* Seattle, WA: International Association for the Study of Pain Press.

The SUPPORT Principle Investigators. (1995). A controlled trial to improve care for seriously ill hospitalized patients. The study to understand prognosis and preferences for outcomes and risks of treatments (SUPPORT). *Journal of American Medical Association*, 274: 1591–1598.

Taddio, A., Katz, I., Ilersich, A. L., & Koren, G. (1997). Neonatal circumcision and pain response during routine vaccination 4 to 6 months later. *Lancet*, 349: 599–603.

Turk, D. C., & Okifiji, A. (1997). What factors affect physicians' decision to prescribe opioids for chronic non-cancer pain patients. *Clinical Journal of Pain*, 13: 330–336.

Uhl, G. R., Sora, I., & Wang, Z. (1999). The μ opiate receptor as a candidate gene for pain: Polymorphisms, variations in expression, nociception, and opiate responses. *Procedings of the National Academy of Sciences*, 96: 7752–7755.

Von Roenn, J. H., Cleeland, C. S., Gonin, R., Hatfield, A. K., & Pandya, D. J. (1993). Physician attitudes and practice in cancer pain management: A survey from the Eastern Cooperative Oncology Group. *Annals of Internal Medicine*, 119: 121–126.

Waller, A., & Caroline, N. (1996). *Handbook of palliative care in cancer.* Butterworth. *Heinmann Medical.* p. 255–257.

World Health Organization (1986). *Cancer Pain Relief.* Geneva, Switzerland: WHO.

Zech, D. F. J., Grond, S., Lynch, J., Hertel, D., & Lehmann, D. (1995). Validation of World Health Organization guidelines for cancer pain relief: A 10 year prospective study. *Pain*, 63: 65–76.

CHAPTER

ISSUES OF SUFFERING AT THE END OF LIFE

Phyllis Taylor

Mr. R called his physician and told him he was thinking of ending his life before the cancer did; he was fearful of dying in pain and of being a burden to his family. A lovely 61-year-old woman called her doctor to talk about dying because the quality of her life was so poor that death seemed preferable to life. Mr. T was convinced that his wife was having an affair after he found himself impotent due to his terminal illness. Mrs. H phoned to say that she and her elderly husband were running out of money because of large medical and drug bills, and that she had just taken an overdose of digoxin but was fearful of ending up in a persistent vegetative state. Mr. P, 77 and dying, said that he felt he was going to go to hell because he had never been baptized.

What do all these individuals have in common? All were terminally ill and all were experiencing suffering related to their illnesses and the impact the illnesses were having on them and their families. This is born out by the statistics coming from Oregon after the passage of the Death with Dignity Act in 1997, which show that the great majority of terminally ill patients' pain was well managed by doctors. In 1998, the first year that there were statistics on the result of the act, 23 terminally ill people received a prescription for lethal medications. Of those, 15 took their own lives, 6 died from their illnesses, and 2 were still alive as of January 1, 1999. What was so striking was that 79% were still ambulatory, 71% were enrolled in a hospice program, and inadequate pain control was mentioned by only 7%. Eighty percent of the individuals said their reason for taking the lethal dose was loss of autonomy secondary to their illness. Fifty-eight percent identified the inability to participate in favored activities as a factor. Fifty-three percent said that loss of bodily functions was intolerable. Thirteen percent said they felt that they were too much of a burden to their families. The median age was 69.

In 1999, there were 27 assisted deaths. The median age was 71. Twenty-one of the 27 patients were in hospice care, and all had health insurance. Seventeen of the 27 patients had cancer; the others had chronic lung disease, AIDS, or amyotrophic lateral sclerosis. In a survey of more than 2,600 Oregon physicians, 5% received a request for lethal prescriptions between November 1997 and February 24, 2000, and that only 1 in 10 requests resulted in a suicide (Associated Press 2000).

Just before Dr. Kevorkian was sentenced to prison, it was reported that he was receiving 1,000 requests per week for assisted dying. Almost all of those requests were because of poor management of physical pain. The contrast between the requests Dr. Kevorkian received and Oregon's experience, where most patients were well managed, highlights the need to address not just physical pain but also suffering at the end of life.

What is suffering? *Webster's New World Dictionary of the American Language* defines it as "the bearing of pain, distress, injury, grief." Dr. Eric J. Cassell (1991) states that suffering is "the state of severe distress associated with events that threaten the intactness of the person." In his books and articles, he has helped many readers understand that suffering is not confined to physical symptoms and that it is ultimately a personal matter. The presence and extent of the suffering can only be known to the sufferer. He also identified that another person's distress increases the suffering of the person who is sick.

When addressing the interface of physical pain and suffering, Cassell (1991) describes the close relationship between pain and suffering. He states that when the pain is overwhelming, there is suffering. When the patient does not believe the pain can be controlled, there is suffering. When the pain is endless, there is suffering, and when the pain is due to some frightening illness, there is suffering. Suffering can also come from a sense of the body being untrustworthy. Making future plans becomes difficult. If there is incontinence or an odorous wound, the humiliation from these can also cause suffering.

Younger (1995, 58), a nurse, wrote an essay on suffering where she describes the alienation that the sufferer feels as a sense of separation from self, others, and transcendent meaning: "Alienation is a sense of homelessness, a lover's quarrel with mankind." She also said, "The care of another redeems the despised self" (p. 67).

Referring to the care of the dying, Quill (1996, 148) said, "Suffering includes psychological, social, spiritual, and existential dimensions that are often intertwined and less amenable to simple interventions than the more physical aspects."

As those who journey with the dying and their families, we are given a unique opportunity to address issues of suffering and to help people find meaning in what they are going through. Some fundamental questions that come from suffering include:

1. Who was I before diagnosis? What did my life mean? Was I selfish? Giving? Did I care for myself? Others?
2. Who am I now that my body has changed? That my activity is less? That I am more dependent than independent?

3. Who will I become? Will I be a burden or blessing to my family and caregivers? Will I be loved or resented?
4. What do I need now? From whom? When?

Underlying all these questions is the fundamental one of whether I am still lovable or of worth to my family, friends, myself and, if spiritual or religious, to God or my Higher Power. In all of these questions, one is coping with multiple losses that have to be grieved.

Loved ones also suffer. Their questions include:

1. Can I provide the kind of care physically, emotionally, and spiritually that my loved one needs?
2. Am I selfish if I want my loved one to live or to die?
3. What do I need to get through this? From whom? When?

Let's look at the types of suffering and interventions that can help.

SPIRITUAL SUFFERING

The word "spiritual" comes from the Latin word *spiritus* which refers to breath, air, or wind. "Spirituality is the dimension of a person that involves one's relationship with self, others, the natural order, and a higher power manifested through creative expressions, familiar rituals, meaningful work, and religious practices. Spirituality involves finding deep meaning in everything including illness and death and living life according to a set of values" (Cohen 1993). "Examples of spiritual needs include hope, meaning in life, and forgiveness" (Wright 1998). Religion is an organized system of beliefs and identification with a religious community. One might not be part of a church, synagogue, mosque, or temple and still be very spiritual.

In working with people at the end of life, it is recommended that there be a dual assessment each time we encounter that person. One question is, "How are you doing in your body?" This lets us know if that person is having pain or other distressing symptoms from their illness, their treatments, or their medications. The other question is, "How are you doing in your spirit?"

In creating a spiritual assessment, Ferszt, Teegen-Case, and Taylor (1999) developed an assessment based on four areas of life. This assessment can be used by all who work with the dying and their families.

- **Connection.** Who are the persons or communities you look to for support? What role do they have in your care? Do you have an image of a power greater than yourself (God, Higher Power, Sacred Spirit)? Has your life situation now affected your feelings about yourself, your faith, or your relationships?
- **Meaning and Joy.** What has been most important in your life? What are you most thankful for? What makes or has made you happy? What do you feel the proudest of in your life?

- **Strength and Comfort.** Is there anything that is comforting to you now? What helped you get through difficult times in the past? Who or what is your source of strength now? Would you like to share any experiences that have shaped your life (or spiritual life), e.g., dreams, visions, turning points?
- **Hope and Concerns.** Is there anything that you hope for? Is there anything that feels unfinished? Is there anything you want? From whom? When?

These questions are meant to be a springboard to conversation. It is important to let the person guide you and to not overwhelm the patient or family with too many questions.

Rituals can be a powerful way of lessening spiritual pain for the patient and the family. Letting families have the option of participating in the care of the body after death can help in the mourning process. It becomes a time of anointing. One mother wanted to help with the preparation of her son's body while the family waited for their pastor to arrive. He was 42 years old and had died of cancer. He looked peaceful except for his eyes which remained open. After washing him tenderly, she showed me a trick for helping the eyes to stay shut. She said she learned this from the elders in her small Southern rural town where she grew up. She turned back her son's upper lid, placed a tiny piece of cotton on the lid and then flipped it back down. The slight pressure and absorptive quality of the cotton resulted in the eyes remaining shut. He then looked like he was asleep. Just after she finished this loving act, their pastor arrived and burst into tears. The family then comforted him. He explained that he had baptized the man as a baby, taught him in Sunday school, and was now having to bury him. The rituals of the care of the body, the comforting of the pastor, and then his comforting of the family helped lessen their suffering.

Another situation involved a Jewish patient. One day Mr. F expressed that he felt he wasn't going to make it. When asked what he still felt was undone, he replied that he had hoped to live for three more months so he could be at his beloved grandson's bar mitzvah. It was suggested that the bar mitzvah be held now in his hospital room. At first he said it couldn't be done, but he was helped to see that the essential parts of the bar mitzvah could be shared at that time. He said he would talk it over with his family. A few days later, in the privacy of his hospital room with his wife, son, daughter-in-law, and grandsons present, the bar mitzvah boy chanted his Torah portion. With the physical help of his son, the grandfather draped his tallis, or prayer shawl, around his shoulder and his grandson's shoulder so they were both covered with this holy material. He then blessed his grandson. That night, after everyone left, he signed his do not resuscitate form and died a few days later with his family by his bedside.

Another example of the importance of ritual to lessen spiritual suffering was taught to a nurse by a 77-year-old man who had no family. The nurse went in one day to assess the patient. When Mr. W was asked, "How are you doing in your body?" he replied he was weak but had no pain. When asked, "How are you doing in your spirit?" he said, "Bad." When asked "How bad?" he replied, "Never been baptized." When asked if he wanted to be baptized, he was delighted. The challenge came in finding a Baptist minister who would do the Baptism, since total body immersion was not possible medically. None could be found. Knowing death would come soon, I searched for any minister to perform the ceremony. One of the other nurses on the unit located her Mennonite pastor. He agreed to perform the service. The "congregation" was the staff on the unit where Mr. W had been over a period of months as his health steadily deteriorated. We sang, poured lots of water on him using a water pitcher, and prayed. The next day he was again assessed. He remained physically comfortable although weak. When asked about his spirit, he said he was better. Two days later he died comfortably in his body and his spirit.

A Muslim woman whose child died wanted the imam from her mosque to come from another city for a ritual washing. The body was taken from the morgue and the imam gently washed the child and prayed over him. He then wrapped him in white cloth. Only at that point was the young mother emotionally and spiritually ready to hold her child and begin the grieving process.

"Respect for human dignity has long been heralded as the overarching principle that should guide the relationship between professionals and the people who seek their services. However, the challenge of exactly how to effect this laudable goal is elusive, especially as professionals come into contact with an increasingly rich mix of people from all parts of the world who seem to differ significantly from the professionals themselves in their beliefs, habits, and lifestyles" (Mondragon 1997, vii). Knowing the diversity of religious and spiritual needs of those we serve can enrich our lives as we help lessen the spiritual suffering experienced by those at the end of life.

Rabbi Harold Kushner once said in addressing the Synagogue Council of America, "People who are hurting, people who see someone they love slipping away from them, want religion, not theology. They don't want to be told about God. They want to experience the care and presence of God in the incarnation of people who care for them."

SOCIAL SUFFERING

Social suffering also needs to be addressed at the end of life. Some situations that cause social suffering are when the person who is ill feels that he or she is a burden to their family, when there are role reversals, when parents watch their children die, when there are unresolved family conflicts, and when there are young children as survivors.

A woman shared that she felt profound sadness because she could no longer go to her church where she was active in the religious and social life of the congregation. She was told the story of a pastor who was diagnosed with amyotrophic lateral sclerosis. He knew enough about the disease to know that in a relatively short period of time, members of his church were going to have to cut his food for him, feed him, and toilet him. What a role reversal this was for a man whose life had been caring for others! However, he came to realize that he gained a great deal of joy when ministering to those in need. He began to understand that if he could learn to receive from others, he would awaken in them the joy he knew so well. By accepting care, he was still giving.

Another man who taught me about social suffering was 52 years old with a diagnosis of lung cancer. When I visited Mr. L in his room, he was staring at his hands. With great urgency he commanded me to look at his hands. I did, but saw nothing unusual. A quick assessment was done to determine cyanotic nail beds or clubbing, but neither was found. I asked him to explain what was wrong with his hands. He replied, "They're clean." He then shared that he had always worked with his hands. No matter how many times he washed them, he could never get all the grease off. His clean hands symbolized that he was no longer the money earner in the family. He had become a burden. He said he felt his wife would be better off if he died quickly so she could get on with her life. Family meetings with his wife began. Helping him feel he was still useful was essential to help lessen the social suffering he was feeling.

Another woman, who had recently transected her spinal cord, also said that she felt totally useless. She couldn't even walk now or help around the house. She was asked to teach the staff about her experience of what it was like to be dying so they could become better nurses and counselors. She responded by saying she would share what it was like to be dying and now a paraplegic. Not only did she teach the staff, but she was also a valuable resource for students. She now had a role that helped lessen her suffering.

One area of great social suffering is the dying of children, no matter what the age. A 70-year-old man who was diagnosed with metastatic cancer said that one area of great suffering for him was what to do with and for his 90-year-old mother. She had moved in with him 10 years earlier when she was widowed. He managed her shopping, and trips to the doctors and the senior citizens center. It was essential for him that there be a plan of care for her in order for him to have any acceptance of his own approaching death.

Another mother yelled at her son, "You are supposed to bury me and now I am going to have to bury you." They both began to cry. Her son, 24, was dying of HIV/AIDS. They both had to cope with the stigma of AIDS, his dying, and the age reversal of how dying ought to be. Talking, crying, and acknowledging the sadness and rage helped both of them during this terribly difficult time.

Situations of conflict in the family also result in social suffering. A woman with a history of alcoholism lay dying in a long-term care facility. All she talked about was her desire to see her two daughters who had not visited her after they admitted her to the home. That was three years ago. Both daughters were contacted; one refused to discuss the matter with the nurse. The other expressed anger at her mother and said she never wanted to see her again.

The nurse then asked if she could call her every few weeks to just give an update on her mother's condition. She did agree to this. As her mother's condition continued to deteriorate, the nurse offered to be with her if she ever did decide to visit. She continued to refuse until the final week of her mother's life. She made one visit, said it was a mistake to come, but then returned on the day the mother died. She ended up telling her comatose mother that she really did love her. There was some closure for both the mother and daughter. The woman's other daughter never did visit, and her suffering continued in the bereavement period in a way that was different than the daughter who visited.

When there are young children who will be survivors, there is also social suffering. We want to protect children from some of the harsh realities of life and yet death enters into their lives frequently. They suffer, and the dying person also suffers since he or she does not want to cause more harm than the illness already does.

What can we do? In the past, it has been found that children do well coping with the dying of an adult if they are included in the process rather than excluded from it. Their imagination is so expansive that what they think must be happening is different from the reality.

The following points are ones that have been found helpful:

- Distinguish "sick" from "sick." There is the "sick" where you get better, and there is the "sick" where you die.
- Explain what they will see if the person looks different from what they are used to.
- Do not pressure them to do anything they do not want to do.
- If the child is coming from a religious family background, talk about how the person will be with God, rather than God loving the person so much that God takes the person back.
- Reassure the child that she or he is not responsible for the illness.

For example, a woman was terminally ill with ovarian cancer. She really wanted to see her three-year-old granddaughter but was fearful the child would be afraid of her. She had lost her hair and had a nasogastric tube. The staff met with the little girl and her mother, the patient's daughter, and explained that grandma was still grandma but she had something in her nose to make her feel better. They did not talk about the grandmother being sick or about God at this first visit. There was a wonderful reunion of the child with her beloved grandmother. These visits spanned three weeks before the woman's death. The only difference the child's parents saw after these visits was that all figures in the child's drawings had nasogastric tubes, including animals. The nasogastric tubes staying in her drawings for two months after her grandmother's death. Both child and grandmother had very special times together.

Another situation involved five girls ranging in age from 6 to 12 years of age whose dad became suddenly ill. He was in the intensive care unit in a coma after complications from abdominal surgery. His young wife asked about bringing in the girls. It was suggested that she ask each child separately if she wanted to visit, so there was little peer pressure. All the children wanted to come. The staff met with them, their mother, and her mother. They were first asked to talk about all the times they had been sick. Each girl did so. The staff then helped them to distinguish the kinds of "sick" they described (such as headaches, stomachaches, colds, and earaches where they felt "yucky" for a short while but then got better) from the kind of "sick" where one dies. So often adults do not explain illness correctly. The children hear that grandpa was sick and he died and now they are sick. In their minds, many fear that they will now die.

The staff then told them that sometimes children feel they are responsible for what has happened. Often children believe that they are at fault because they have done things that are not generally approved of, such as lying, cheating, or fighting with friends or siblings, or heard an adult say, "You'll be the death of me yet," and then the person died. After reassuring them that they did not cause their father to be sick, the staff began to explain about what they would see when they went into the intensive care unit. Every piece of equipment was described to lessen their anxiety. They went in as a group. Three of the girls left after a few minutes with their grandmother and another nurse. Two wanted to stay and hold their dad's hands. No one was forced to do anything.

That night their father died. The staff met with the children, who attended a parochial school, and talked about how their father was with God, rather than taken back by God. Again, experience suggests that younger children often think of a hand coming from the sky to take people back. They are also taught that God loves them. Comments such as "God loved Daddy and took him back. Remember God loves you" can result in the child thinking, "God loved Daddy and look what happened. I don't want God's love."

The entire school staff and children were present at the funeral. There were many tears, but it also meant that when the bereaved children returned to school they returned to a community of people who had entered into their grief (Taylor 1996).

We cannot always end social suffering, but we can definitely help lessen this type of suffering. Using a team approach can help the terminally ill person and his or her family recognize the areas that are creating suffering and find ways to address each concern.

SEXUALITY SUFFERING

"Sexuality is an important part of our everyday life. Feelings about sexuality affect our zest for living, our self-image, and our relationships with others. . . . Sexuality is one aspect of our need for closeness, touch, playfulness, caring, and pleasure. Even when sex becomes impractical, such as during a severe or terminal illness, physical expression of caring remains an important way of sharing closeness" (Schover 1994, 1–2).

Sexuality refers to everything that makes us masculine and feminine, our sexual identity. Sex is the physical activity stemming from biologic desires or the desire to reproduce. When there is illness, there is an assault on how we feel about our bodies. This area of suffering is often not addressed, either because it is assumed that people with life-threatening illnesses are not concerned about sexuality and sex or because caregivers are uncomfortable discussing it.

"The dying process and human sexuality do have common elements. For one, if either is to be a 'good' or rewarding process, open communication is almost always essential" (Gideon and Taylor 1981). Out of this realization, Gideon and Taylor developed "A Sexual Bill of Rights for Dying Persons." It states: "All people have the right to

1. be a sexual person, physically, emotionally, spiritually and socially;
2. know that intercourse and sexuality are different phenomena;
3. counseling either with your sexual partner present or alone;
4. information that will help in accommodating physical changes happening in the body;
5. be in charge of his or her own body;
6. state sexual needs and negotiate the meeting of those needs;
7. confidentiality;
8. forms of pleasuring other than intercourse;
9. information regarding the use of physical aids to enhance physical sexual activities;
10. express sexuality regardless of hospitalization or institutionalization;
11. practice own sexual lifestyle, express sexual orientation and sexual needs, and be respected as a person while doing so;
12. risk self and partner's getting hurt;
13. bear or father children within full understanding between two parents;
14. communicate with own children regarding physical illness and sexual identity and growth;
15. open communication with sexual partner and a communication system that allows for the expression of physical needs that might otherwise seem to be expressions of 'negative feelings'."

Examples of the need to address sexuality include the need to have one's hair done or to have access to wigs or toupees, to be bathed, to be shaved, to have excellent mouth care, and to be afforded privacy when the body is exposed. It also involves the need for touch. One couple had both been diagnosed with cancer. During one long period of hospitalization for the wife, who had leukemia, she was in a room on the oncology floor. A few weeks after her admission, her husband was admitted to the pulmonary floor with lung cancer. When asked about putting them in the same room, the staff said they felt that would be unwise since one might die and that might be too upsetting to the survivor. However, the experts in addressing the staff's fears were the couple, so each was asked what they wanted. They both said they wanted to be together. This eased some of the staff's concerns. However, when there was a request to rearrange the room so they could hold hands, the reply was that it could not be done. It was suggested that there was no reason why that had to be the case, and the staff was shown how the bedside table could be moved to the outsides of the beds so that the arrangement would be bedside table, bed, bed, bedside table. This finally was allowed, and the couple had a week together holding hands while they watched TV or just were quiet. He died as they held hands. During the bereavement period, she often expressed appreciation for the chance to touch her husband of so many years.

Another woman shared that she felt ugly, not just because her belly was swollen by tumor and ascites, but because her hair looked bad. While using a rescue dose of morphine to stop breakthrough pain, she had her hair washed and styled by a beautician. Three days later she died feeling much more comfortable about how she looked.

Another couple expressed the desire to cuddle. They were not interested in "making love" but in being able to lie side by side again without causing additional pain for the man, who was dying of leukemia. It was decided that they could be in the same bed, touching at times but moving apart when the pressure of her body became burdensome. For another couple, they wanted to try to "make love." Using illustrations they were given, they experimented with what position would be comfortable for them (Arthritis Foundation 1982).

It is important to address the area of sexuality suffering. A woman angrily said that her husband was "dead" for her and their children, although his body was still alive in a nursing home. She shared that his brain tumor had stripped away his ability to function as a dentist and a breadwinner for their family. As the tumor grew, he could no longer play with his three young sons. The final insult to his sense of self was when they tried to "make love." The disease and his medications had rendered him impotent. No one told them that would happen. Through tears and rage, she shared how night after night he tried to be the husband he once was. Finally, he stopped, withdrew and died in his spirit. She said he felt that he was a failure as a dentist, a father, a husband, and a man. She stated that if anyone had told them this would happen, they could have talked about their needs in terms of sexuality and sex, and obtained help to work out their feelings and concerns. I agreed that the health community had failed them and began to look at addressing sexuality suffering regardless of one's age, diagnosis, or prognosis.

It is necessary to find a way to make it safe for patients and family members to raise these concerns and to educate them about sex and sexuality. If we are not comfortable ourselves, there are many people in the health community who are able to work with individuals and couples. The American Cancer Society is a good resource, as are groups like the American Association of Sex Educators, Counselors, and Therapists.

FINANCIAL SUFFERING

This area is often the hardest to address because of the reality of the cost of health care today. The cost of health insurance and medications often forces people to make decisions about food and shelter or going to the doctor and getting the drugs prescribed. More than 44 million people in the United States are currently uninsured (Holahan and Brennan 2000).

When people are admitted to the hospital or come in for medical procedures, they should be asked not only if they have health insurance, but also if they have a prescription plan. If they do not have insurance or a prescription plan, a social worker should be called immediately to see what resources are available to those we serve. A discharge plan cannot be complete and the assumption made that the patient has the financial means to fill the prescriptions ordered. Many pharmaceutical companies have an indigent program that can be used to get some of the medications people need. Our congressional representatives and senators and the general public should be informed of what our patients are experiencing. They can spur the need for changes in the health care system so financial suffering can be reduced, if not eliminated. People can be referred at the end of life to hospice programs, where the costs for staff, equipment, supplies, and medications related to the terminal diagnosis are paid for by the hospice. This reduces the financial suffering most people experience during this very difficult time.

The need to address this form of suffering was graphically illustrated to me when a nurse friend, who had congestive heart failure and who was now terminally ill, called to say she had just taken an overdose of her cardiac medications. She did so because the costs of her doctor visits and medications were depleting the small savings she and her 75-year-old husband had built up over many years. She saw no options of leaving him with money to get into a life care or assisted living community except to stop the drain on their finances by ending her life. She did die and her husband did get the care he needed at the end of his life, but at what cost!

SUMMARY

All of the areas of suffering addressed in this chapter involve loss and grief. There is the loss of health, with the sense that the body is untrustworthy. There is the loss of spontaneity and the ability to plan for the future. There is a loss of a sense of usefulness as the illness changes the roles one had in the family and in society. For some there is a loss of a belief in the rightness of the universe. As we journey with those we care for, we can help them work through some of the tasks of grief identified by Dr. J. William Worden in an address given at the 9th American Association of Retired Persons, Widowed

Persons Service Conference in October, 1986. He identified the tasks of grief listed below:

- to accept the reality of the loss
- to experience the pain of grief
- to adjust to the new reality
- to invest in the present and future and withdraw emotional energy from the past reality

In the introduction to a book written by Viktor E. Frankl (1963, xi), a Holocaust survivor, Dr. Gordon W. Allport states, "To live is to suffer, to survive is to find meaning in the suffering. If there is a purpose in life at all, there must be a purpose in suffering and in dying. But no man can tell another what this purpose is. Each must find out for himself, and must accept the responsibility that his answer prescribes. If he succeeds he will continue to grow in spite of all indignities. Frankl is fond of quoting Nietzche, 'He who has a why to live can bear with almost any how.' What alone remains is 'the last of human freedoms'—the ability to 'choose one's attitude in a given set of circumstances.' "

The word *compassion* has its roots in old French where it means "to suffer with." As we address the spiritual, social, sexuality, and financial suffering experienced by patients and those who love them, we can allow our compassion to grow. As Dr. Ira Byock (1996, 252) writes, "We may not have answers for the existential questions of life and death any more than the person dying. We may not be able to assuage all feelings of regret or fears of the unknown. But it is not our solutions that matter. The role of the clinical team is to stand by the patient, steadfastly providing meticulous physical care and psychological support, while people strive to discover their own answers."

We can help people find support groups where they can borrow strength from others. We can help people stay in the present, letting go of the past with its reality of what he or she used to do or be and grieving those losses. We can help them learn to adjust to changes and to redefine what is of value. That involves learning that you are not what you do but who you are. We can help patients find meaning in who they are now and find hope even in the midst of dying. Norman Cousins (1972, 133) said it well when he said, "Death is not the ultimate tragedy of life. The ultimate tragedy is depersonalization—dying in an alien and sterile area, separated from the spiritual nourishment that comes from being able to reach out to a loving hand, separated from a desire to experience the things that make life worth living, separated from hope." As caregivers we can hold out a compassionate hand during the journey at the end of life and lessen the suffering felt by the patient and the family.

REFERENCES

Associated Press, "Assisted Suicide: Oregon law problems studied." *Star Tribune* 2000 February 24: A14.

Arthritis Foundation. (1982). *Arthritis: Living and loving: Information about sex*, 8–9. Available from the Arthritis Foundation. Louisiana Chapter, 15254 Old Hammond Hwy. Baton Rouge, LA 70816.

Byock, I. R. (1996). The nature of suffering and the nature of opportunity at the end of life. *Clinics in Geriatric Medicine*, 12:(2), 252.

Cassell, E. J. (1991). *The nature of suffering and the goals of medicine*. New York: Oxford University Press.

Cohen, M. (1993). Introduction: Spirituality, quality of life, and nursing care. Quality of life: A nursing challenge. *Spiritual Well Being*, 2(3), 47–49.

Cousins, N. (1972). *Anatomy of an illness as perceived by the patient*. New York: Norton & Co.

Ferszt, G. G., Teegen-Case, S., & Taylor, P. B. (1999). *Spiritual assessment tool*. Unpublished manuscript.

Frankl, V. E. (1963). *Man's search for meaning*. New York: Pocket Books.

Gideon, M. C., & Taylor, P. B. (1981). A sexual bill of rights for dying persons. *Death Education*, 4, 304.

Holahan, J., & Brennan, N. (2000). Who are the adult uninsured? (On-line). *Urban Institute Working Paper*. Washington, DC: The Urban Institute. Available from: http://newfederalism.urban.org/pdf/b14.pdf.

Mondragon, D. (1997). *Religious values of the terminally ill: A handbook for healthcare professionals*. Scranton, PA: University of Scranton Press.

Quill, T. E. (1996). *A midwife through the dying process*. Baltimore, MD: The John Hopkins University Press.

Schover, L. R. (1994). *Sexuality and cancer*. American Cancer Society. pp. 1–2.

Taylor, P. B. (1996). Fostering farewell: Giving children the chance to let go. *Nursing 96*, 26(1), 54–57.

Webster's New World Dictionary of the American Language. 2nd ed.(1972). Cleveland, OH: William Collins and World Publishing Co.

Wright, K. B. (1998). Professional, ethical and legal implications for spiritual care in nursing. *Image: Journal of Nursing Scholarship*, 30(1), 81.

Younger, J. B. (1995). The alienation of the sufferer. *Advances in Nursing Science*, 17(4), 58, 67.

CHAPTER

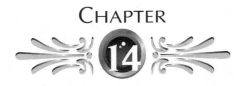

PSYCHOSOCIAL ISSUES IN PALLIATIVE CARE: A MATTER OF ACCEPTANCE

Michael T. Landry and Heidi T. Landry

"Some people are so afraid to die that they never begin to live."

Henry Jackson Van Dyke

One of the most challenging and meaningful aspects of nursing is providing care when cure is no longer a viable option. This becomes especially apparent when one considers the wide range of psychological responses that are expressed by the patient, caregiver, and nurse when the patient has a terminal prognosis. In her landmark work on death and dying, Kubler-Ross (1975) provides several categories of conditions that the nurse might encounter when providing palliative patient care: denial (or shock), anger, bargaining, depression, and acceptance. These stages have as an underlying theme the degree to which patients are able to psychologically accept their own mortality.

This chapter will explore the psychosocial issues that influence the care of the dying patient. First, the importance of the nurse's own feelings regarding death will be discussed, because providing psychosocial care involves the therapeutic use of self. Second, because the nurse relates to the patient through communication, those factors that influence communication with the terminally ill patient will be considered. Third, the five Kubler-Ross stages, along with the nursing process, will be utilized as a guide for the nurse providing care for the dying patient. The final section of this chapter will be devoted to other psychosocial considerations that impact the patient and the care of the patient.

THERAPEUTIC USE OF SELF: THE ROLE OF THE NURSE

"When one reaches out to help another, one touches the face of God."

Walt Whitman

One of the major facets of palliative care for the nurse is therapeutic use of self. The nurse provides care through therapeutic use of self, allowing the patient to receive compassion, support, and comfort through human contact. By "being there" for the patient, the nurse conveys the message that the patient is an important, unique fellow human being. A study by Rittman, et al. (1997) indicates that there are four psychosocial themes for the nurse in the nurse-patient relationship during palliative care: knowing the patient, preserving hope, easing the struggle, and providing for privacy.

The prior experiences of the nurse can affect this relationship. When caring for a terminally ill patient, the nurse may become acutely aware of his or her own mortality. The nurse may recall the death of family and friends, and even experience feelings of sadness, loss, anger, depression, and helplessness that accompanied those events. These are common examples of counter-transference, a psychological process in which the experiences of caring for a patient invoke memories from the nurse's past.

If the nurse's prior experiences with death were negative, serious psychological difficulties may face the nurse when caring for the dying patient. For example, during childhood, a nurse had a grandmother who died at home following a very lengthy and very painful illness. Because of this nurse's unresolved, painful memories of that event, she found it impossible to care for a patient who was dying at home. Studies indicate that nursing students experience fear, sadness, frustration, and anxiety when caring for dying patients (Beck 1997). Boyle and Carter (1998) note that death anxiety, or anxiety related to discussing and coping with death, can impact nursing care for the terminally ill.

Therefore, prior to caring for the patient who is dying, the nurse should reflect on personal feelings regarding death (Harper 1997, O'Gorman 1998). A few questions are listed below to help in this self-evaluation. Ideally, after contemplating such issues and coming to terms with prior life experiences, the nurse should be able to develop the ability to be focused on and entirely empathetic with the patient while providing palliative care. At the same time, the nurse needs to develop strategies for leaving these feelings with the patient to prevent the potential for nurse burnout.

The reflection questions are:

1. What have my experiences with death been like in the past?
2. What meaning do I attach to death and to the dying process?
3. What are my religious and spiritual views of death?

4. How comfortable am I with talking about death and dying?
5. How would I react and how would I feel if I were told I have six months to live?

COMMUNICATION WITH THOSE WHO ARE DYING

"There is only one good rule for being a good talker; learn to listen."

Christopher Darlington Morley

One of the greatest sources of discomfort for the novice nurse may be in the area of speaking with a dying patient. This is perhaps in part due to the fact that death and dying are typically topics that are not discussed openly in our culture. O'Gorman (1998) contends that in the first half of the 20th century, society lost sight of the importance of rituals and education associated with death and dying, leaving patients and health care professionals less able to cope with death.

Initiating and maintaining open lines of communication can enhance care and promote end of life decision making (Basile 1998). The nurse may be the best person to initiate end of life care discussion with the patient (Goetschius 1997). Faulkner and Regnard (1994) note that patients need an environment that allows them to disclose and talk through their concerns and options. Research indicates that better communication is needed so that patients can have more optimal pain management (Fine and Busch 1998).

Pasacreta and Pickett (1998) note that supportive psychotherapeutic measures help to minimize distress, enhance feelings of control, and improve quality of life. Dean (1998) reports that communication is an area of primary concern when considering occupational stress in hospice nurses. Nurses block open communication by verbalizing their discomfort and inadequacy through interference, denial, unrealistic optimism, resistance, and anger (McGrath, et al. 1999). The most important aspect of communication with the dying patient is to listen.

PSYCHOLOGICAL RESPONSES OF THE DYING PATIENT

Denial

"We are slow to believe that which if believed would hurt our feelings."

Ovid

Denial is powerful. Denial, or the inability or unwillingness to acknowledge events or what is lacking in our lives, is an ego defense mechanism. In a simplistic view of Freudian thought, this denial results because of the anxiety caused by the conflict between our superego and ego. Because as humans we do not want to die, we tend to never think about death, almost to the point of developing a false sense of immortality guided by the idealism of our superego. Then, when we have to face death, our ego, or our perception of what is reality, is unable to handle this, and so we become very anxious. The defense mechanism of denial helps to lower this anxiety, protecting the ego so that we can continue to function. In the context of social learning theory, because we are taught to fear death, we develop great anxiety when faced with a terminal prognosis. In either case, denial is an indication that the patient is experiencing an unacceptable level of anxiety.

Health care professionals typically view denial as a negative or unhealthy coping mechanism. Denial inhibits one from seeking needed assistance. For example, the chemically dependent patient in denial is unwilling to admit to having a problem and thus is prevented from beginning the rehabilitation process. However, denial in the terminally ill patient indicates that the patient is not yet psychologically prepared for the inevitable (Davidhizar and Gigar 1998), and needs more time in coming to grips with the finality of the diagnosis. While veracity needs to be at the core of the nurse's interactions with the patient (Ross, et al. 1992), the nurse does not need to destroy the patient's protective denial process. The patient must be allowed to work through this phase at his or her own pace.

Assessment.   On assessment, the patient in denial demonstrates an unwillingness to agree with the prospect of death. The focus of the patient is on seeking a cure, as opposed to palliative care. Symptoms may be minimized, and the patient may talk about "beating" the illness. Long-term plans continue to be made for activities to be undertaken once a recovery is made. The patient may refuse to participate in his or her care. The patient will view it as unnecessary to make plans to finalize wills and other such matters of a personal or business nature. In essence, the patient communicates a lack of understanding of the terminal nature of his illness. The patient may appear to be happy or confident, despite having tremendously high levels of anxiety. The patient may seek second opinions and resort to the use of home remedies.

Intervention.   The nurse should allow the patient to verbalize feelings, while avoiding confrontation. The patient will need encouragement to comply with medical treatment. Patient education on diagnosis is important. The patient's significant others should be included in discussions and should receive psychosocial support as well. The patient should be connected with pastoral care and social services. The best therapeutic approach for the nurse is being there for the patient. The nurse should answer the patient's questions as honestly as possible and reinforce that the prognosis is limited. Allowing questions and answering truthfully will establish a therapeutic relationship. When the patient talks about beating the illness or about recovery, the nurse can use silence and reflection to allow the patient to verbalize these feelings. The nurse can assist the patient by encouraging a focus on pleasant memories and past accomplishments.

Patient Outcomes.   Denial may present itself in the initial stages of death. Patient outcomes for denial include the ability to verbalize feelings, level of anxiety, and physical symptoms. The patient's willingness to discuss the prospect of death and remain compliant with those treatments that add to their quality of life indicates movement toward the ultimate outcome of acceptance (Table 14–1).

Anger

> *"Men often make up in wrath what they want in reason."*
>
> William Alger

Anger is a normal human emotion. There is nothing intrinsically wrong with anger. When used constructively, anger can greatly mobilize one's energy to accomplish great things. In this sense, anger is a necessary emotion for the patient to develop the strength and courage needed to cope with his prognosis. When anger is expressed by the patient in a destructive manner, it can pose a threat to the therapeutic relationship. The nurse should realize that in struggling with the dying process, the patient may exhibit anger and frustration at any time.

Assessment.   The nurse and family may become targets for the patient's anger. The patient may strike out without provocation and verbalize rage and frustration, saying hurtful things or acting thoughtlessly towards loved ones, even blaming them for the illness. The patient may be moody or irritable, or throw things at caregivers. The patient may be unwilling to discuss feelings. Because of the heightened level of energy, there is a greater potential for self-harm or suicide.

Intervention.   The nurse needs to approach the patient in a calm, nondefensive, nonthreatening manner. Usually the nurse is not the cause of the patient's anger but may bear the brunt of it, such that limit-setting may be needed. The patient should be encouraged to vent his feelings, and the lines of communication between the patient and family need to be kept open. The patient's family should be educated on the causes of anger and be supported to not take the patient's outbursts personally. Keeping the patient as comfortable as possible can reduce anger related to physiological pain. Positive reinforcement for appropriate venting of anger is recommended. The nurse should assess for suicidal ideations and implement suicide precautions when needed.

Patient Outcomes.   The goal for angry patients is that they do nothing to harm themselves or others. Patient outcomes include the ability to verbalize feelings and identify sources of anger, as well as to develop improved coping strategies (Table 14–1).

Bargaining

> *"It is never too late with us, so long as we are aware of our faults and bear them impatiently."*
>
> Friedrich Heinrich Jacobi

TABLE 14–1 PALLIATIVE CARE: A PSYCHOSOCIAL NURSING CARE PLAN

STAGE	ASSESSMENT	PATIENT OUTCOMES	NURSING INTERVENTIONS
Denial	• Minimizes symptoms • Refuses to participate in care • Inappropriate affect • Seeks home remedies • Speaks of cure and not care • Has long-range plans • Refuses to accept diagnosis • Refuses to discuss diagnosis	• Verbalizes decreased anxiety • Verbalizes symptoms • Willing to talk about diagnosis • Compliance with treatments • More short-term focused • Makes plans for death (wills, etc)	• Allow verbalization of feelings • Avoid patient confrontation • Encourage compliance • Educate on diagnosis • Include family in discussions • Communicate honestly and empathetically with patient • Establish rapport with patient • "Be there" for the patient • Connect with pastoral care and social services
Anger	• Verbally assaults caregivers • Throws things • Moody and irritability • Impulsive • Blames others for illness • Unwilling to discuss feelings • Potential for self-harm, suicidal	• Decreased outbursts of anger • Verbalizes feelings appropriately • Identifies sources of anger • Improved coping strategies • Free of self-harm	• Use calm approach • Educate family on causes of anger • Provide positive feedback when patient can control anger • Use limit setting • Mediate between patient and family • Support to other caregivers

Bargaining	• Verbalizes promises in the form of "If I live I will…." • Patient may be very introspective • Highly manipulative	• Verbalizes feelings • Increased short-term focus • Decreased incidence of use of manipulation as a coping device	• Use calm, firm approach • Encourage verbalization of feelings • Encourage patient to live for today
Depression	• Lack of energy • Sad, crying, hopelessness • Verbalizes feelings of isolation or of being abandoned • Verbalizes no reason to live • Needy	• Patient will have increased energy • Verbalize feelings • Decreased episodes of crying • Verbalizes positive feelings • Participates in treatment	• Be there for patient • Encourage verbalization of feelings • Reminiscence: Have patient recall accomplishments and prior pleasurable events • Appropriate use of humor • Diversions: movies, music, reading, visitors
Acceptance	• Verbalizes acceptance of prognosis • Prepares for death (wills, etc) • Verbalizes need for care, not cure • Participates in treatment	• Patient will continue to verbalize feelings	• Encourage verbalization of feelings • Assist patient to focus on the present • Continued use of diversional activities

Bargaining represents a condition in which the patient has ambivalence regarding the acceptance of the prognosis. On the one hand, there is still an element of denial, as patients feel they can negotiate for more time. The patients partially accept their condition, in that they may say they know they will die but are just not ready yet to do so. In this condition, patients are slowly relinquishing control over their lives. Patients need psychosocial support with this struggle during this phase.

Assessment.   Patients in this phase may become highly introspective as they negotiate for more time or another chance. They may become very manipulative, displaying a lot of attention-seeking behaviors. The classic symptom at this stage is that the patient will make promises in the form of, "If I live until _____ , I will do _____ ."

Intervention.   The nurse should use a calm, firm approach with the patient who is in the bargaining stage. The patient should be encouraged to continue verbalization of feelings. Assistance should be provided to reorient the patient to a focus on the present, an encouragement to live for today. Reminiscence can be highly productive at this stage in helping the patient to recall past accomplishments and pleasurable experiences and memories.

Patient Outcomes.   It is critical at this stage that the patient be able to continue verbalizing feelings. The patient should have decreased use of manipulation. An increased ability to focus on today and living in the present is a goal for the patient who is bargaining (Table 14–1).

Depression

"What we call despair is often only the painful eagerness of unfed hope."

George Eliot

It has been estimated that more than one-fourth of terminally ill patients suffer from depression. Patients grieve for the loss of their own lives, loved ones, control, and need for future plans (Slaughter et al. 1999). Loneliness, a subjective and individualized experience, characterized by loss (Brown and McKenna 1999), often is associated with depression. Depression, panic attacks, and anxiety often precede the knowledge of terminal diagnosis in pancreatic cancer, suggesting that at least in some cases, these conditions may be secondary to the illness itself, rather than being related to receiving a terminal diagnosis (Passik and Roth 1999).

Assessment.   The depressed patient presents with low energy levels, below what is normally expected by the patient's physiological status. The patient may verbalize feelings of loneliness, isolation, abandonment, or hopelessness. The patient may be nonverbal or have frequent episodes of crying and long periods of sadness. There may be a generalized lack of will toward living, and the patient may verbalize "giving up" on living.

Intervention.   Being there for the dying patient is critical during this time of despair and depression. The patient should be encouraged to verbalize feelings. Reminiscence is used to assist the patient in recalling past accomplishments and pleasurable memories. Humor can be used when appropriate. Diversional activities such as movies, reading, and visitors can be used during this time. Prayer and meditation can also be encouraged. The challenge is to assist the patient in finding meaningful activities that promote quality of life. Caregivers need extra psychosocial support when the patient is depressed. The nurse should notify the physician so that evaluation for antidepressant medications can be made.

Patient Outcomes.   Patient goals include increased energy levels and increased participation in care. Episodes of crying and sadness diminish as the patient begins to accept the prognosis. The patient will verbalize positive aspects of life. The patient will seek out interactions with family and friends as isolation decreases.

Acceptance

> *"Men fear death, as it is unquestionably the greatest evil, and yet no man knows that it may not be the greatest good."*
>
> William Milford

The acceptance phase indicates that the patient has psychologically come to terms with the prognosis. However, research indicates that the will to live may be highly unstable among the terminally ill (Chochinov, et al. 1999). Continued support is needed to ensure that the patient's quality of life is not compromised. Storytelling through reminiscence and life review can be cathartic and assist the patient in making meaning of his or her life (Brady 1999). Life review therapy can greatly increase the empowerment experienced in the terminally ill (McDougall, Blixen, & Suen 1997).

Assessment.   The patient begins to verbalize an acceptance of the prognosis. Focus shifts from seeking a cure to obtaining needed care. The patient begins to prepare for death in terms of saying goodbye to friends and family, as well as finalizing personal business, such as wills. Some patients will make their own funeral arrangements as acceptance increases. The patient is compliant with treatment. The patient's focus also shifts away from self and more on others.

Intervention.   The nurse can assist the patient by encouraging verbalization of feelings. Encouragement can continue to focus the patient on the present. Diversional and reminiscence activities can continue to be used during this phase. These interventions can improve the quality of life for the dying patient.

Patient Outcomes.   The goal of this phase is for the patient to continue to face death with an attitude of acceptance. The patient should continue to verbalize feelings and find meaning and quality in life.

SPECIAL CIRCUMSTANCES

The Uninformed Patient

There are times when the patient's family members are aware of the patient's terminal prognosis, and yet the patient is not given this information. In this situation, family members do not want the patient to know that he or she is dying. The rationale family members give for this is that they feel the patient will be unable to psychologically cope with the prospect of death. This situation can be avoided by first informing the patient of the condition and then communicating this to family members. In the meantime, nurses are caught between the wishes of the family and the patient's right to know. This ethical dilemma can be resolved through being a patient advocate and encouraging the physician to notify the patient, and by educating the family in the psychological responses patients experience when given a terminal prognosis. Family members need to be confronted when this situation arises to promote open and honest communication between the health care team and the patient and family. Successful resolution of this situation requires tremendous patience and effort.

The Exhausted Family

Family members are at risk for a decrease in physical and psychological well-being as a result of the stress associated with caring for a terminally ill patient (Chan and Chang 1999). Often in practice we find elderly spouses as primary caregivers for those who are dying. Often these caregivers have health problems of their own. These caregivers may experience serious limitations on their lifestyles (Davis, Cowley, and Ryland 1996). Patients may outlive their terminal diagnosis, to the point that it may deplete the family of its psychological resources and ability to care for the patient. Clumpus and Hill (1999) note four major psychosocial nursing needs of the family: (a) the nurse being there for the patient and caregiver, (b) having the nurse to talk to, (c) a need for information, and (d) having someone treat them well. Many caregivers report that the psychosocial support offered by the nurse is the most important aspect of the palliative care provided.

SUMMARY

> "A joyful heart is good medicine."
>
> *Proverbs* 17:22

Nursing's greatest role continues to be that of patient advocate. In the care of the dying patient, this includes that commitment to never abandon the patient. It includes initiating communication between patient, caregivers, staff, and the physician. It centers on promotion of the good death. The good death is one in which there is awareness, acceptance, and preparation for death by all concerned (McNamara, Waddell, and Colvin 1995). It is also important to assist patients in finding meaning in their suffering experiences (Pollock and Sands 1997).

Studies indicate that patients can focus on the quality of living rather than on dying in the living–dying interval, that time period between receiving a terminal prognosis and death itself (Engle, Fox-Hill, and Graney 1998). Marrone (1999) notes that the ability to redefine meaning in our lives, while dealing with profound loss, can greatly add to the quality of our life. A positive approach to palliative care can help the individual and family to approach this last stage of life with hope and fulfillment. Enabling can help the person remain involved in key decisions, while mediacy can ensure that the death occurs in the most appropriate setting for the individual (Russell and Sanders 1998).

Caring for the dying patient can invoke the nurse's own sense of mortality. The psychological responses of the patient and family to the terminal diagnosis can be very difficult to deal with. Communication remains the most effective tool the nurse can use to support the patient and family throughout the dying process. Humor, when used judiciously and appropriately, can greatly enhance this process. The nurse should do everything possible to enhance the patient's quality of life and to ultimately assist the patient in the good death. The nurse should never underestimate the impact and the importance that being there for the patient has on enhancing the joy and quality of life of the terminally ill.

REFERENCES

Basile, C. M. (1998). Advance directives an advocacy in end-of-life decisions. *Nurse Practitioner*, 23(5), 44–6, 54, 57–60.

Beck, C. T. (1997). Nursing students' experiences caring for dying patients. *Journal of Nursing Education*, 36(9), 408–415.

Boyle, M., & Carter, D. E. (1998). Literature review. Death anxiety amongst nurses. *International Journal of Palliative Nursing*, 4(1), 37–43.

Brady, E. M. (1999). Stories at the hour of our death. *Home Healthcare Nurse*, 17(3), 176–180.

Brown, R., & McKenna, H. P. (1999). Concept of loneliness in dying patients. *International Journal of Palliative Nursing*, 5(2), 90–4, 96–7.

Chan, C. W. H., & Chang, A. M. (1999). Stress associated with tasks for family caregivers of patients with cancer in Hong Kong. *Cancer Nursing*, 22(4), 260–265.

Chochinov, H. M., Tataryn, D., Clinch, J. J., & Dudgeon, D. (1999). Will to live in the terminally ill. *The Lancet*, 354(9181), 816–819.

Clumpus, L., & Hill, A. (1999). Clinical audit. Exploring the views of carers of cancer patients in an inner city locality. *International Journal of Palliative Nursing*, 5(3), 116–123.

Davidhizar, R., & Gigar, J. N. (1998). Patients' use of denial: Coping with the unacceptable. *Nursing Standard*, 12(43), 44–46.

Davis, B. D., Cowley, S. A., & Ryland, R. K. (1996). The effects of terminal illness on patients and their carers. *Journal of Advanced Nursing*, 22(3), 512–520.

Dean, R. A. (1998). Occupational stress in hospice care: Causes and coping strategies. *American Journal of Hospice & Palliative Care*, 15(3), 151–154.

Engle, V. F., Fox-Hill, E., & Graney, M. J. (1998). The experience of living-dying in a nursing home: Self-reports of black and white older adults. *Journal of the American Geriatrics Society*, 46(9), 1091–1096.

Faulkner, A., & Regnard, C. (1994). Handling difficult questions in palliative care: A flow diagram. *Palliative Medicine*, 8(3), 245–250.

Fine, P. G., & Busch, M. A. (1998). Characterization of breakthrough pain by hospice patients and their caregivers. *Journal of Pain & Symptom Management*, 16(3), 179–183.

Goetschius, S. K. (1997). Families and end-of-life care: How do we meet their needs? *Journal of Gerontological Nursing*, 23(3), 43–56.

Harper, B. C. (1997). Growth in caring and professional ethics in hospice. *Hospice Journal*, 12(2), 65–70.

Kubler-Ross, E. (1975). *Death: The final stage of growth*. Englewood Cliffs, N.J.: Prentice Hall, Inc.

Marrone, R. (1999). Dying, mourning, and spirituality: A psychological perspective. *Death Studies*, 23(6), 495–519.

McDougall, G. J., Blixen, C. E., & Suen, L. (1997). The process and outcome of life review psychotherapy with depressed homebound older adults. *Nursing Research*, 46(5), 277–283.

McGrath, P., Yates, P., Clinton, M., & Hart, G. (1999). What should I say? Qualitative findings on dilemmas in palliative care nursing. *Hospice Journal: Physical, Psychosocial, & Pastoral Care of the Dying*, 14(2), 17–33.

McNamara, B., Waddell, C., & Colvin, M. (1995). Threats to the good death: The cultural context of stress. *Sociology of Health & Illness*, 17(2), 222–244.

O'Gorman, S. M. (1998). Death and dying in contemporary society: An evaluation of current attitudes and the rituals associated with death and dying and their relevance to recent understandings of health and healing. *Journal of Advanced Nursing*, 27(6), 1127–1135.

Pasacreta, J. V., & Pickett, M. (1998). Psychosocial aspects of palliative care. *Source Seminars in Oncology Nursing*, 14(2), 110–120.

Passik, S. D., & Roth, A. J. (1999). Anxiety symptoms and panic attacks preceding pancreatic cancer diagnosis. *Psycho-Oncology*, 8(3), 268–272.

Pollock, S. E., & Sands, D. (1997). Adaptation to suffering . . . meaning and implications for nursing. *Clinical Nursing Research*, 6(2), 171–185.

Rittman, M., Paige, P., Rivera, J., Sutphin, L., & Godown, I. (1997). Phenomenological study of nurses caring for dying patients. *Cancer Nursing*, 20(2), 115–119.

Ross, D. M., Peteet, J. R., Medeiros, C., Walsh-Burke, K., & Rieker, P. (1992). Difference between nurses' and physicians' approach to denial in oncology. *Cancer Nursing*, 15(6), 422–428.

Russell, P., & Sanders, R. (1998). Clinical palliative care: Promoting the concept of a healthy death. *British Journal of Nursing*, 7(5), 256–261.

Slaughter, J. R., Beck, D. A., Johnston, S., Holmes, S. E., & McDonald, A. (1999). Anticipatory grief and depression in terminal illness. *Annals of Long-Term Care*, 7(8), 299–304.

CHAPTER

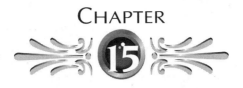

SPIRITUAL PERSPECTIVES IN
END OF LIFE CARE

Douglas Smith

The intent of this chapter is to sensitize nurses to the spiritual needs and concerns of patients. We will explore five major spiritual or religious perspectives, exploring their attitudes toward sickness, death, afterlife, and mourning. Although only five perspectives will be explored, this chapter seeks to persuade nurses of the importance of a patient's spiritual or religious background, whatever that background might be. Two caveats: (1) The following are merely brief summaries. Any summary involves generalizations, and any generalization is not true for all people at all times. We must be open to varieties of expressions within each perspective. (2) Any person writing about a perspective from outside that perspective (me) cannot be as accurate as someone writing from within that perspective. My hope is that this chapter will move nurses to do further research on those who have actually lived within these perspectives.

THE HINDU PERSPECTIVE

The Hindu faith is often considered the oldest of organized religions. However, one thing makes it decidedly different from most other organized religions: It is not focused upon one individual personality or one well-defined set of sacred writings. There are many exemplary models of the Hindu faith and many sets of sacred writings. Knowing how much variety there is in Christianity (which is clearly focused on one person and one well-defined set of sacred writings), it is easy to imagine the great amount of variety within Hinduism—and there is a great amount of variety.

One aspect of the Hindu faith that is often misunderstood by those outside the faith is the Hindu emphasis on our present reality; the Hindu faith is often erroneously thought of as being overly mystical, too oriented beyond this world. That is far from the case. There is a saying within Hinduism: One who has no "here" will certainly have no "hereafter."

However, the emphasis that the Hindu faith places upon present reality is not one that glorifies the present. Hindus believe that no matter what our goals in this life—whether they be fame, wealth, or even just being the most caring nurse imaginable—we will all eventually get to a point in our lives in which we will feel there must be something more than just this life. The Hindu believes in the "more" of reincarnation.

For the Hindu, all of us have led countless lives before this one and we will most likely lead countless lives after this one. Who we are now is a product of what we have done and said before now—both in this life and in previous ones. Who we will be in the future is a product of what we are doing and saying now. That is a profound emphasis on the present. We end up being the architects of our own fate, and no one can undo anything we do, and no one can erase anything we say.

For the Hindu, God is both internal and external, within every person and transcending every person. Hinduism teaches that the main purpose of our existence is to become aware of that divine core, the Self. In this life we are to also seek an awareness of that essence of God that transcends all personal existence.

In the health care environment, Hindus prefer to receive their care from caregivers of the same sex. A Hindu woman would most likely prefer to have her nurse, her social worker, and even her medical technician be women.

Another important consideration in caring for Hindus is being aware of the importance of jewelry. Often each item of jewelry received by a woman—necklaces, amulets, bracelets—is associated with a specific blessing that has been given to this woman. If a nurse removes that item of jewelry, that blessing has been removed. We need to allow Hindus the option of retaining their jewelry throughout the health care environment—except at the moment of death: Hindus often feel that any jewelry worn at the moment of death restricts the soul's passage onto the next life. So we loosen or release the jewelry at that moment.

As death is near, we can bring comfort to our Hindu patients by doing some positive life review. "I would be honored to hear about some of the things you've done to contribute to the well-being of your community." "Please share with me some of the ways you have helped your family." Processing such things will allow these patients to go into death with some assurances that their next life will be a good one.

Sometimes as death is near, fellow Hindus will be brought in to do singing and chanting. Not only are the words of these songs and chants important, but the tone is important as well—giving the dying person a calm and clear mind. This calm and clear mind is important because the last thoughts of a Hindu are often thought of as the most prescriptive as to what their next life will be. So we want to set as an important goal the calming of this person, giving this person the ability to think clearly. Hallucinating is the worst thing a Hindu could be doing at the moment of death; a Hindu might often prefer some pain and a somewhat clear mind over hallucinating with no pain.

If we have questions as to the wishes of the dying person or the wishes of the family, one member of the family has usually been appointed to answer all the questions—usually the oldest son. Appointing one person as representative is a great practice that I wish all other faiths would adopt.

Once the death has occurred, the family will often want to be the ones to prepare the body for cremation, which will occur as soon as possible, hopefully within 24 hours of the death. For the Hindu, the body is relatively unimportant; the individual soul, which has no beginning or end, is far more important than the temporal body.

In attending a Hindu funeral, expect an open casket. Wearing white is more appropriate than black. Flowers may be taken to a home. Comfort can be given to the family by recounting the good deeds of the person who has died.

THE BUDDHIST PERSPECTIVE

Most Buddhists center their faith around four "noble truths." These are the truths that need to be processed for a Buddhist to attain enlightenment:

1. Suffering exists. It permeates all that we experience; it is interwoven with everything there is.
2. The cause of that suffering is our continual manipulations of the world to meet our ends. We suffer because of our cravings, our unhealthy desires, and our placing of our own agendas at the expense of everyone else's agenda.
3. We can eliminate being overpowered by that suffering by eliminating our self-centered manipulations of the world. We eliminate our being victimized by suffering by eliminating our cravings, our unhealthy desires, and our placing of our own agendas at the expense of everyone else's agenda.
4. The prescription for eliminating the overpowering quality of suffering is the eightfold path: right knowledge, right aspiration, right speech, right behavior, right livelihood, right effort, right mindfulness, and right absorption—in other words, right everything. We need to eliminate our unhealthy desires and self-centered manipulations throughout our entire lives, our inner and outer selves.

With the Buddhist faith (as we saw with the Hindu faith and will see with all other faiths), there can be an immense amount of variety. Oftentimes with Buddhists, there is not only variety within the faith but also varieties in combining the Buddhist faith with the Christian faith. Many Buddhist immigrants who were sponsored by Christian congregations to come to this country might regularly attend the worship services of the congregations that sponsored them; however, when death enters the picture, these families might also want to rely heavily upon their Buddhist traditions and practices. They often might want to contact a Buddhist monk or nun to help them during this time, as well as the pastor from their Christian congregation.

When it comes to death, most Buddhists have, at one and the same time, an ultimate concern with death and no concern whatsoever. In order to understand this dichotomous marriage of viewpoints, a student once approached the Buddha asking, "What happens after death?" The Buddha answered with a parable. A man was walking down the road, minding his own business, when an arrow flew through the sky and lodged itself in the man's back. The Buddha asked, "Now is that man going to sit down and wonder how far that arrow flew, or is he going to think about what kind of feather is at the end of that arrow to make it go so straight, or is he going to try to visualize the stance of the archer before the arrow was let go? No. The man is going to try to remove the arrow from his back. The same with you: You work on removing suffering and the rest will take care of itself." In other words, don't be concerned with what happens after death; be concerned with what is happening here and now.

Another student once approached the Buddhist teacher Master Hakuin with a similar question: "What happens to the enlightened man after death and what happens to the unenlightened man?" Hakuin said, "Why are you asking me?" "You're an enlightened man," responded the student. "But I'm not a dead one," said Hakuin. The Buddhist must be continually aware of the impermanence of life, but not dwell upon what happens after this life.

As caregivers of Buddhists we need to be careful of our verbalizations of someone's prognosis. For many Buddhists to talk about death with the dying is to evoke death, to hasten it. Therefore it is unadvisable to talk directly to the dying person about his or her death. It is sometimes not even advisable to talk directly with the spouse of the dying person. Speaking to the children or some other relative might be a better choice.

For most Buddhists, death is not seen as some "moment" as it is in the typical Western mind. For the Western mind there is this moment, before which the person was alive and after which the person is dead. For the Buddhist, all is a "process." So, at the moment of death, we need to observe a period of respect as the person is going through the process of leaving this existence and entering another one. Observing a period of at least 10 minutes where we do not move the body or talk around it would be a respectful thing to do.

According to much of Buddhist belief, people go through a series of reincarnations until they are finally liberated from this world of illusions and selfish cravings and manipulations. This final state of freedom is called nirvana.

In attending a Buddhist funeral, expect an open casket. It is appropriate to view the body, for this is a reminder of life's impermanence. We are to bow slightly toward the body as a sign of appreciation for its lesson of impermanence.

Sending flowers to the funeral would be appropriate. Oftentimes the family would recommend a charity for donations.

THE JEWISH PERSPECTIVE

Here we have much variety again. There are three major traditions within Judaism: Reform, Conservative, and Orthodox. However, there can be an immense amount of variety even within each of these traditions.

There are several ways of portraying the general flavor of each of these traditions. Demographically, in this country, about 6% of the Jews would label themselves Orthodox, 42% Reform, 40% Conservative, and 2% Reconstructionist or other. Liturgically, the Orthodox worship entirely in Hebrew, the Reform mostly English and some Hebrew, and the Conservative are somewhere between Orthodox and Reform. The Orthodox put a very high value on historical customs, the Reform interpret historical customs through individual conscience and contemporary philosophy, and the Conservative are somewhere between the two. Regarding the ordination of women, the Reform tradition started the practice in 1972, the Conservative in 1985, and the Orthodox have yet to do such.

Important for all three of those traditions is the belief that God has made a covenant with Israel. This covenant states that the Jews are a "chosen" people. Being "chosen" is not so much a privilege as an obligation to bring God's message to the world.

Although there can certainly be summaries of the Jewish faith—the Shema ("Hear O Israel, the Eternal is our God, the Eternal is One") and the words of Micah: "Do justice, love goodness, and walk humbly with your God"—the faith is often not considered a "creedal" religion: Doctrines can be tried, tested, and then rejected. For example, beliefs in "Satan" and "original sin" were once strong elements within the Jewish faith but have now generally been discarded.

The Jewish community certainly has a comprehensive view of suffering. We need only read the Book of Job or the Book of Psalms to realize that. Suffering can be a punishing event. Suffering can be a teaching event. Suffering can be a redemptive event. And it can be all three at once.

When it comes to suffering, Jews also are often concerned with the "why" of suffering: coming to some intellectual understanding of why suffering exists.

Once a death has occurred, the family will often want the burial to occur as soon as possible, hopefully within 24 hours. Many times someone from the Jewish community will wash and prepare the body for the burial.

At a funeral there is most often an emphasis on simplicity and modesty. The funeral is not a time for economic competition, emphasizing that we came into this life as equals and we leave as equals. Usually there is a plain wooden casket, which remains closed. Flowers are discouraged.

The Jewish funeral is often focused on processing the sadness of the loss. The atmosphere is somber. Dark, conservative clothes are often worn.

Probably of all the spiritual perspectives that we are examining in this chapter, the Jewish one seems to be the most receptive to people outside of that faith participating in the funeral service, especially at that moment when people get in line to place dirt in the grave—anyone can get in that line. That act is filled with meaning; not only symbolizing the finality of death, but also representing the last loving act we can do for a person (helping this person to be buried), a pure loving act, done without expectation of anything in return.

If someone wanted to do something for the family, a gift to a charity recommended by the family would be a good gesture. A note or letter of remembrance would be very appropriate. A gift of food (if proper food) would be nice.

There are several periods of mourning within the Jewish perspective. A concentrated period of mourning immediately after the death, called shiva, lasts three to seven days, depending upon when the death occurred and to which of the three traditions the family belongs. There are also some observances done the first month, some for a year, and some on each anniversary.

When it comes to afterlife, there can be many beliefs within the Jewish community, from the belief in no afterlife to belief in resurrection of the soul to belief in bodily resurrection. Most Jews would probably summarize their beliefs by simply saying, "It is in God's hands, and I trust God."

THE CHRISTIAN PERSPECTIVE

Even though we are now looking at a faith that is clearly focused on one individual and one well-defined set of sacred writings, there is an immense amount of variety once again. There are, however, two central doctrines of which probably all Christians can agree. The first doctrine is that, that which is wrong in our world, that which is amiss, that which is tainted is our own fault; people have messed up what God has created as good. That doctrine, however, is always paired up with a second one that proclaims that, that which has been made wrong is made right, that which is amiss is straightened out again, that which is tainted is cleansed anew, through the person of Jesus.

In ministering to Christians, sometimes a hymnal can be a more effective tool for ministry than Scripture or prayer. When it comes to Scripture, there have been so many different translations of the Christian Bible that it is very likely that a nurse's chosen translation is not the patient's chosen translation; what might be the comforting words of the twenty-third Psalm for one person might be quite uncomfortable for another. What used to be a common shared prayer among all Christians, the Lord's Prayer, is no longer said the same way by all Christians; it still begins with the word "our" but ends with a cacophony of some people saying "debts," some "trespasses," and some "sins." However, there has been little attempt to change the words to the hymns. Chances are likely that a patient might be familiar with a different translation of the Christian Bible than the nurse, and chances are likely that a patient might say the Lord's Prayer in a different way than the nurse, but chances are great that they can share the same words to the hymn "Amazing Grace."

When a Christian becomes seriously ill, we need to realize that many expressions of Christianity have a service for the blessing of the sick. Roman Catholics, Episcopalians, Lutherans, and Methodists all have services for blessing people at the onset of serious illnesses. Nurses might need to contact appropriate clergy if the family or patient is in need of such a service.

Probably the most amount of disagreement among Christians centers on what happens to people after they die; there is a very long continuum of beliefs. At one end of the continuum are Christians who state that there will be very few in heaven, and at the other end of the continuum are Christians who say there will be many; some Christians even say that all people (Christian and non-Christian) will somehow be reunited with God in heaven. It is important to realize that it is not as if one of these positions has support in the Christian Bible and the other not; they both have scriptural basis. One side points to passages talking about "separating the sheep from the goats," "gathering up the wheat and burning up the chaff," and "entering by the narrow gate"; the other side points to passages talking about "as in Adam all die, so in Christ shall all be made alive" and "Jesus came into the world to save the world."

Nurses must be very careful in assuming where someone is on this continuum, for there have been some dramatic changes within many Christian traditions as far as their beliefs on who will be with God after death. The Roman Catholic Church has made some of the most dramatic changes. We do not have to go too many years back to remember that someone who committed suicide was not buried by the Roman Catholic Church—even if it was a Roman Catholic. However, today many Roman Catholic theologians are talking about the possibility of universal salvation, all people being united with God in heaven (Catholic and Protestant, Christian and non-Christian). This trend toward that end of the continuum has been occurring within many of the mainline denominations within Christianity. This is why in recent times we've seen Christian funeral services becoming more and more celebratory—expressions of the conviction that this person is in a better place no matter who this person has been.

That said, it is important for us to realize that a person's faith (whether they are Christian or non-Christian) can give that person a peaceful mindset when going into death or a fearful one. People can also go back and forth between peacefulness and fear. With all faiths (and this cannot be overemphasized), we need to be open to a variety of expressions, interpretations, and attitudes.

THE MUSLIM PERSPECTIVE

The Muslim faith, in all its many varieties of expression, centers on five "pillars" of the faith:

1. The Muslim creed, which is very succinct: "There is one God, Allah, and Mohammed is his prophet."
2. The practice of prayer. Here is an area where we can certainly admire this faith: Five times daily Muslims all around the world are praying.

3. The practice of charity. Whatever has been given to the Muslim is expected to be shared. In whatever way the Muslim believer has been blessed, he or she must bless others.
4. The observance of Ramadan, a month of fasting and other special observances commemorating the month in which Mohammed received his commission from Allah.
5. The visit to Mecca. The believer in Islam must visit Mecca, the place in which Mohammed received his commission.

Muslim children are taught from a very young age to believe in Allah, to practice the faith, and practice charity so that they will have a place in the Garden of Paradise; do not believe in Allah and do not practice charity and they will not have a place.

As was important for Hindus, so with Muslims: Caregivers should be of the same sex as the patient. A Muslim woman will want a woman for a nurse.

Also of importance for Muslim women is that the body be fully clothed. If hospitals do not have hospital gowns that go all the way to the floor and to the ends of the wrists, they should allow Muslim women to bring appropriate clothing from home. The face will often be covered; the amount of covering depends upon which Muslim tradition the woman belongs. Some women might have a thin veil, some a thick mesh, and some even a metal plate around the face so that neither wind nor hand can brush it aside.

When death is near, someone is often brought in to read from Muslim Scripture (the Koran) at the bedside. In fact, there are some people whose profession it is to read the Koran at the bedside of the sick and dying.

When death occurs, Muslims give great importance to a person being buried whole. This is because of the belief in the resurrection of the body. If a Muslim man or woman has had an amputation sometime during his or her life, that body part is often retained for the burial. Also, because of this belief, organ donations and autopsies will not be requested by a Muslim.

After the death, the family might want to prepare the body for burial. Muslims will usually want the body to be buried within 24 hours after the death.

A great practice among Muslims is the keeping of company with the bereaved. For that first 24 hours after the death, the bereaved are not left alone. Someone is present waiting to be of service to the bereaved in whatever capacity is desired.

If a nurse wishes to visit the home of the bereaved, he or she may shake hands or hug and kiss the family members of the same sex. Talking quietly with the bereaved or sharing silence is the usual practice. Selections from the Koran are often read in the home for the benefit of family and visitors.

For the Muslim, afterlife may or may not be a place of spiritual contentment and physical pleasures. That afterlife is preceded by the Day of Decision, or the Day of Reckoning, in which people will be judged as to whether they are fitting for the Garden of Paradise or banished to hell. Those who go to the Garden of Paradise will enter a state of perpetual peace and bliss; those who go to hell will suffer eternal torment and torture.

SUMMARY

We have seen a variety of spiritual perspectives, and we have acknowledged variety within each of those perspectives. In the midst of all of that variety, nurses might want to use the following guidelines in addressing the spiritual needs of patients:

1. Acquire knowledge of various spiritual beliefs and practices.
2. Show respect for those beliefs and practices.
3. Make accommodation for those beliefs and practices.
4. Help others in acquiring knowledge, showing respect, and making accommodation.

Unit V

Patient Centered Care

Critical Thinking Activities
1. Differentiate symptoms of nerve, bone, and soft tissue pain
2. List intrinsic and extrinsic factors that impede pain management
3. Compare and contrast acute and chronic pain
4. List outcomes of effective pain management
5. Differentiate between hospice care and hospital care
6. Give examples of four types of suffering experienced by the dying
7. Defend the premise that the family is the ideal unit of care in hospice and palliative care
8. List specific assessment, interventions, and expected outcomes relative to the psychological needs of the dying
9. Compare and contrast differences among religious faiths relative to end of life care

Teaching-Learning Exercises
1. Prioritize nursing interventions in physical, psychosocial, and spiritual components of patient care
2. Write a critical path for pain and suffering at the end of life
3. Write a comparison paper related to hospice and acute care

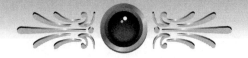

UNIT VI

COMMUNICATION

Learning Objectives

1. Identify principles of therapeutic communication
2. Describe the role of the nurse in communicating with the dying and caregivers
3. Discuss verbal and nonverbal communication techniques
4. Identify characteristics of a therapeutic relationship
5. Discuss the role of the nurse in interpreting metaphors expressed by the dying person
6. Discuss the importance of listening
7. Identify resources to enhance communication efforts of professional caregivers

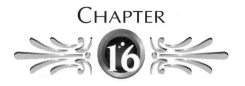

COMMUNICATING WITH THE DYING PATIENT

Belinda Poor and Elizabeth Gary

One of the most important aspects of caring for the dying patient is the development of a therapeutic relationship between the nurse and the patient. Therefore, an examination of components of effective therapeutic communication is necessary. Characteristics of the therapeutic relationship are (1) a patient-centered approach, and (2) empowerment of the patient (Arnold 1999).

PATIENT-CENTERED CARE

As suggested by the title, a patient-centered approach means that the patient's needs and feelings are at the center of any communication. The patient must feel comfortable in the communication in order to share experiences and the meaning of these experiences with the nurse (Arnold 1999). A nurse's first encounter with a patient will probably be an introduction visit only. Many subsequent visits will be required to develop open communication.

It is important to recognize that each patient responds differently to nurses. Not every patient will communicate feelings and needs. It is the responsibility of the nurse to keep the opportunity for communication open. Sometimes the patient may not be ready to share emotions at the particular time the nurse tries to stimulate conversation. This rejection is not personal and the nurse should allow the patient private time and offer to return at another time. This offers respect for the patient's feelings and the need to be alone (Arnold 1999).

EMPOWERMENT

Empowerment is defined as "enabling people to choose to take control over and make decisions about their lives. It is also a process which values all those involved" (Rodwell 1996, 309). Nurses empower patients to make decisions regarding their lives every day, by teaching them about different options they have in choosing treatment and helping them set goals.

Empowerment encourages patients to take maximum control of their lives. It builds on patients' strengths. It serves the purpose of allowing patients to assume responsibility for their own health. Empowering patients helps to enhance their self esteem (Boggs 1999).

CONCEPTS OF THE THERAPEUTIC RELATIONSHIP

Other than the characteristics of patient-centered care and empowerment, there are five concepts that are the basis of therapeutic relationships: caring, trust, empathy, mutuality, and confidentiality.

Caring

Caring is not a new concept in nursing. Florence Nightingale first demonstrated caring in her work with soldiers in the Crimean War. Watson (1988) defines caring as an interpersonal phenomenon and uses this concept as the foundation of her nursing theory. She identified 10 "carative factors" relating to caring. These factors "affirm the subjectivity of persons and leads to positive change for the welfare of others and allows the nurse to benefit and grow" (pp. 74–75). These factors are:

- humanistic-altruistic system of values
- faith-hope
- sensitivity to self and others
- helping-trusting human care relationship
- expressing of positive and negative feelings
- problem-solving caring process
- transpersonal teaching-learning
- supportive, protective, and/or corrective mental, physical, societal, and spiritual environment
- human needs assistance
- existential-phenomenological spiritual forces

The caring nurse assists the patient in developing to the greatest potential and gives the patient the freedom to make choices. Caring contributes to the growth of trust. The nurse must recognize that the patient is an individual and not a diagnosis. The nurse must also respect the patient.

Family members also need to feel a sense of caring from the nurse. Families that are providing care to a family member who is dying sometimes express fear and concern about what is happening to their loved one. The nurse is the person who spends the most time and communicates with the family. An honest, caring approach is the best way to assist the family.

Trust

Trust is the "assured belief that other individuals are capable of assisting in times of distress and will probably do so" (Travelbee 1971, 80). Trust may appear as attitudes, beliefs, and behaviors. A therapeutic relationship always begins with trust. The nurse can help the patient to develop trust. Consistency and reliability are important characteristics in the development of trust (Sundeen, et al. 1998). Do not offer to do something that you as a nurse cannot complete. Be very specific about what the nurse will be able to do. For example, if the nurse tells a patient or caregiver to call if they need anything at all, that nurse must be available for any need that the patient or family may have. If this happens often, it can be detrimental to the nurse-patient trust relationship being developed.

Honesty is invaluable in developing trust. As nurses are faced with questions from patients or families, correct, accurate answers are essential. If the nurse does not know the answer to a question, the nurse should admit that and offer to try to find the correct answer. Most often patients know their conditions and are waiting to talk to someone about it. If the nurse is not completely honest, the patient will know that. This will not allow the patient to develop trust in that nurse.

Empathy

Empathy is the ability of a person to perceive and understand another person's feelings and emotions accurately. Empathetic nurses are able to identify or communicate the meanings of feelings through verbal or nonverbal behavior. They can identify and feel the patient's emotions but at the same time maintain their own identity. If nurses overidentify with the feelings of the patient, they lose objectivity and the ability to help the patient. The nurse must remember that the patient's feelings belong to the patient and not the nurse (Boggs 1999).

Mutuality

Mutuality is simple sharing with another person. In this nurse-patient relationship, the two identify and agree on the patient's health problems and means to resolve them, working together to enrich the patient's health status. In mutuality, the patient is involved in all aspects of developing the unique individualized nursing plan of care and thus all phases of the nursing process (Boggs, 1999). The nurse should be truly sensitive to the patient's feelings, and accept and respect the patient's lifestyle.

Confidentiality

Confidentiality is not only an ethical responsibility in health care but also a legal issue. Patient information, including history, current problems, treatment plans, and prognosis, is strictly confidential and can only be shared with members of the health care team that provides care to the patient. In the nurse-patient relationship, the patient trusts the nurse with intimate information and expects the nurse to protect his or her right to privacy. Only pertinent information necessary to plan the patient's care should be kept. This information is not to be shared with friends, family, or health care providers not directly involved in care.

THERAPEUTIC COMMUNICATION

Establishing a therapeutic relationship with a dying patient is a privilege for the nurse. Therefore the relationship must be open, honest, and sincere. This must be accomplished through therapeutic communication, the purpose of which is to assist the patients in more effectively coping in relationships with others (Boggs 1999).

Peplau (1960) described the importance of therapeutic conversation as a method of making the illness bearable and promoting the natural healing powers of a person. It also allows the nurse the opportunity to become a companion on the illness journey and help the patient to achieve well-being through communication (Pearson, Borbasi, and Walsh 1997). Expressing problems, feelings, and emotions allows the patient to discover problem-solving methods related to health and receive feedback in a caring manner. This allows the patient to discover meaning in suffering and determine what is truly important in life (Boggs 1999). Table 16–1 lists techniques to apply in a therapeutic conversation.

Listening

The most important and effective technique in therapeutic communication is *listening*. The only way nurses can identify patients' needs is to incorporate active listening, a technique that gives them the ability to allow a patient to express thoughts, feelings, and emotions. This technique requires that the nurse be able to

- hear what the patient says
- understand the meaning of the message
- provide the patient with feedback regarding the message (Arnold 1999)

Active listening requires critical thinking to gain a clear understanding of the patient's perspective. The nurse should utilize the tone in the patient's voice, the pauses in the conversation, and their own intuition in understanding the patient's message, and request feedback from the patient to determine if these observations are accurate. Active listening results in less misunderstandings, effective use of time, and more accurate information (Arnold 1999).

As the relationship continues to develop, the patient may become weaker and experience more physical changes and problems. It is important to keep the physical problems, such as pain, to a minimum to allow the patient to be

TABLE 16–1	COMMUNICATION TECHNIQUES TO APPLY IN A THERAPEUTIC CONVERSATION

1. Always start initial contact on a formal note. Introduce yourself and give your credentials.
2. Use direct eye contact.
3. Use good posture, leaning torso slightly toward patient. Position yourself on same level as the patient.
4. Create the right setting. Find a private, comfortable place to have a conversation.
5. Use open gestures and open-ended questions.
6. Use nonverbal cues such as smiling and nodding.
7. Respond empathetically with active listening.
8. Follow the patient's lead concerning receptiveness to discuss diagnosis or prognosis. Use minimal cues.
9. Use vocabulary that the patient can understand.
10. Keep messages clear, concise, and honest.
11. Nonverbal messages should support verbal messages.
12. Ask the patient for verbal feedback to validate understanding.

able to focus on any conversations. It is also of utmost importance to include family or significant others in as much of the conversation as possible.

The nurse should remember that discussing physical changes and the approaching death with the patient is very difficult. Nurses may be the very people that patients confide in when they feel like they are not doing well. The nurse may have to answer very difficult questions such as, "How much longer do I have?" The nurse must feel comfortable discussing issues about death and dying in order to answer these questions in an honest, caring manner. This in turn will provide much needed support to the patient.

NONVERBAL COMMUNICATION

Sending and receiving messages in a variety of ways without the use of words can be intentional and nonintentional. Examples of nonverbal communication that are recognized may include dress, body movement, emotional state, posture, gestures, facial expressions, eye contact, and touch. The culture of the person you are caring for will dictate some of the proper and acceptable nonverbal communication.

Proper, professional dress is required in the profession of nursing. Even when you are visiting patients in their homes, you should be dressed appropriately. Usually your employer will have a dress code policy. It is the nurse's professional responsibility to dress appropriately when approaching a patient or family members.

Body movement can indicate attitude and is part of your message. Are you facing the person you are speaking to? Are you leaning toward the person or away from the person? Your posture is part of your body movement. Are you rigid? Are you slouching?

Emotional state is important in nonverbal communication. Are you relaxed? Are you in a hurry? Are you nervous or uncomfortable? Are you jiggling coins in your pocket? Are you gazing at the television or staring outside? Are you bored? All of these are important aspects that are interpreted by the patient. Patients have expressed at times that the nurse was very kind and caring because of the tears that were shed during a touching moment. These moments are precious to the patient and family and relay an important message.

Gestures are important in caring for the dying patient and family. Nurses should use open, relaxed gestures when in their presence, keeping in mind the culture of the patient and family. What is acceptable in the United States is not always accepted in other countries. For example, when pointing, Americans use the index finger, Germans use the little finger, and Japanese the entire hand.

Facial expressions provide clues to our own feelings. Although facial expressions are identical from culture to culture, their meaning is different. For example, some see animated expressions as a sign of a lack of control, too much smiling is viewed as a sign of shallowness, and women smile more than men.

Eye contact and gaze show respect in some cultures but not in others. Western cultures view direct eye contact as positive, Arabic cultures believe eye contact shows interest and allows them to understand the truthfulness of the other person, whereas in Japan, Africa, Latin American, and the Caribbean, eye contact is avoided to show respect. In the United States, eye contact delineates the degree of attention, impacts persuasion, helps to control interaction, transfers emotion, and allows for the surveillance of impressions of others.

The basic message of touch is to affect or control an exchange of information. Touch can be used to protect, support, or disapprove. Different cultures view touch differently. In the United States, a handshake, a hug, or a kiss is common. Cultures with a high level of emotional restraint have little public touch, such as English, German, Scandinavian, and Chinese. Cultures that advocate a high level of emotion such as Latino, Middle East, and Jewish accept and enjoy frequent touches.

Just as the nurse can interpret nonverbal communication in the patient and family members, they too can interpret our nonverbal communication. Maintain awareness of the messages you are sending, since these messages can make a very big difference in the relationship with the patient and their journey to a peaceful death.

UNDERSTANDING METAPHORS

As the illness progresses and the patient approaches death, conversations change. Patients may appear to be confused or make no sense. Family, friends, and health care providers who are not experienced in caring for the dying may label these irrational conversations as "confusion" or "hallucinations." But they may not be.

The dying person may instead be trying to give us information about what is being experienced. In order to understand and comprehend these messages, you must listen closely and gather information about the metaphors they express. Our understanding of the messages may relieve the dying person's anxiety or stress. Also, the family and friends can develop more comprehension about what the patient is experiencing in the dying process and what they can do to help the patient to a peaceful death. Health care professionals who understand these messages will be able to provide better care to the dying and achieve a sense of satisfaction. Callanan and Kelley (1992) have identified this experience as "nearing death awareness." They have categorized these messages into two groups: attempts to describe what a dying person is experiencing, and requests for what the dying need for a peaceful death.

In an attempt to describe what a dying person is experiencing, the dying may describe a glance of another world and those who are there. The description may be very vague but the dying will describe with "amazement" and "astonishment" the peace and beauty in this other place. The dying may also talk with or be in the presence of people we cannot see, often people they have known in their lives. They may also see or speak to a spiritual figure. This may make them feel very peaceful and loved. They may also feel a gentle serenity during these experiences. The dying will sometimes review their lives. This process helps them find meaning in their lives and an understanding of the meaning. Once patients realize that they are dying, they focus their concern on family and friends left behind. At this point, the dying person does not seem to fear death (Callanan and Kelley 1992).

The second category consists of the need for reconciliation of personal, spiritual, or moral relationships, and removing some barrier to allow for peace.

To understand the message, the nurse should ask the patient questions about the things they are experiencing. The following are true accounts of patients who have had experiences and how the nurse was instrumental in deciphering these messages. These accounts of patients' experiences will help the student to develop insight so they may recognize messages from the dying. (Fictional names have been substituted to protect confidentiality of the patients.)

Presence of Someone Not Alive

Pop.   At the age of 45, Pop (affectionately named by his two toddler grand-children) was diagnosed with advanced arteriosclerosis and renal failure. Af-ter one kidney was removed and one leg was amputated, he proceeded with his life in a normal fashion. He had a great four years before he finally became ill enough to approach dying. He was hospitalized for the last three weeks of his life. During this time he made peace with his wife and children. He visited with some of his siblings. Two days before he died, he began a conversation with his mother. They planned a trip to Amsterdam. He smiled and even laughed a little as he carried on this conversation. He was at peace and very comfortable during this time. It is important to note that Pop's mother had died 18 years earlier, and it is suspected that she died of the same illness. Pop died in 1978. As a family member, I attributed his conversation to confusion secondary to renal failure at that time. Today, being able to understand that Pop wasn't alone when he died and that he felt a great sense of peace because of his mother's presence, allows me a certain sense of comfort and tranquility concerning his death.

Steven.   The hospice nurse was called to Steven's home. He was a hospice patient with colon cancer. He was very near death. His family was very dis-traught and requested that the nurse sedate him. When the nurse arrived, she found Steven sitting up in bed talking to someone sitting on the bed. (The nurse could not see this person sitting on the bed.) In his conversation, he mentioned the name "T-Boy." Steven's hands were moving across the bed as if he was passing something out. He did not appear to be in any emotional or physical distress. In fact, he appeared very happy and content. The family ex-plained that T-Boy was a beloved nephew and had been killed in an automo-bile accident two years previously. One of Steven and T-Boy's favorite activi-ties was playing a local card game called bouree. The nurse explained that the patient was comfortable and displayed no fear. She also told the family that these conversations occurred often in this stage of the dying process. This helped the family to accept Steven's behavior, and they even referred to this behavior as a blessing.

Monique.   Monique was a 32-year-old African American mother of two young children. She survived her breast cancer after two years of chemotherapy and radiation. During that time, she became extremely ill and was sent home to die. Instead, she overcame the illness. After recuperating, Monique related a story about a beautiful, gentle "woman" in a white flowing gown who stood by her bed the entire time she was ill. The woman looked at her constantly and smiled at her. Monique said that the woman gave her a sense of tranquility and peace and alleviated any fear that she had. Several months later, Monique became much weaker, and hospice was consulted. As death became imminent, the hospice nurse visited often. During a visit in the last few days of Monique's life, the nurse asked her if the beautiful woman was with her.

Monique smiled and had a dreamy, peaceful expression on her face when she replied that the woman had been with her for several days. Monique never became uncomfortable and eventually died very peacefully with her children at her bedside.

Naomi.   My first hospice patient was Naomi, a 69-year-old mother of three dying of pancreatic cancer. I visited them with a preceptor. The daughters were very loving and had been taking turns caring for their mother. The father was disabled and could not assist very much. I listened along with the oldest daughter as my preceptor answered questions the family asked. At this time, Naomi was comatose and unresponsive. The daughter informed us that the last words she could understand her mother to say was something concerning angels. The preceptor explained to the family that angels are recurring themes in conversations with the dying. The daughter stated that her mother had a peaceful and contented manner about her and had not experienced any agitation or anxiety during this time. Naomi died the next morning. When I arrived, the daughters were gathered at the kitchen table talking about the angels they had seen the night before. They were grateful that the angels had come for their mother. As a scientific nurse, I decided that this was a group hysterical reaction and the family may need some serious counseling. Little did I know, the angel theme recurred fairly often. I came to realize that there is an entity that appears to the patient. The patients may gesture, pat hands, stroke hair, or cradle something in their arms. This is the only time I have had family members visualize angels. That vision brought this family serenity and peace in saying goodbye to their mother.

Preparing for Travel or Change

John.   John was a 55-year-old truck driver. He was married and had three children, a son and two daughters. John was diagnosed with colon cancer with liver metastasis. He underwent chemotherapy with very poor results. Within two months, John was very near death. As he neared death, he began stating that he had to follow the truck route to get to the "new place." He also stated that he would not be returning. Once the nurse helped the family to understand what he was saying, they were able to let John go. John and the family were able to experience a peaceful death.

A Place that Only They Can See

Jimmy.   Jimmy, a four year old, lived with his parents and an eight-year-old brother, when he was diagnosed with a neuroblastoma. He underwent chemotherapy for a year and finally a bone marrow transplant, after which he was in remission. Within a few months, however, the cancer had reoccurred. Chemotherapy was again reinstituted as the primary treatment. Jimmy became very weak and had more intense side effects from the treatment. His parents were offered another bone marrow transplant but were warned that the chances of survival were less than 10%. After much discussion concerning the side effects and possible toxic effects, the decision to stop treatment was made. Jimmy was very instrumental in making the decision. He went home and for several months was very active. He helped his mother plant flowers in the garden and tended the flowers through the spring. During the summer, the temperature soared. Unfortunately the flowers that Jimmy planted with his mother died, unable to survive the heat. As August approached, Jimmy became very weak. By the second week of August, he was dying. During the dying process, Jimmy repeatedly told his mother that he had to go to his new house, the house with the beautiful flowers. Jimmy was telling his mother that he was going to a peaceful place, a new house with beautiful flowers. Despite the pain associated with grief, Jimmy's mother had a sense of comfort about his death.

Knowledge of When They Will Die

Joey.   Joey was a 28 year old with a wife, Janet, but no children. They had been married for three years when they decided to begin their family. After trying for six months, they decided to see a physician. The diagnostic studies revealed non-Hodgkins lymphoma. Joey and Janet were devastated. Joey was referred to a medical oncologist who immediately began chemotherapy. Joey completed the chemotherapy and did rather well for about a year. During a routine examination by the oncologist, it was discovered that Joey's lymphoma recurred. After another round of aggressive treatment, Joey, Janet, and the oncologist decided that hospice was a better option. Joey was admitted to the hospice program in March. He declined very rapidly. By July 1, he was very near death. In one conversation with Janet, Joey expressed his desire to "just get the dying part over with." Janet asked Joey to "hang on" until July 4 when his parents would be there. Joey told Janet that he would not be around for July 4. Janet listened to Joey's message and immediately told his parents what he said; they arrived about six hours before he died—on July 3. They were able to spend time with Joey before he died and help Janet provide care during his last hours. This allowed Joey a peaceful death, and his parents and Janet were able to bring about a sense of satisfaction and fulfillment in providing care to Joey.

Claire.   The hospice doctor and nurse visited Claire on a Friday morning. She appeared very near death. The doctor explained what probably would happen in the next 24 to 48 hours. On Monday, the nurse called and was surprised that Claire was still alive. In the background, she could hear party sounds. The son told the nurse that she would not believe what was going on, but she was welcome to visit any time. Upon arrival, the nurse saw that the house was full of friends and family. She said that she had not seen so many people at Claire's home before. Claire was propped up in bed, makeup on, not a hair out of place, telling jokes. A birthday party for Claire was indeed in progress.

Claire's vital signs were good and she denied any pain or discomfort. Her son said that this party had been going on since Saturday. Claire said that she had a dream in which she could see that she was wrapped up in a blanket and taken out through the window and placed in a hearse. Before she arrived at the funeral home, her husband, who had died two months earlier, told her that she could not join him yet because the funeral home was busy and the tomb was not ready. But then he said that everything would be ready in 10 days. Her son told the nurse that unknown to Claire, work had been done on the tomb and the mortar was still wet. Also the funeral home in the small town was indeed very busy and could not have handled another death that weekend. Claire had a pleasant week with her family. She died a few minutes before the start of the 11th day.

Need for Reconciliation of Person, Spiritual, or Moral Relationships

Joseph.   Joseph was a 79-year-old man married to Rose, and they had six children. Joseph was diagnosed with prostate cancer with bone metastasis. He was quickly approaching death and was admitted to the hospital to die. Rose was with Joseph every minute. He became very restless and unsettled. Joseph was a spiritual man but had not been to church in several years. During a conversation with Joseph's nurse, Rose mentioned this to the nurse and told her that this was something that really worried him. The nurse quickly checked his records and found that he was Catholic and that he had not seen a priest since he became ill. The nurse called pastoral services and relayed this information. Not only did the priest see Joseph, but he also said Mass in the room for Joseph and his family. Joseph became calm and relaxed. He died peacefully a few days later, with Rose at his side.

Sophie.   Sophie was an 84 year old with no major health problems. She cared for herself and a pet Pekinese. Sophie brought her Pekinese to the veterinarian and left him to be groomed. While she was backing out of the parking lot, a car slammed into the left side of her car. Emergency surgery was performed, but Sophie developed severe complications, and it soon became apparent that she would not survive. The physician insisted that Sophie continue to be ventilated so the family could visit before she died. She was bleeding from every orifice, her heart rhythm was agonal, and her pupils were dilated and fixed. The nurse strategically placed towels to hide the blood so the family could see her. Sophie's two sons, grandchildren, and siblings took turns visiting. Her chaplain arrived and all the family gathered around her to pray. The chaplain prayed and began to sing a hymn very softly near her ear while he put his hand on her forehead. Just as the chaplain finished the song, Sophie died. Her granddaughter leaned over and kissed Sophie's forehead and said, "You were waiting to be blessed and for us to be here." The family tearfully and peacefully left the hospital.

Removing a Barrier to Allow for Peace

Sarah.   Sarah was a 55-year-old woman who had never been married. She had lived with her homosexual significant other (Donna) for the last 18 years and her dog named Blue. Sarah drove a tractor-trailer cross-country with Blue for 25 years until she was diagnosed with sarcoma of the left hip. She underwent aggressive treatment for several months with very little improvement in combating the disease. Sarah eventually became a hospice patient and moved in with her sister (Ann) and her family. Once Sarah's pain and symptoms were controlled, she began to enjoy her time there. Ann and her family were very supportive and also enjoyed her being in their home. But Ann could not accept Sarah's lifestyle and would not let Donna visit Sarah. As Sarah's health declined and she neared death, she became more and more restless. Even constant around-the-clock sedation did not relieve her restlessness. One day while the nurse was visiting, Sarah said that she could see her mother at the top of the mountain but she couldn't reach her because of the boulders in the way. The nurse explored this a little more and asked Sarah what boulders were in the way and what did she need to get around the boulders. Her only reply was "Donna." The nurse talked to Ann and explained that Sarah was miserable and really needed to see Donna. When she told Ann that this pain caused as much discomfort to Sarah as the cancer pain did, Ann relented. Donna was called immediately and arrived at their home within 30 minutes. Sarah became very calm and died peacefully within a week. During the last days of Sarah's life, Donna continued to visit during the day and helped Ann care for Sarah. During these days, Donna and Ann became friends. At Sarah's funeral they provided support for each other. Donna still visits Ann, her family, and Blue occasionally. Sarah needed Ann's cooperation and she needed reconciliation between the important members of her family before she died. The nurse was instrumental in helping her achieve this goal by listening and understanding the message sent.

Luke.   Luke and Elaine lived in a small home next to a wooded area. They fed birds, rabbits, and squirrels, which provided many hours of enjoyment for them. Luke had been diagnosed with lung cancer during the prior year. One of Luke's great pleasures was to put food out for the wild rabbits that lived in the woods. Over the years, the rabbits fed closer and closer to the home. Luke became weaker from his illness but continued to feed the rabbits. Eventually Luke became too ill to feed the rabbits, so Elaine would feed them for him. As he approached death, he became very restless and anxious. Elaine assured him that she would continue to feed his rabbits. Elaine and the family gathered at the bedside to say goodbye as Luke was dying. A granddaughter happened to look out of a window. The yard was full of rabbits facing the window to Luke's bedroom. Imagine looking out of your bedroom at twilight and seeing all of those rabbits on your lawn just staring back at you! When Luke's granddaughter told everyone about the rabbits in the yard, Luke's breathing changed. He died moments later. The granddaughter again looked out of the window and the rabbits were disappearing into the woods. They had said goodbye also.

IMPORTANT COMMUNICATION STRATEGIES FOR CAREGIVERS AT DEATH

It is very difficult to be a caregiver, a family member, or significant other and wait for a loved one to die. Oftentimes the dying person holds onto life even when the quality of life is very poor. This is painful for the caregiver, family members, and significant other to endure because they want the patient to experience a peaceful death. The nurse should examine the environment. Are they talking about the patient where the patient may hear them? Just because the patient is in a coma and cannot verbally respond does not mean that they can't hear what is being discussed. A good rule to follow would be to limit discussion to things you would only want the patient to hear. It would be ideal if the last words the dying person heard were from important people in their life saying, "I/we love you," or "Now you can have peace," or "We will miss you," rather than hearing the family divide up the patient's personal belongings. These patients know they are dying and do not need constant reminding from family and friends.

If the patient is not experiencing physical discomfort, then look for some spiritual problem. The patient usually is not experiencing fear but is concerned about the people being left behind. Sometimes family and friends need to give the patient permission to die or they may need to know that someone will be helping the family get through the experience. Families and friends will need help with this as it is very hard to say these things. Give them suggestions on how to phrase statements such as, "I hate that this is happening, but I don't want to see you endure anymore than you already have. You can go if you are ready. The family will help each other and we will be all right." These types of statements convey love, caring, support, and regret. Patients will relax and die peacefully when the family allows them to.

SUMMARY

Communication is the most important aspect in a relationship. It is how we express our feelings and emotions and how we get feedback from others. Both verbal and nonverbal communication are essential in the therapeutic relationship between the patient and nurse. The nurse has a responsibility to foster this relationship and promote therapeutic communication with the dying patient. This may be the very thing that allows a person to die peacefully and with dignity.

REFERENCES

Arnold, E. (1999). Structuring the relationship. In E. Arnold and K. U. Boggs (Eds.), *Interpersonal Relationships: Professional Communication Skills for Nurses* (3rd ed., pp. 80–106). Philadelphia, PA: W.B. Saunders Company.

Boggs, K. U. (1999). Bridges and barriers in the therapeutic relationship. In E. Arnold and K. U. Boggs (Eds.), *Interpersonal Relationships: Professional Communication Skills for Nurses* (3rd ed. pp. 107–126). Philadelphia, PA: W.B. Saunders Company.

Callanan, M., & Kelley, P. (1992). *Final gifts: Understanding the special awareness, needs, and communication of the dying.* New York: Bantam Books.

Pearson, A., Borbasi, S., & Walsh, K. (1997). Practicing nursing therapeutically through acting as a skilled companion on the illness journey. *Advanced Practice Nursing Quarterly, 3*(1), 46–52.

Peplau, H. (1960). Talking with patients. *American Journal of Nursing, 60*(7), 964–966.

Rodwell, C. (1996). An analysis of the concept of empowerment. *Journal of Advanced Nursing, 23*(2), 305–313.

Sundeen, S. J., Stuart, G. W., Rankin, E. A. D., & Cohen, S. A. (1998). *Nurse-client interaction: Implementing the nursing process.* St. Louis, MO: Mosby, Inc.

Travelbee, J. (1971). *Interpersonal aspects of nursing.* Philadelphia, PA: F. A. Davis Company.

Watson, J. (1988). *Nursing: Human science and human care.* New York: National League for Nursing.

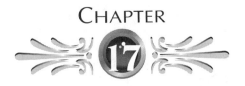

COMMUNICATION WITH DYING PATIENTS AND FAMILY MEMBERS: A BODY, MIND, AND SPIRIT APPROACH

Karen Borne

Dearest Lord, may I see you today and every day in the person of your sick, and whilst nursing them minister unto you.

Though you hide yourself behind the unattractive disguise of the irritable, the exacting, the unreasonable, may I still recognize you and say: "Jesus, my patient, how sweet it is to serve you."

Lord, give me this seeing faith, then my work will never be monotonous. I will ever find joy in humoring the fancies and gratifying the wishes of all poor sufferers. . . .

Sweetest Lord, make me appreciative of the dignity of my high vocation and its many responsibilities. Never permit me to disgrace it by giving way to coldness, unkindness, or impatience. . . .

Lord, increase my faith, bless my efforts and work, now and for evermore.

Daily prayer of Mother Teresa of Calcutta

The resurgence of religion and spirituality in the late 20th century has expanded the role of health care professionals to include caring for the "total person"—not just physical needs, but spiritual and emotional needs as well. Caring for a patient's body, mind, and spirit becomes of paramount importance as the patient nears the end of life, especially when he has opted for palliative care.

Palliative care, or comfort care, is a relatively modern concept in Western medicine. The dictionary defines palliative as "to relieve the symptoms or effects of without curing, as a disease; alleviate; mitigate." Palliative care provides relief to a terminally ill person usually by managing symptoms or pain but without seeking a cure. True palliative care also addresses the patient's emotional, mental, and spiritual needs, as well as the needs of loved ones. The emphasis is on quality of life rather than on death.

Whole books can and have been written on the concept of total person care for the terminal patient. As with other kinds of care, clear, compassionate communication with patients and family members is vital. In this chapter we will discuss the special needs that dying patients and their families have for in-depth communication, and describe the elements of effective communication at this time of transition for patients and their loved ones.

THE NEED FOR COMPASSIONATE COMMUNICATION—JANE'S STORY

Jane lost three loved ones within a five-year period. Her father died of cancer in 1994, her brother suffered a lengthy and painful death due to bone cancer in 1997, and her mother died from Alzheimer's disease in 1999. As the primary caregiver for all three patients, she dealt with health care professionals in hospitals, hospices, assisted living centers, and home health agencies.

Jane found the level of care in hospitals to be inferior. Shorthanded, overworked staff had little time to give patients the necessary attention. Laws prevent patients from being restrained to keep them from getting out of bed or pulling out IVs and catheters. As a result, the level of such incidents in hospitals is much higher than in private care facilities.

The staff at the assisted living residence was also limited. Yet they wanted to keep Jane's mother in the facility until they absolutely could no longer care for her. Family members were led to believe she was being cared for properly, when actually the level of care required was far greater than the facility could offer. Oftentimes, the patient suffered as a result.

Jane's experience with hospice was superior. "Hospice staffers were most informed and professional with regard to terminally ill people, the family, and the level of care required in the final weeks or months," she said. "What sets hospice apart from other health care providers is an unconditional concern for the patient's comfort and peace of mind. The hospice staff pulls out all stops to make sure the family is kept informed of the patient's condition and any changes that indicate finality. They work closely with the family to educate them, especially if the family members have never experienced the death of a loved one. There are many signs indicating when death is near, and hospice makes the family aware of those signs and prepares them to accept the ensuing death."

While electing to have live-in home health care providers was not something Jane took on lightly, she found the experience rewarding. During her mother's last three weeks, she had two exceptional caregivers. Although they were not RNs, they were experienced in caring for the terminally ill and dealing with the family. "They were attentive to Mother's needs. They kept her clean, well groomed, and fed to the extent she would eat. They spent much time by her bedside, assuring her she was loved and had lived a long and happy life. They listened when she wanted to talk, held her hand, and sang to and with her. These people were essentially strangers to Mother at first, but she came to know, love, and trust them. Of course, she had a favorite, and when she slipped into a coma approximately 12 hours prior to her death, she would not die until her favorite arrived to see her off. Then she died within an hour or so of her favorite's arrival."

According to Jane, the key to being a good health care professional is not the level of medical care administered, but the level of emotional and spiritual care given by spending time with the patient and showing concern for the family. "Caring for a terminally ill patient requires you to assume the role of the patient's best friend, the last link here on earth, apart from the family," she said. "The caregiver must assure the dying person that his family will be okay, and that it is okay for the patient to die. Otherwise, the patient views dying as doing an injustice to the family he has loved all his life."

Jane's story is an excellent example of the inherent value of communication as a part of palliative care. Notice the phrases she used about her positive experiences:

- "unconditional concern for the patient's comfort and peace of mind"
- "family is kept informed of the patient's condition"
- "work closely with the family to educate them"
- "prepares them to accept the ensuing death"
- "attentive to Mother's needs"
- "spent much time by her bedside, assuring her she was loved"
- "listened when she wanted to talk, held her hand"

Interestingly enough, Jane did not once mention curing the patient or prolonging life.

THE CONSEQUENCES OF POOR COMMUNICATION—ANN'S STORY

Ann is a 38-year-old woman who has undergone numerous surgeries on her shoulders, back, and reproductive system. After her back surgery, she became addicted to painkillers and was admitted to rehabilitation. As a result, her physicians became very cautious when prescribing pain medication, even to the point of denying her medications when they believed she was displaying addictive behavior.

After Ann's most recent surgery, a hysterectomy, she received only limited pain medication. Angry and perplexed, she felt betrayed and abandoned by her physician and the hospital staff, who she thought were overreacting and unwilling to accommodate her needs. According to Ann, the nurses were "unwilling to communicate" with her and even referred to her as "hysterical." In fact, her most painful memory is her sense that "no one would listen or empathize" with what she was going through.

Unfortunately, this experience has impacted her life far more than a typical unpleasant memory. She now fears future hospitalizations and dwells on her mortality and the possibility of pain associated with dying. She even has panic and anxiety attacks due to her experience.

Ann's story illustrates the importance of not jumping to conclusions about a patient's condition or needs. Although she survived her surgery and is doing well physically, the trauma of facing a painful surgery and recovery period with inadequate medication has had long-term psychological consequences—which could have been avoided with a little caring, empathetic communication.

TOOLS FOR EFFECTIVE COMMUNICATION

Try Therapeutic Listening.   The first step in communicating effectively with your patient is to listen. We all know how frustrating it is to pour out our hearts to someone and know they haven't heard a word we've said. How many wives have experienced the total frustration of talking to their husbands through the morning newspaper? Think how much more frustrating it must be for a dying person to speak to a preoccupied nurse.

Early in my training at Texas Children's Hospital, I visited Susan, a 10-year-old girl with end-stage cystic fibrosis. Although I knew she had lived most of her life in and out of the hospital, I wasn't aware how near death she was. I decided to "cheer her up" by playing a board game with her in her room. I noticed that she was extremely short-tempered (she threw a tantrum when I won the game), and she was abrupt and even rude to the aide who brought her lunch tray. I was ill-prepared to deal with such an angry little girl, and I became irritated and left her room, vowing never to return. Two weeks later, I was stunned to learn that Susan had passed away. I experienced a wide range of emotions, from inadequacy (I should have known what to say or do to make her life better) to guilt (Why wasn't I more understanding? How could I have been so judgmental?).

As this example shows, listening, really listening, is not that easy. I have spent 16 years of my professional life as a human resource recruiter and have interviewed hundreds of people. Yet after I finished my training as a chaplain (and learned from my experience with patients like Susan), my recruits began telling me they had never met a recruiter like me before. When asked why, they replied, "Because you really listen to me. I no longer feel like just a number."

This is active listening. It is more than just hearing and it requires more skill. The active listener is aware of feelings without losing the thread of the conversation.

One of the most important listening skills I learned in the chaplain training program was this: You can't listen to someone if you are talking all the time. The first rule of active, therapeutic listening is to stop talking.

Here are some other steps you can take to make your listening easier and more effective:

1. Focus on the person speaking. Even if your time is limited, you must learn to take your mind off the dozens of tasks awaiting you, set the needs of your other patients aside, and forget about your tired feet and aching back—even for a moment—while you focus on one patient or family member.
2. Eliminate distractions. Nothing is worse than trying to talk to someone who is reading or watching television. A dying patient may be too weak to speak loudly enough to be heard over the interference. Ask permission to turn off the radio, TV, etc. If the room is full of visitors, come back at another time.
3. Create a supportive environment. Give up any judgments you may have about the patient, the condition, the clinical severity of the symptoms, or anything else that may affect your ability to hear the patient's concerns. Offer your unconditional acceptance and caring. You may not agree with the person, but you can respect how he feels.
4. Sit at eye level. If the person speaking is in bed, bring a chair to the bedside so you are not hovering above him. Most caregivers avoid actually sitting on the patient's bed to avoid the risk of pulling out tubes, etc. Use common sense.
5. Listen to understand the person, not just the problem. The dying patient needs you to understand him as a person, not as a "case" or a set of symptoms. You may not be able to solve the patient's problem— you may not even be able to make him feel better—but you can listen and show him that you understand.

As an active listener, you can become a catalyst for the patient to grow and learn new things about himself. Active listening shows the patient that you have connected with his emotions and moods. This sense of connection allows the patient to feel free to go deeper into the emotional/spiritual realm where true healing can take place.

Adopt the Patient's Point of View. You'll be a more effective communicator if you can see things from the patient's and family's point of view. Only then can you begin to establish the level of trust required to get them to openly communicate their needs. The following list offers suggestions for nurses to incorporate in their care of the dying:

*   Focus on patient's diagnosis symptoms.
*   Focus on the patient in a holistic manner (physical, mental, emotional, spiritual aspects).
*   Focus on overall daily care of the patient.
*   Focus on promoting comfort in the patient's environment.

- Focus on caregiver needs.
- Focus on multidisciplinary team approach with patient, family, and caregivers.
- Focus on nurse advocacy roles.

Try to put yourself in your patient's world. This new point of view will make you a more effective communicator and also a more effective nurse.

Offer Empathy, Not Sympathy. Just because you adopt the patient's point of view doesn't mean you should be sympathetic. It is important to distinguish between empathy and sympathy.

Sympathy means being affected by or having the same feelings as the patient. You may experience your patient's sense of loss, anger, fear, or sadness, and this might make you feel as if you are connecting with your patient. However, as a result you may both be hurting and you may be rendered ineffective, which will not help your patient in the long run.

Empathy means grasping the content of the problem and the patient's feelings without becoming caught up in those feelings. You can be understanding yet objective at the same time. Empathy will allow you to guide patients in coming up with their own solution or answer.

Table 17–1 identifies responses that indicate feelings of sympathy and empathy.

Several circumstances require particularly empathetic responses (Stephen Ministry Training Manual 1991, 186):

1. Responding to a care receiver's denial of death

    Care Receiver: "I know somebody got the test results mixed up. That's the only logical explanation for it."

    Caregiver: "It sure would be great if you found out that they made a mistake."

TABLE 17–1 RESPONSES THAT INDICATE FEELINGS OF SYMPATHY AND EMPATHY

WHEN I FEEL SYMPATHY . . .	WHEN I SHOW EMPATHY. . . .
I fix, protect, rescue, control, carry the other person's feelings, don't listen.	I encourage, share, confront, am sensitive to the other person's feelings, listen.
I feel tired, anxious, fearful, liable.	I feel relaxed, free, high self-esteem.
I am concerned with solutions, answers, being right, details, performance.	I am concerned with feelings, relationships, communicating, sharing myself, the person.
I am a manipulator.	I am a helper-guide.
I expect the person to live up to my expectations, and I feel compelled to stay in control of the situation.	I expect the person to be responsible for himself and his own actions, and I can trust and let go.

Care Receiver: "This can't be happening to me. I'm only 40 years old. I've got a lot of years left."

Caregiver: "You don't expect news like this when you're still in your prime."

2. Responding to the care receiver's anger

Care Receiver: "Why do you bother coming here? I don't need to see you. I'm fed up with this."

Caregiver: "You're pretty angry and fed up with the situation you're in. It must be a very difficult time for you right now."

3. Accepting the care receiver's concern without "playing along" or arguing

Care Receiver: "If you ask me, God is no better than the devil. God enjoys seeing people suffer. I've got no use for a God who causes so much pain."

Caregiver: "Well, for one reason or another, God certainly allows some terrible things to happen. There's no doubt about that."

Care Receiver: "It says in the Bible that God is love. I find that pretty hard to swallow right now. If God really loved us, He wouldn't let things like this happen."

Caregiver: "With some of the things that happen on this earth, it can seem like God isn't around. But I still have faith in a loving God."

Encourage Honest Sharing. If you follow the guidelines discussed so far, you will probably find that your patient is much more willing to open up and share real concerns, private fears, and deepest needs. The following techniques will help you probe further (Stephen Ministry Training Manual 1991, 23):

1. Ask open-ended questions. How did you feel about that? How are you feeling right now? What's going on inside of you? How do you feel about that deep down? When open-ended questions don't work, try more specific closed questions that focus on the patient's feelings, such as: Are you feeling angry right now? Did you feel frustrated at that point?

2. Listen for the message, not the words. Is your patient communicating physical, emotional, or spiritual messages? Become accustomed to identifying key words or phrases (p. 27):

   * Physically oriented words: alert, alive, aroused, beat, breathless, cold, comfortable, energetic, hungry, hot, hurt, ill, jittery, lethargic, listless, nervous, relaxed, shaky, sick, sleepy, stiff, tense, warm, weak, well, wide-awake

   * Emotionally oriented words: afraid, aggravated, agitated, alarmed, angry, annoyed, anxious, bitter, calm, confused, distraught, embarrassed, excited, frightened, frustrated, glad, grieved, happy, horrified, hurt, miserable, resentful, sad, scared, tense, terrified, upset

- Spiritually oriented words: alive, awakened, committed, dead, despairing, detached, downhearted, empty, fearful, guilty, helpless, hopeful, hopeless, insecure, joyful, lonely, lost, loving, peaceful, powerless, redeemed, repentant, secure, strong, thankful, touched, unsure, whole

3. Reflect or "mirror" the person's feelings. Show the person that you understand by responding with a nonjudgmental statement that reflects those feelings (p. 23):

Care Receiver: "I'm so down. I just have so many bills to pay."

Caregiver: "You're feeling pretty depressed about your money problems."

Care Receiver: "I'm sick and tired of this hospital! When will I ever get out?"

Caregiver: "It really must be frustrating for you to be in the hospital."

Care Receiver: "Ever since I've been here, I've been on a strict diet—1,000 calories a day with no sweets and no spices of any kind."

Caregiver: "That does sound like a pretty strict diet. That must be quite a change from your regular eating habits."

This type of reassurance is equally effective with family members. In response to a relative's concern—whether expressed verbally or not—you can mirror feelings like this (p. 173):

Caregiver: "It sounds like you are afraid of what may happen to your wife in surgery tomorrow. You know, there's nothing wrong with having such fears in a situation like this. In fact, it's quite natural. If you'd like to talk about it, I'm willing to listen."

Caregiver: "You say you're feeling calm, but you've been pacing the floor. You know, even the strongest parent feels worried at a time like this."

These techniques for encouraging honest sharing aren't designed to force the person to open up. When you combine these methods with genuine empathy and active listening, you not only let the person know you understand and care, you also leave the door open for further discussion.

Patience, Patience, Patience.   Of course you're in a hurry. (Aren't we all?) If you know you are going to be involved in a meaningful conversation with someone, plan your time accordingly. Glancing at your watch every few minutes will not encourage someone to really open up to you. Sharing your time and undivided attention may do more to foster effective communication than any other skill or technique you could master.

Utilize All the Resources Available to You.   Communicating effectively with dying patients and their families is a huge responsibility. As a nurse involved with those patients on a daily basis, you are in an excellent position to understand and empathize with their feelings, encourage them to face fears and prepare for death, and help them to learn and grown from these experiences. Fortunately, you are not alone in this effort.

In *The Healing Power of Faith—Science Explores Medicine's Last Great Frontier,* Dr. Harold G. Koenig explores the power of faith in healing. According to his research, when older people were asked what enabled them to cope with their illness, between 24% and 42% mentioned religion; 70% of those who used religious coping said they used it to a large extent. Hospitalized patients who used religion to cope showed the lowest levels of depression, indicating that they were coping well with the stress of their illness. Orthopedic patients who received chaplain visits required 66% less pain medication, made two-thirds fewer calls on the nursing staff, and were discharged two days earlier than patients with similar diagnoses who received no chaplain visits.

Koenig (1999 page 118) reported that "severely ill patients who trust in God and pray acquire an indirect sense of control over their illness. This is probably because they are certain God is personally interested in them and answers their prayers." When religious people suffer severe illness, many angrily blame God while others turn to God for comfort. Koenig found that the angry responses usually were resolved, and people found comfort in their faith.

As an active, empathetic listener for your patients, you should be aware of and sensitive to their religious beliefs and need for spiritual counsel. Religious views are intimately connected with attitudes about death and suffering. It is imperative that you understand the patient's thinking if you are to minister effectively.

You may even want to read up on the wide variety of beliefs among the world's religions. This background will help you become a more effective communicator in a multicultural society. Whether your patient is a Christian who believes his soul is going to heaven or a Hindu who believes in reincarnation—and whether or not you agree with those beliefs—you want to be able to understand the spiritual concerns as death nears. When the time is right, you may want to offer to contact the hospital chaplain or the religious leader of the patient's choice.

Nurses must attend to the spiritual needs as well as the physical and psychological needs of patients and families. Palliative care for dying patients should use a multidisciplinary approach. In today's environment of managed care and short staffing, it is vital to use all the resources available to you.

REFERENCES

Koenig, H. G. (1999). *The healing power of faith—Science explores medicine's last great frontier.* New York: Simon & Schuster.

Stephen Ministry training manual. (1991). St. Louis, MO: Stephen Ministries, Inc.

CHAPTER 18

COMMUNICATING END OF LIFE ISSUES AMONG PROFESSIONALS

Camille Claibourne

We are all going to die. When and how are the only questions that are unanswerable and mysterious. Death is not a fun topic, often not easy to approach, and more often resisted until it is absolutely necessary. This chapter will examine ways that we can increase the opportunity to dialogue about the end of life, in order to improve patient care, increase advanced death planning, and further the discourse in society regarding death.

Death is not an easy subject for many reasons. Traditionally, textbooks for nursing and medical students contain very little information regarding this topic. In fact, a recent presenter in Portland, Oregon, stated that the nursing and medical textbooks allocated 2% to 5% of information on end of life and death discussions. With the growing number of patients dying in hospitals, we need more education in traditional programs. Simply stated, we have been trained to save lives. Death discussions often only happen when a terminal illness diagnosis has been established and we are forced to talk about it.

The U.S. population is living longer, as medical and technological advances identify methods to prolong life. The average life span has almost doubled in the past century and the 1990 U.S. Census Bureau identified 37,000 centenarians, a number predicted to double in 2000 (Perls and Silver 1999). Biotechnology and technological advances create a discourse within society about the ethics of extending life. In addition, health care consumers are becoming concerned with these changes, as the need to "control" their own lives increases. The mixture of these changes in the postmodern era creates opportunities for dialogue and discussion about life and death. Life and its extension is the by-product of many of these advances in health care. In addition, the aging of society coupled with technology is a recipe for end of life and death discussions.

Death is the term that should be used instead of an antonym that describes death. We often hear terms such as "passed away," "gone away," "gone to heaven," or other phrases that describe a process instead of the truthful statement: He or she died. Health care professionals should be the model in this regard by clearly communicating what subject matter we are talking about. By using the term *death*, we are clearly directing a conversation to the matter at hand. Knowing when and how to communicate end of life issues is both an art and a science. The person, environment, and significant other must all be balanced with the health needs of the dying patient. Some of the questions examined in this chapter are:

- How do we promote patient care at the end of life?
- What are some of the fears or obstacles that are barriers to discussions about death?
- What are effective ways to communicate end of life concerns?
- How can health care professionals role model a healthy life and healthy death?

With these questions in mind, ideas and thoughts will be presented to improve the discussions. Society needs a better understanding about death as technological advancements continue to focus on life extension and support. Rarely is a patient classified as "natural death," leading the health care industry to continually try to find a cure to treat a disease. This chapter will provide a foundation of information that can be used to better train our health care professionals to be more informed about death. Research in death and dying support systems identifies an additional benefit when one seriously contemplates his own mortality and communicates those thoughts to another; the result is an appreciation for life itself (Claiborne 2000). Life becomes the benefit in talking about death.

HOW DO WE PROMOTE PATIENT CARE AT THE END OF LIFE?

The most important step is to keep the patient as the center of all concerns and conversations. Each health professional caring for a patient at the end of life needs to know the following:

- What is the patient's condition?
- What does the patient know and understand of the condition?
- What does the family know and understand of the condition?
- What are the patient's and family's major concerns?
- What are the needs of the patient in order to promote quality, comfort, and compassion?

Communication breakdowns can occur if not all caregivers—professionals, laypersons, and families—are not aligned with the understanding of knowledge and information about the patient's condition. Often the diagnosis of a terminal illness does not come with a standard timeframe when death will occur. In addition, there is frequently a denial of the diagnosis. Therefore, an accurate assessment is the first step to plan appropriate care.

After initial patient assessment and chart review, the aforementioned questions can be answered. If there are any unanswered questions, it is important to speak with the physician to identify a plan for communication to the patient and significant others. For many reasons, the discussions about terminal illness and death are timed to the patient's psychological stability and physical condition. As a health team, we develop the plan for communication together that is individualized for the patient. Some organizations recommend a family conference to discuss options and make decisions. These conferences are an opportunity to bring all the caregivers together to discuss the needs of the patient and the plan of care. This is all done with the patient's needs as the center of discussion.

The Patient's Bill of Rights (Department of Health and Human Services 2000) clearly states that patients have the right to information regarding their condition, therefore they have the right to all information regarding their condition. A nurse is an advocate for the patient to ensure that his or her rights are honored. The health care professional has a responsibility to ensure this right is upheld while maintaining an environment of care, compassion, and sensitivity.

Many organizations have strived to improve patient care in the dying phase. In the late 1980s, the Robert Wood Johnson Foundation contributed $28 million to fund the SUPPORT study. SUPPORT stands for the study to understand prognosis and preferences for outcomes and risks of treatment, and it was intended to achieve a clearer understanding of the character of dying in American hospitals. The study enrolled 9,000 patients suffering from life-threatening illnesses in five U.S. teaching hospitals (Moskowitz and Nelson 1995). New programs for training, both public and professional, resulted from this study.

In addition, other projects such as Death in America (George Soro's Open Society Institute in New York) also spent $15 million to help reconceptualize the experience of dying through research, scholarship, the arts and humanities, and education. Thousands of programs across the country are emerging to talk about this important topic.

The Internet has an enormous amount of information about dying, death, and related subjects. A number of topic-related web sites were found using the Microsoft search engine (January, 2000):

Keyword	Matches
Hospice	93
Palliative care	17
Pain	783
Cancer pain	32
Terminally ill	38
Bereavement	20
Cancer	2,336

This brief list indicates the availability of information on these delicate subjects.

Information is power and the information age has brought new technology to access and share information. Pereira and Bruera (1998) published an article identifying the World Wide Web as a valuable source of information for medical and health-related issues. As with all information sources, it is important to know the advantages and disadvantages.

The advantages are ease of use, ease of publishing and editing, inexpensive publishings, and access. The disadvantages are lack of peer review process, uncontrolled publishing, legal and ethical issues, conflict of interest, language barriers, and lack of Internet access. Patients and families may use this source and it is critical that the practitioner understands its applicability.

There are many sources of data such as community brochures, funeral homes, hospice organizations and others that publish information regarding care of and for the dying. The patient and family need help from the health care practitioner to ensure that the information they read is reliable and valid.

In addition, most hospitals have an ethics committee. This committee is composed of multidisciplinary members trained in end of life issues. Any family member, patient, or health care practitioner can access the ethics committee for counsel. This resource is often an opportunity to discuss options with a health care provider not directly responsible for care and who provides an objective opinion in relation to end of life options.

WHAT ARE SOME OF THE FEARS AND BARRIERS TO DISCUSSIONS ABOUT DEATH?

There are many fears and barriers to the topic of death. If you want to stop a group conversation abruptly, ask the following question: "Hey everyone, what are your plans for death?" I recently tried that at a graduate seminar in Washington to engage the group in a dialogue about death planning. The verbal (lack of) and nonverbal response validated the difficult nature of this topic. We have been taught to talk about life, to save lives, to think life, and so it is contrary, except for the dying, to find this topic engaging.

The first barrier to overcome is your own fears regarding death. Ask yourself the following:

- If I could live one more day, month, or year, what would I change?
- Do I have any regrets?
- Are there any people I have not connected with in my life?
- What are my life priorities?

These are the types of questions your dying patient will ask himself, and unless you are comfortable with your own mortality, you may not be as empathic as necessary. Stephen Levine (1997) experimented with this concept. His book, A *Year To Live*, describes the thoughts and actions of someone with a 12-month life expectancy. Though some of us will travel this route quite differently, the book presents a structure for some of the delicate issues one may think about. The topics range from relationship mending to funeral planning.

Scientific Western medicine celebrates the capacity of technological and biomedical devices to overcome life-threatening illness. Therefore, professionalism in a biomedical tradition is oriented to the preservation of life. The physician or nurse may have an overwhelming desire to take action to cure the problem instead of dealing with the emotional aspects a dying patient may evoke (Marshall 1995). To overcome this barrier one must remain as objective as possible.

In addition to structural or systemic problems that limit discussions about death, there are also human issues. In the United States, we are distanced from intimacy with the death process (Marshall, 1995). The patient is often hospitalized near death and placed in a highly technological environment. This further isolates the patient from family and loved ones. This makes discussions more difficult and can present barriers to decisions because of the critical nature of symptoms and emotions involved.

Death itself is fearful, as one thinks of pain and suffering. It is critical to talk about the fears of death so the practitioner can assist in planning for pain, suffering, hospice, or home care. One barrier is a lack of understanding about palliative care and pain control. Palliative care is becoming widely accepted as an approach to managing terminal illness by focusing on symptom control and comfort care rather than a cure or life prolongation. Palliative care teams, composed of physicians, nurses, social workers, and pastoral care, can be consulted to better explain how a patient and family can have their needs met and concerns heard.

Some patients express the fear of losing control over decisions or body functions. Identify what decisions they value and how they can maintain as much control as possible. This process will enhance patient dignity.

Another barrier is a lack of understanding regarding living wills and advanced directives. It is critical for the health care workers to know the difference and be able to explain them to the patient and or family. If you are not familiar, there are attorneys available through the ethics committee or community organizations. It is also important to know when these documents can be executed. Each state has laws that determine when and how a terminal illness is documented.

Last year I had the opportunity to be at the bedside of two women dying of breast cancer. One patient died at home and the other died in the hospital. In the months prior to their deaths, numerous discussions about death, afterlife, pain, suffering, care of their spouses after death, children, grandchildren, and memories of life took place. The many discussions that these women had with loved ones, health care providers, and friends assisted them in a peaceful death. In both cases, an overwhelming crowd of loved ones surrounded them at the final hour, those people who had walked the death process with them. I believe, in each case, the fears of death were overcome by healthy dialogue during the dying process.

Death talk is not easy; the biggest fear is starting the conversation. However, the result is a conversation of intimacy and understanding. It is an opportunity to discuss emotional feelings and express gratitude. These conversations are often critical to the healing process and can create personal transformation for anyone involved.

WHAT ARE EFFECTIVE WAYS TO COMMUNICATE END OF LIFE CONCERNS?

The best way to communicate these issues is proactively when death is not pending. First, it begins with you. Have you thought about death? Will you be an organ donor? Have you told your loved ones what you want should a tragic death occur? Not all of us will have time, like some terminally ill patients to discuss plans. Do you have a living will? What about advanced directives should you become hospitalized? It amazes me how few of the health practitioners I associate with plan ahead for death. Start today and communicate your wishes to your family and or significant others. Discuss this topic in class and in your workplace.

Secondly, assist those around you to answer the same questions. Your comfort level in discussing death is important in training and educating others. Support community-based education that answers questions regarding the difference between living wills and advanced directives. If your community does not have any programs, set one up. Organizations that support the grieving, funeral homes, and hospice organizations are good resources for creating this type of forum. Laypeople are hungry for this information, with all the publicity over physician-assisted suicide in the last few years.

The next step is to be a patient advocate for this topic. Let the patients know their options and don't assume they understand it all. One daughter called me a few months ago and did not realize that every hospitalized patient gets resuscitated if they had a cardiac or respiratory arrest. She did not know about a DNR (do not resuscitate) order. This family needed a serious conversation about options for their elderly family member. People need to understand the health care environment in hospitals and our resources and how we respond to emergent conditions.

Lastly, treat this topic with respect and dignity. Unless you are dying, you do not completely understand the patient's view. Listen with your ears, eyes, and heart. Listen to their concerns, stories, and thoughts. Listen and be with them so that you can fully be present in their plan of care. Listening is a great way to communicate your interest and concern to the patient.

HOW CAN WE ROLE MODEL A HEALTHY LIFE AND HEALTHY DEATH?

Educating yourself about end of life issues is a good start. However, reading alone won't change your behavior. Medical sociologists teach three ways to change professional behavior (Anna 1995):

1. Convince the profession that it is in its best interest to change.
2. Change the norms of the profession.
3. Change the incentives.

The health care profession needs to understand two basic things. One, consumers want choice, and Americans seem to understand this by their support of physician-assisted suicide. Let's help the consumer in learning advanced life-planning strategies. Secondly, the cost of care for the dying is exorbitant. Most families and patients do not know their insurance limits or out-of-pocket expenses in case of accident or tragedy. This lack of understanding insurance limits could lead to prolonged futile care. If we could limit futile care, we could fund more proactively in areas such as immunizations, vaccines, and disease prevention.

Changing the norms of the profession can happen with a commitment to new processes and systems regarding end of life. Hospitalized patients deserve the conversation about their health status. If the patient has a terminal or irreversible condition, it is important to talk about options as soon as possible following the diagnosis. If we don't make that an everyday occurrence, we may not change.

Changing the incentive in health care is about reimbursement. Many lobbyists are working on new bills to extend hospice and add palliative care for a reimbursement benefit. As legislators support the physician in end of life or palliative care, the result could mean less pain and suffering for the dying. The litigious nature of society is always a concern for the health care practitioner, which further complicates decisions. The physician is often placed in a position of being in between knowing the best clinical decision and the family's wishes. If the wants and needs are aligned, there is less chance for conflict and potential lawsuits.

Palliative care is an umbrella term for end of life care. In the last five years, palliative care has become more common in hospitals and communities; however, it is still not well understood. The goal of palliative care is the well being of the patient (Bruera and Pereira 1998). Another definition is "the active total (physical, emotional, social, and spiritual) care of patients with life-threatening illness and the support of their family and friends" (WHO 1990).

Palliative care does not hasten death and in fact could prolong life. The goal of palliative care is to maintain optimal quality of life. Palliative care is often associated with terms like care, compassion, and recognition of values, pain control, dignity, and cultural sensitivity.

Palliative care teams may exist within a hospital or an outside agency. The team members may include registered nurses, pastoral care, social workers, case managers, physicians, and volunteers. Each member is trained in end of life care and advanced life planning so that other health care professionals may consult him or her when necessary. A study regarding end of life decision making by Fins, et al. (1999, 12) identified some key strategies for hospitals to improve end of life care. These are:

- Increase the comfort care plans for patients who die in hospitals.
- Closely approximate the proportion of comfort care to that of patients who have DNR orders and are identified as dying.
- Make more timely end of life decisions early in the hospital admission.
- Increase the proportion of patients who are appropriately withdrawn from life-sustaining treatments.
- Provide more coherent comfort care plan.
- Expand the proportion of terminally ill patients discharged to home hospice.

This list is a comprehensive plan to change death support systems in a very positive direction. Death support systems are family, home health, acute care hospitals, emergency care, nursing homes, hospice, and palliative care homes. All of these systems must improve their level of understanding about death. This will assist the communication as a patient transfers to different levels of care.

Death can provide an opportunity for growth and change. Celebrating one's purpose and contribution is a tribute to all who have gone before us. Each of us has the opportunity to create meaning in this sometimes tragic event. Health care professionals can make the difference. Communication is key to successful planning and care for this special group in society, the dying.

REFERENCES

Anna, G. J. (1995). How we lie. Special Supplement, *Hastings Center Report* 25, (6, Special Supplement), 12–14.

Bruera, E., & Pereira, J. (1998). Recent developments in palliative cancer care. *Acta Oncologica* 37(7/8), pp. 749–757. Oslo, Norway: Scandinavian University Press.

Claiborne, C. (2000). [Death Support Systems]. Unpublished data.

Department of Health and Human Services. (2000). *Medicare conditions of participation: Patient rights*. 482.13. Washington, DC: Author and U.S. Government.

Fins, J. J., Miller, F. G., Acres, C. A., Bacchetta, M. D., Huzzard, L. L., & Raplcin, D. D. (1999). End of life decision making in the hospital: Current practice and future prospects. *Journal of Pain and Symptom Management* 17 (1), 6–15.

Levine, S. (1997). *A year to live*. New York: Bell Tower, pp. 169–175.

Marshall, P. A. (1995). The SUPPORT study: Who's talking? *Hastings Center Report* 25 (6, Special Supplement), 9–11.

Moskowitz, E. H., and Nelson, J. L. (1995). Dying well in the hospital: The lessons of support. *Hastings Center Report* 25 (6, Special Supplement), 3–6.

Pereira, J., & Bruera, E. (1998). The internet as a resource for palliative care and hospice: A review and proposal. *Journal of Pain and Symptom Management*, 16 (1), 59–68.

Perls, T., & Silver, M. H. (1999). *Living to 100: Lessons in living to your maximum potential at any age*. New York: Basic Books.

World Health Organization. (1990). *Cancer pain relief and palliative care*. WHO, Geneva Switzerland. Technical Report Series II. 804.

UNIT VI

COMMUNICATION

Critical Thinking Activities
1. Differentiate between empathy and sympathy
2. List criteria to evaluate effective communication
3. Develop guidelines to assess problems in communication

Teaching-Learning Exercises
1. Interview a palliative care or hospice nurse
2. Interview a patient with a life-limiting illness
3. Role-play communication on the first visit with a patient who has just been informed that he has six months to live
4. Role-play communication efforts of professional nurses

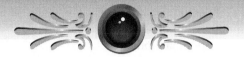

UNIT VII

MANAGEMENT OF SPECIFIC TERMINAL ILLNESSES

Learning Objectives
1. Identify measures to support the dying and family or caregivers with role changes, task reassignments, and changes in social customs
2. Recognize symptoms of loneliness as a result of separation and pending loss
3. Identify symptoms of increased stress and anxiety relative to illness outcomes
4. Identify physical, psychological, social, financial, and spiritual resource support systems for the dying and their caregivers
5. Identify coping skills of the dying and their caregivers
6. Identify signs and symptoms of respiratory and cardiovascular problems that are common sequelae of advanced cancer and cancer treatment
7. Describe guidelines for skin assessment relative to terminal illnesses, particularly in patients dying of cancer and AIDS
8. Describe guidelines for oral assessment relative to end of life and terminal illnesses
9. List measures to prevent oral problems at the end of life
10. List nursing interventions to alleviate symptoms of nausea, vomiting, dysphagia, anorexia, constipation, diarrhea, and bowel obstruction
11. Discuss impact of terminal illness and pending death on human sexuality
12. Discuss the importance in preventing complications in care of the terminal cancer patient

13. Discuss common characteristics and problems associated with neurologic terminal illnesses
14. Describe guidelines for assessing suicidal thoughts, intentions, and behavior among terminal patients
15. List nursing interventions to support families and significant others coping with a suicide death

CHAPTER 19

CARE OF THE DYING
CANCER PATIENT

Dr. Melinda Oberleitner

INTRODUCTION AND OVERVIEW

Despite significant advances in cancer screening, detection, treatment, and survival in recent years, the American Cancer Society (ACS) estimates that 552,200 Americans will die from cancer in 2000. This translates to more than 1,500 people per day dying from cancer. In the United States, cancer is second only to heart disease as a leading cause of death with 1 in every 4 deaths caused by cancer. Cancer remains primarily a disease of adults middle age and older. Approximately 80% of all cancers are diagnosed in adults age 55 and older. Although cancer mortality rates have begun to decline, as Americans live longer it is projected that cancer will continue to be a significant cause of morbidity and mortality (ACS 2000).

Survival rates from cancer vary depending on cancer type and stage of the cancer at the time of diagnosis. For example, the five-year relative survival rate for localized breast cancer today is 96%. However, if a woman is diagnosed at a later stage when distant metastasis is present at the time of diagnosis, the five-year survival rate drops precipitously to 21%. The largest cancer killer of Americans, lung cancer, accounts for 28% of all cancer deaths. The five-year relative survival rate for all stages of lung cancer remains a dismal 14%. For all cancers combined, the current five-year relative survival rate is 59% (ACS 2000).

Goals of cancer care today include achieving a cure for some types of cancer such as acute lymphocytic leukemia in children and Hodgkin's lymphoma, controlling cancer, or offering palliative or end of life care if cure or control of the cancer is not possible. In recent years, several national organizations representing cancer care professionals including the American Society of Clinical Oncology (ASCO) and the Oncology Nursing Society (ONS) have developed recommendations and position papers related to end of life care of the cancer patient. The ONS position statement on end of life care was developed and published in collaboration with the Association of Oncology Social Work

(Table 19–1). The ONS-AOSW statement provides a framework for nurses, social workers, and other health care professionals in improving the care of the dying cancer patient and focuses on symptom management, cultural variations in death and dying, decision making and choice, and the rights of patients and families in end of life decisions.

Care of the dying cancer patient is often complex, with a multitude of physical and psychosocial issues to be addressed. This chapter will address selected issues in the physical care that are likely to affect most terminal cancer patients—the management of pain, opioid-induced constipation, dyspnea, and anorexia-cachexia. Implications for nursing practice based on the most current research related to each individual topic will also be presented.

TABLE 19–1   Oncology Nursing Society and Association of Oncology Social Work Joint Position on End of Life Care

---

The increasing awareness of deficiencies in care at the end of life and the growing conviction that steps to improve care are essential led the Oncology Nursing Society (ONS) and the Association of Oncology Social Work (AOSW) to promulgate a position on end of life care. The position of the ONS and AOSW is that people with catastrophic, potentially fatal illnesses and those close to them should be able to expect and receive reliable, skillful, and supportive care.

It is the position of the ONS and AOSW that:

- Nurses, social workers, and other health care professionals must improve care of the dying patient using prevailing knowledge effectively to identify and relieve symptoms associated with the end of life experience.
- Nurses, social workers, and other health care professionals must recognize the spiritual component of patient and family care and make resources available to those who wish them and in the form desired.
- All curricula and continuing education programming must initiate changes to cultivate practitioners who exhibit appropriate and nonjudgmental attitudes, knowledge, and skills to provide end of life care. This must include information on the spiritual/religious aspects of care, clinical practice issues, patient advocacy, as well as ethics and patient rights.
- Graduate and continuing education programs must be developed to create end of life experts in sufficient numbers to provide consultation and support to patients, families, and caregivers.
- It must be recognized that suffering is an interpretive process, framed within a cultural context, and unique to each individual. Thus, nurses, social workers, and other health care professionals must be sensitized to the diversity of experience inherent in end of life care.
- Biomedical, clinical, and behavioral research must be strengthened to provide a foundation for evidence-based practice and to define and measure outcomes other than death.

TABLE 19-1   CONTINUED

- Nurses and social workers must work with policymakers, consumer advocate groups, and licensing and regulatory agencies to revise and enhance mechanisms for financing care and to simplify ponderous regulations including drug prescription laws that impede relief of pain and suffering.

- Health care professionals must render culturally sensitive end of life care. Patients and families must be informed of the diagnosis, prognosis, risks, and benefits of proposed treatments within the context of their culture and be allowed to make choices, based on this information, to include nontreatment.

- The capacity for autonomous patient and medical decision making must be extended through the use of advanced care directives. All patients and families must have the right to accurate information related to advanced care planning and end of life decision making to minimize psychological distress.

Background:

Technological advances in health care practices have institutionalized death and, in some cases, prolonged suffering. Improving care at the end of life requires supportive federal and state policies, including financial policies. At the community level, the response has been to implement the hospice model to improve the quality of life for the dying and those close to them.

The developing specialty of palliative care speaks to the response to these concerns by health care professionals and has helped to focus research on the physical, psychological, and spiritual issues related to potentially fatal illnesses. Professional caregivers must take responsibility to develop those skills that will protect them from depersonalization and dehumanizing detachment by confronting their own discomfort with death.

Family/caregivers must be able to access the health care system to meet their needs in providing end of life care, with the focus on quality living.

ONS Board of Directors Approved 10/98
Used with permission of the Oncology Nursing Press

ISSUES IN THE PHYSICAL CARE OF THE PATIENT DYING WITH CANCER

Pain Management

When discussing cancer in relation to either themselves, family members, or friends, many people conjure up the image of the dying cancer patient as is often portrayed on television. That image is typically of someone who is alone in a hospital room writhing in uncontrolled pain. To many, pain is the most feared symptom associated with cancer. The reality is that today cancer pain can be controlled by relatively simple measures, in up to 90% of cancer patients (Jacox, et al. 1994).

Pain from cancer can be either acute or chronic and is caused by a variety of biophysiologic mechanisms, including tumor infiltration of bones such as the vertebrae or long bones and infiltration of nerve pathways which can lead to, for example, spinal cord compression. Examples of visceral pain from cancer spread include pain from peritoneal irritation, obstruction, metabolic disturbances, and alterations in mucosal integrity. Pain associated with cancer can also be treatment related. Pain can result from diagnostic procedures such as bone marrow aspiration or spinal taps, or from surgical procedures such as mastectomy that are intended to remove or ameliorate the cancer. A range of cancer pain syndromes exist that are the result of surgery, chemotherapy, or radiation therapy (Cunningham, Thorpe, & Ruger 1998).

In 1994, the Agency for Health Care Policy and Research (now the Agency for Health Care Research and Quality) released the publication *Management of Cancer Pain—Clinical Practice Guideline Number 9*. This document provided much needed direction to health care professionals related to the assessment and treatment of cancer-related pain (Jacox, et al. 1994). According to the guidelines, which are based on the World Health Organization's analgesic ladder, the treatment of moderate to severe cancer pain, as is often encountered in the terminal phase of the illness, requires the use of opioid agonist medications including morphine, fentanyl, and hydrocodone. Partial agonists and mixed agonist-antagonist drugs have limited application in treating chronic and moderate to severe cancer pain and should not be used. The pure agonist opioid, meperidine, should be avoided in treating severe and chronic cancer pain. Meperidine is metabolized to the metabolite normeperidine, which in some individuals with compromised excretory capacity can lead to central nervous system toxicity.

Routes of administration and formulations of pain medications available to patients with advanced cancer are numerous. Routes of administration include oral (the preferred route), parenteral, subcutaneous, rectal, sublingual, transdermal, buccal, epidural, and nasal. Administration of pain medications via the intramuscular route in cancer patients is discouraged due to unpredictable absorption, the often long-term nature of treatment, pain caused by injection, risk of bleeding if thrombocytopenia is present, and because cachexia or muscle wasting is often present in advanced cancer. Formulations include short-, intermediate-, or long-acting (sustained release) preparations. The intermediate- and sustained-release formulations allow the patient to receive "around-the-clock" dosing, with short-acting medications available to treat breakthrough pain. The daily dose of narcotic analgesic is titrated upward to achieve pain relief to the patient's satisfaction. There is no maximum or ceiling dose of the pure agonist opioids such as morphine. The use of placebos to treat cancer pain is unwarranted and is considered unethical.

The most common side effects of opioid analgesics, particularly in the opioid naive patient, include opioid-induced constipation, nausea, vomiting, somnolence, and unsteadiness. Respiratory depression is a rare side effect. Tolerance, physiologic dependence, and psychologic dependence are phenomena associated with opioid use. Tolerance is the patient's need for increasingly higher doses of a drug to achieve the original analgesic effect. Physiologic dependence is the state in which physical symptoms such as abdominal cramping, agitation, and return of the pain will occur if the drug is withdrawn abruptly or if an antagonist is administered. Psychologic dependence, or addiction, is often feared by patients being treated with narcotic analgesics. Psychologic dependence is extremely rare in individuals being treated for cancer who have been prescribed opioids, occurring in less than 1% of all patients treated (Paice 1999).

Adjuvant medications are often incorporated into the daily pain management of the patient with advanced cancer. These adjuvants include corticosteroids, antidepressants (to provide analgesia independent of their mood-elevating effects), anticonvulsants, local anesthetics, and others. Side effects of the adjuvants are numerous and vary depending on the drug group. For example, side effects of NSAIDs include gastrointestinal upset and ulceration, while corticosteroid effects include fluid retention and mood changes.

Pain from metastasis to the bone is often present in the terminal cancer patient. Some of the most frequently occurring cancers—breast, prostate, and lung—are tumors which commonly metastasize to the bone. Most patients who die of breast or lung cancer will have experienced bone metastasis prior to the time of death (Mundy 1997). The pain associated with bone metastasis is described as dull, intermittent pain that becomes progressively severe. The pain is unrelenting and is often worse at night and upon movement (Struthers, Mayer, and Fisher 1998). Associated with bone metastases are pathologic fracture, hypercalcemia, spinal cord compression, and anemia (Welch-McCaffery 1988).

The diagnosis of bone metastasis includes clinical evaluation utilizing bone scans and x-rays to determine the precise location of metastasis. Computed tomography (CT) and magnetic resonance imaging (MRI) may also be useful in isolating abnormalities in bone. Serologic testing to include serum calcium, alkaline phosphatase, and complete blood count may assist in determining the presence of bone metastasis. The triad of serum calcium levels greater than 11 mg/dL, hemoglobin level less than 10 g/dL, and alkaline phosphatase greater than 115 mU/mL, may signal bone involvement by the cancer (Struthers, Mayer, and Fisher 1998).

Bone metastases may be treated using an array of modalities including pharmacologic therapy, surgery, radiation therapy, chemotherapy, hormone therapy, and the use of bisphosphonates. Pharmacologic therapy includes the use of nonsteroidal anti-inflammatory drugs (NSAIDs) and opioid analgesics titrated to effect as recommended by the World Health Organization's analgesic ladder. If the bone pain is local, radiation therapy may be recommended along with corticosteroids. Radiation therapy is very effective in relieving pain from bone metastases and also exerts local control of the tumor (Struthers, Mayer, and Fisher 1998). To treat diffuse bone pain bisphosphonates, drugs which inhibit bone dissolution are added to local radiation therapy and corticosteroid therapy (Nguyen, Zekry, and Bruera 2000). Nonpharmacologic approaches to managing bone pain include physical modalities such as immobilization, application of heat and cold, massage, relaxation, and use of therapeutic surfaces such as air mattresses and air flow beds.

Opioid-Induced Constipation

Unfortunately constipation is a very common and predictable side effect of treatment with opioid analgesics. Opioids decrease peristalsis by not propelling food forward in the colon which results in constipation. Patients seldom develop tolerance to constipation from narcotic analgesic treatment, and the effects of opioids related to constipation are dose dependent (Bisanz 1997). Adjuvant drugs such as anticonvulsants and antidepressants used in cancer pain management have also been implicated in causing constipation. Compounding the problem is the increased age of many cancer patients. Decreased motility of the large intestine, which occurs as a function of aging, is a primary cause of constipation. Because patients with advanced cancer are treated with large and often escalating doses of opioid analgesics, rigorous attention must be paid to preventing opioid-induced constipation at the inception of the narcotic therapeutic regimen. Cameron (1992, 375) recommends, "The objective for patients should be prevention of constipation from narcotics rather than treatment for established constipation."

Measures to prevent or alleviate constipation include increasing fluid intake to 1.5 to 2 liters per day if the patient is able to tolerate the fluid, and increasing daily fiber and activity levels. However, according to Levy (1991), these measures are unlikely to be successful unless combined with laxative intake in cancer patients receiving opioid analgesics. Bulk laxatives containing fiber and psyllium should not be used unless fluid intake is adequate. Inadequate fluid intake combined with increased fiber or psyllium intake results in "rock-hard" stool (Kedziera 1999, 13). Other types of laxatives that may be prescribed include large bowel stimulants such as senna and cascara, osmotic laxatives which include lactulose and sorbitol, and detergent laxatives which contain docusate. Products such as mineral oil are lubricants which aid in reducing friction during defecation.

Robinson, et al. (2000) reported the results of successful protocol development to prevent opioid-induced constipation in patients with cancer on a 28-bed oncology unit at a Midwestern hospital. The protocol includes the use of two Senokot-S® (Purdue Frederick Co., Norwalk, Conn.) tablets at the hour of sleep beginning on day one of opioid use. If the patient's bowel pattern is unchanged the next day and subsequent days, the patient is to continue the previous day's laxative therapy. If the patient has no bowel movement, 30 cc of Milk of Magnesia USP (Pharmaceutical Associates, Inc., Greenville, S.C.) is added the next day and the Senokot S® is increased daily up to four tablets three times per day. At this point, if the patient has not had a bowel movement, impaction should be ruled out unless the patient's absolute neutrophil count or platelet count are decreased. The protocol then outlines further interventions based on whether an impaction is present or not. Nonpharmacological interventions such as increasing fluid intake, increasing intake of high fiber foods, exercise, and providing private, quiet time for defecation after breakfast are also included in the protocol.

Dyspnea

Dyspnea, difficult or labored breathing, is a common problem encountered by patients with advanced cancer. Heyse-Moore, Ross, and Mulee (1991) concluded that 70% of cancer patients in the last six weeks of life experience dyspnea. Dyspnea is a frightening symptom not only to the patient, but to family and caregivers as well who often feel helpless in dealing with the problem.

Cancer patients with primary or metastatic lung cancer are at high risk for the development of dyspnea. Other causes of dyspnea in the cancer patient include congestive heart failure, asthma, anxiety, chemotherapy-induced pulmonary toxicities, radiation-induced pneumonitis, airway obstruction by the tumor, and anorexia-cachexia syndrome.

Management of dyspnea involves identifying the etiology if possible and instituting appropriate treatment. Medical interventions which may be used to treat or manage dyspnea include red blood cell transfusions, treatment of pneumonia, radiation therapy or chemotherapy for tumor control, and thora- or paracentesis. Other less invasive strategies to manage dyspnea include pursed-lip breathing and utilization of positioning techniques which increase ventilatory capacity. The best such position is leaning forward with arms braced on a chair or knees and upper body supported (Harwood 1999).

Management of severe dyspnea in the terminal stages includes positioning, oxygen therapy, relaxation techniques, and use of narcotics such as morphine. Morphine or hydromorphone administered by nebulizer has been beneficial in treating dyspnea in some studies. Other drugs that have been utilized to treat dyspnea and the associated anxiety in advanced cancer are midazolam, chlorpromazine, and dexamethasone (Abrahm 1998).

Anorexia-Cachexia

Nutritional alterations can occur at any point during the cancer continuum, i.e., prior to diagnosis or during treatment, and are very common during the terminal phase of the disease. In fact one of the "warning signs" of cancer is unintentional weight loss of greater than 10% of body weight in the previous six months. Those individuals who have lost 10% or more of body weight prior to diagnosis often do not live as long as those patients who were diagnosed with the same type of cancer, at the same stage of diagnosis, who had not lost weight (Ottery 1995).

According to Wilkes (1999), etiologic factors related to weight loss in cancer patients include location, stage, and size of the tumor; type and side effects of treatments for cancer; decreased dietary intake in the face of increased nutritional requirements; increased excretion of nutrients; malabsorption; and abnormal nutrient utilization. Other factors that may lead to weight loss in cancer patients include early satiety, the feeling of being full even after eating only very small amounts, taste changes associated with chemotherapy or tumor byproducts, food aversions, nausea and vomiting, fatigue, and lack of appetite or anorexia. Anorexia may be the result of physiological factors such as those described previously, psychological factors such as depression or anxiety, or from a combination of physiological and psychological factors.

Medications which have been used to treat the anorexia in cancer and other terminal illnesses such as AIDS include megestrol acetate, dexamethasone, metoclopramide, and delta-9-tetrahydrocannibinol. Corticosteroids have been proven to be effective for appetite stimulation only in the short term (Meares 2000).

In advanced cancer, cachexia, or muscle wasting can occur. Cachexia is a disorder of advanced protein-calorie malnutrition. The incidence of cachexia is not the same across cancers. For example, it is common among patients with advanced lung cancer but occurs more infrequently in breast cancer patients (Grant and Rivera 1995). Although the etiology of cachexia is not yet fully understood, it is different from starvation (Whitman 2000). In starvation the body compensates for decreased nutrient intake by decreasing or slowing metabolism. Although there is decreased intake in cachexia, metabolism is not slowed, resulting in the breakdown of lean tissue and lean body mass as a result of disruption of fat and carbohydrate metabolism.

Cachexia can be classified as either primary or secondary, depending on etiology (Cunningham and Bell 2000). Determination of the classification is important when prescribing intervention options. Primary cachexia is the most common cause of death in cancer. It is most often seen in cancer patients but can also be observed in life-threatening conditions such as trauma and sepsis. Involuntary weight loss, anorexia, and tissue wasting culminating in death characterize primary cachexia. Secondary cachexia occurs as a result of functional inability to ingest or digest nutrients—caused by, for example, obstruction by tumor and malabsorption.

According to Meares (2000), there is no direct evidence in the literature or in clinical studies that the anorexia-cachexia cancer syndrome can be cured, arrested, or reversed. Instead, interventions should be aimed at improving appetite and intake only as they relate to enhancing the quality of life of the patient.

Of particular concern to many family and professional caregivers is the state of terminal dehydration in the patient with terminal cancer. Over time the patient refuses to ingest either food or fluids. Nutrient and fluid cessation can lead to symptoms in the patient including thirst, dry mouth, weakness, fatigue, muscle cramps, and other symptoms reflective of cessation of intake. There is controversy in clinical practice as to whether terminal dehydration should be prevented or treated. Proponents of not treating the dehydration point to reduction in airway secretions, which may relieve the patient's sensation of drowning and which may help relieve dyspnea in the patient's terminal phase, as well as a decrease in incontinence, vomiting, choking and coughing (Meares 2000). It is postulated that the increased production of ketones and endorphins as a result of terminal dehydration leads to naturally occurring analgesic and anesthetic effects. Advocates of preventing or treating dehydration in the dying patient believe that administration of fluids may help the patient to gain a sense of well-being from the correction of fluid and electrolyte imbalance.

For family members, the distinction between cachexia and starvation may not be evident (Holden 1991). Holden interviewed 14 patients and their caregivers about the cessation of food and fluid intake during the terminal phase of the disease. The greatest impact of cessation of eating and drinking occurred in the female caregivers who had held the role of food preparer for the patient prior to the illness. In a study conducted on 32 inpatients receiving palliative care from admission to death, McCann, Hall, and Groth-Juncker (1994, 1265) reported "lack of food and fluids sufficient to replete losses did not cause them (the patient) suffering, and (some patients) experienced abdominal discomfort and nausea when they ate to please their families."

Meares (1997, 1755) conducted qualitative research to explore the meaning of nutrition cessation in 12 adult in-home hospice patients with cancer, as described by their female primary caregivers following the patients' deaths. The overall theme that emerged was the female caregivers believed nutrition cessation was a naturally occurring event and was not physically painful to the patient. Of particular note in this study was many of the caregivers were unaware that intake cessation is expected or "normal" for patients in the terminal phase of illness and would have considered that information helpful had they received it from a health care professional during the caregiving period prior to the patient's death.

SUMMARY

Prior to the passage of the Patient Self-Determination Act of 1991, many cancer patients, even those in the terminal stages, died in hospitals as "full codes." That means, even though there was no longer any hope of cure or even of controlling the cancer—and even if being "coded" was against the patient's wishes—the patient was subjected to full cardiopulmonary resuscitation. Today cancer patients have the choice of dying with dignity in their homes surrounded by family and friends or in hospitals or other institutions where their wishes about how they want to die must be respected. With the renewed interest in providing humane, respectful end of life care, it is hoped that all cancer patients will experience a peaceful, pain-free death in the surrounding of their choice. Nurses play a crucial role in choreographing the quality of that final experience.

REFERENCES

Abrahm, J. L. (1998). Promoting symptom control in palliative care. *Seminars in Oncology Nursing*, 14(2), 95–109.

American Cancer Society (2000). *Facts and figures.* Atlanta, GA: Author.

Bisanz, A. (1997). Managing bowel elimination problems in patients with cancer. *Oncology Nursing Forum*, 24(4), 679–688.

Cameron, J. C. (1992). Constipation related to narcotic therapy. A protocol for nurses and patients. *Cancer Nursing*, 15, 372–377.

Cunningham, R. S., & Bell, R. (2000). Nutrition in cancer: An overview. *Seminars in Oncology Nursing*, 16(2), 90–98.

Cunningham, M. L., Ruger, T., & Thorpe, D. M. (1998). Assessment of pain syndromes in cancer patients. *Strategies for Pain Management*, 1(1), 2–16.

Grant, M., & Rivera, L. (1995). Anorexia, cachexia, and dysphagia: The symptom experience. *Seminars in Oncology Nursing*, 11(4), 266–271.

Harwood, K. V. (1999). Dyspnea. In C. H. Yarbro, M. H. Frogge, & M. Goodman (Eds.), *Cancer symptom management* (pp. 45–57). Boston: Jones and Bartlett Publishers.

Heyse-Moore, L. H., Ross, V., & Mulee, M. (1991). How much of a problem is dyspnea and advanced cancer? *Palliative Medicine*, Vol. 5, pp. 27–33.

Holden, C. M. (1991). Anorexia in the terminally ill cancer patient: The emotional impact on the patient and family. *Hospice Journal*, 7(3), 73–84.

Jacox, A., Carr, D. B., & Payne, R., (1994). *Management of cancer pain: Clinical practice guideline no.* 9. (AHCPR Publication No. 94-0592). Rockville, MD: Agency for Health Care Policy and Research, Public Health Service, U.S. Department of Health and Human Services.

Kedziera, P. L. (1999). Management of analgesic side effects. In M. L. Cunningham, D. M. Thorpe, & T. F. Ruger, *Strategies for pain management*, 2(1), 1–14.

Levy, M. H. (1991). Constipation and diarrhea in cancer patients. *Cancer Bulletin*, 43, 412–422.

McCann, R. M., Hall, W. J., & Groth-Juncker, A. (1994). Comfort care for terminally ill patients. JAMA, 272, 1263–1266.

Meares, C. J. (1997). Primary caregiver perceptions of intake cessation in patients who are terminally ill. *Oncology Nursing Forum*, 24(10), 1751–1757.

Meares, C. J. (2000). Nutritional issues in palliative care. *Seminars in Oncology Nursing*, 16(2), 135–145.

Mundy, G. R. (1997). Mechanisms of bone metastasis. *Cancer*, 80 (Suppl.), 1546–1555.

Nguyen, P., Zekry, H., & Bruera, E. (2000). Cancer pain assessment and palliative care management. *Oncology*, 3, 135–140.

Ottery, F. D. (1995). Supportive nutrition to prevent cachexia and support quality of life. *Seminars in Oncology*, 22 (Suppl.), 98–111.

Paice, J. A. (1999). Pain. In C. Henke, M. H. Frogge, & M. Goodman, (Ed.), *Cancer symptom management* (pp. 118–147). Boston: Jones and Bartlett Publishers.

Robinson, C. B., Fritch, M., & Hullett, L., Petersen, M. A., Sikkema, S., Thenninck, L., and Timmer, K. (2000). Development of a protocol to prevent opioid induced constipation in patients with cancer: A research utilization project. *Clinical Journal of Oncology Nursing, 4*(2), 79–84.

Struthers, C., Mayer, D., & Fisher, G., (1998). Nursing management of the patient with bone metastases. *Seminars in Oncology Nursing, 14*(3), 199–209.

Welch-McCaffery, D. (1988). Metastatic bone cancer. *Cancer Nursing, 11,* 103–111.

Whitman, M. M. (2000). The starving patient: Supportive care for people with cancer. *Clinical Journal of Oncology Nursing, 4*(3), 121–125.

Wilkes, G. M. (1999). *Cancer and HIV clinical nutrition: Pocket guide* (2nd ed.). Boston: Jones and Bartlett.

CHAPTER

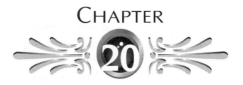

CARDIOVASCULAR AND PULMONARY DISORDERS

Marlene Foreman

INTRODUCTION AND OVERVIEW

Cardiovascular and respiratory disorders are difficult to manage because of the long-term illness and the variable end of life trajectories. It is difficult to predict with any certainty whether any particular exacerbation will result in death. The individual and the family are constantly vigilant for any signs of impending death while attempting to live as normally as possible within the limitations imposed by the illness. Typically, these disorders have a prolonged and protracted illness and end-stage interval. However, the actual death event may be sudden or there may be a "death watch" lasting several days to weeks. The cardiac and pulmonary systems are so closely related that both are often involved regardless of the primary underlying disorder. For this reason, this chapter will often interweave the information that is common to both systems.

PATHOPHYSIOLOGY OF CARDIOVASCULAR DISORDERS

The common knowledge that all death is the result of cardiac arrest is true, but all deaths are not the result of primary cardiac or vascular disorders. The pathophysiology of cardiovascular disorders involves problems of circulatory control, alterations in blood flow, and heart failure, which affect oxygen transport to vital organs and ultimately death at the cellular level. It is important to know human anatomy and physiology of the heart, lungs, and blood circulation to relate to the pathophysiology.

To review basic principles of blood circulation, it is important to realize that the major components are volume, pressure, and flow. Blood volume means the amount of blood measured in milliliters that is contained within the vascular system. Blood that is in the body but not within the vascular system does

261

not contribute to blood volume. This is apparent in situations in which there is hemorrhage within the body. The blood is not within the vascular system and the blood pressure drops accordingly. Blood volume that is reduced slowly is compensated for by the body and tolerated by the individual better than a sudden loss of large volumes of blood which rapidly produces shock. Blood pressure consists of five components: blood volume, blood viscosity, diameter of the lumen of the vessels, elasticity of the vessel walls, and force of contraction of the heart pump.

Blood viscosity or density is the concentration of formed particles, blood cells, and other solids in relation to the plasma or fluid component of blood. Thick blood has more formed particles than thin blood when the plasma component remains constant. The diameter of the lumen of the blood vessels may be narrowed by atherosclerosis (fatty plaques), tumors compressing the exterior of the vessel, or activation of the sympathetic nervous system which results in vasoconstriction. Damage to the autonomic or peripheral nervous system may result in vasodilation. It takes less pressure to force blood through the dilated vessels, but the perceived volume of blood will be decreased because of the reduction in pressure.

When there is vasodilation, there is also a reduction in cardiac output. Pulse rate varies to compensate for volume and pressure deficits. The lower the perceived volume and pressure of blood flow, the higher the pulse rate. For example, if the heart is unable to pump the blood with sufficient force, the blood pressure will decrease and the heart rate will increase to compensate. The blood vessels will constrict in response to the decrease in blood pressure to assure sufficient flow to vital organs at the expense of peripheral circulation and other organs. Blood may also pool in the peripheral circulation on standing which may induce orthostatic hypotension.

The elasticity of the vessel wall may be altered by arteriosclerosis (hardening of the arteries), one of the consequences of aging. The force of contraction of the heart pump may be decreased in cardiomyopathies (diseases which affect heart muscle). Cardiac muscle hypertrophy, necrosis, aneurism, or electrical failure, as well as atrial and ventricular dysrhythmias, will affect heart pump action and cardiac output. The force, pressure, or flow of blood through the vascular bed is affected by the ability of the heart to push blood through the system as well as the ability of the vascular system to get sufficient volume back to the heart and the heart to retrieve that blood volume. Therefore, blood flow is dependent on the heart muscle pump action, blood viscosity that affects ease of flow, and vessel diameter and integrity.

There are also mechanisms by which blood flows from the arterial system through the capillaries and tissues to the venous system. One of these mechanisms is hydrostatic pressure and another is oncotic or colloidal pressure. The force of blood from the heart to the arterial circulation pushes fluid through the capillaries, cells, and interstitial spaces. Oncotic pressure, primarily proteins within the venous system draw the fluid back into the vessels. A reduction in dietary protein would result in decreased fluid return to the venous end, edema, and reduced amount of blood return to the heart. The lymphatic system is an alternate route by which proteins, waste products, and fluid is returned to the venous system. Blockage of the lymphatic system interrupts this process.

PATHOPHYSIOLOGY OF THE PULMONARY SYSTEM

Pathophysiology of the pulmonary system may involve the pulmonary system, musculoskeletal system, nervous system, or cardiac system, all of which create problems in gas exchange. The physiologic basis for respirations is that the body needs oxygen to live and needs to eliminate carbon dioxide and other gaseous wastes. The heart and lungs work together to provide the body with adequate oxygen. The lungs are an important mechanism in maintaining acid-base balance within the body. The air passages from the nose to the lungs must be able to move air from the atmosphere to the alveoli where the exchange takes place. The method of air movement relies on an intact airway, ability of the muscles of respiration to move air into and out of the lungs, and the coordination of the alveoli and the capillary circulation of blood to facilitate the exchange.

Adequate blood flow and an adequate amount of hemoglobin within the blood is necessary to carry the oxygen to the tissues. Anemias alter the ability of the blood to circulate oxygen through the tissues. Air is introduced into the pulmonary system through the nose, mouth, or tracheostomy and passes into the main bronchus. The air passages end in the alveoli. Constriction of these smaller air passages by asthma or tumor limits the amount of air reaching the alveola and the amount of air returning to the main airways. Alteration in alveolar function by chronic obstructive pulmonary diseases, mucus, or tumors decrease the ability of the lungs to move air and to exchange oxygen and carbon dioxide. Increased or decreased blood pressure alters this exchange also. Abnormal collection of fluid in the pleural spaces decreases lung mobility and gas exchange. Acute anxiety and other emotional states decrease pulmonary function.

Intact muscles and nerves responsible for chest wall movement, diaphramatic excursion, and accessory muscle activity are a necessary component of respiratory effort. It is necessary to have intact connections to the respiratory center in the central nervous system pons and medulla to breathe. Central chemoreceptors in the medulla identify carbon dioxide levels in the blood by measuring hydrogen ions in the cerebrospinal fluid. They alter respiratory rate and depth accordingly, increasing the rate and depth as carbon dioxide rises. Persons with chronically high carbon dioxide levels do not respond to this stimulus.

Peripheral chemoreceptors located in the carotid and aortic arteries monitor carbon dioxide also, but are more sensitive to monitoring arterial blood oxygen concentrations. Therefore, decreased oxygen levels (hypoxia) is the main stimulus for respiratory effort in individuals with chronic pulmonary diseases and resultant carbon dioxide retention (hypercapnea). These individuals will respond to high doses of supplemental oxygen with respiratory depression. Several types of lung receptors regulate inspiration and expiration, breathing patterns, sighing and yawning, and work of breathing (Porth 1994). They react to airway resistance, irritants, bronchial muscle tone, and lung inflation. The cough reflex, a primary respiratory system defense mechanism, protects the lungs from irritants and rids it of collected secretions. Any central or local interruption of cough effort results in retained secretions and noisy breathing.

PHYSIOLOGIC CHANGES IN CARDIOVASCULAR DISORDERS

Cardiac disorders such as cardiomyopathies and heart failure create long-term deficits that culminate in the end-stage, terminal phase, which is no longer amenable to medical interventions. It is at this point that palliative care is the most viable alternative. Palliative care is aimed at symptom relief rather than management of the underlying disease process.

Impaired tissue perfusion is related to pathologic changes in the ability of the heart muscle to pump effectively, to fill adequately, or to exert enough force to maintain peripheral circulation. Medications that may improve cardiac and circulatory function for a time are listed in Table 20–1. Further diagnostic studies are not only futile, but may contribute to increased suffering and, potentially, death. It may be helpful for the individual to keep the head of the bed elevated or sleep on several pillows. Some actually sleep better in a recliner than in bed. A hospital bed may improve the ability to maintain adequate elevation of the head and thorax to allow maximum comfort. Congestive heart failure may lead to the inability to lie on the left side without a feeling of breathlessness and a need to sit up to breathe (orthopnea). These elevated positions reduce the pressure on the diaphragm and decrease venous return by pooling blood in the lower extremities, thereby decreasing cardiac workload.

Activity intolerance and the altered ability to independently maintain activities of daily living is related to the weakness, fatigue, and inadequate circulatory effort of the failing heart. It becomes increasingly necessary to limit activities and obtain assistance in hygiene, dressing, and cooking. It is important to maintain some activity as long as possible, even if frequent rest periods and naps are required to maintain energy levels. As the disease progresses, even eating and rising from bed becomes too much exertion.

As activities become more limited, social isolation ensues as the individual is unable to attend social events, church activities, and family functions. Portable oxygen and the use of wheelchairs or scooters may prolong the day that activities outside the home become impossible. The individual who is

TABLE 20–1	MEDICATIONS USED IN CARDIOVASCULAR DISEASES
Digoxin	
Anti-Arrhythmics	
Ace Inhibitors	
Beta Adrenergic Antagonists	
Vasodilators	
Calcium Channel Blockers	
Diuretics	
Nitrates	
Vasopressors	

confined to the home has already lost workplace relationships and casual acquaintances related to leisure activities. It is important for family and friends to remain connected by going to the home and visit or assist with personal and home care activities.

The individual living with chronic disease and impending death must acknowledge the spiritual meaning of life and death. It is difficult to comprehend that life will go on even when you become nonexistent in this world. Most people have difficulty with the concept of not being, even when they hold the belief that life will continue in some form in a spiritual realm. It is important for the individual and family to acknowledge and work through the emotional and spiritual impact of end-stage cardiovascular disorders. Unresolved anger, anxiety, and depression increase the physiological responses to stress (rapid pulse, increased blood pressure from vasoconstriction, and edema from retained fluids), which cause further deterioration of cardiac status.

The individual, family, and health care team must work together to develop goals for an acceptable plan of care. The individual and the nurse may have different values related to priority needs. It is important to acknowledge and work with priority needs identified by the individual. The baseline medication regime should be maintained as long as the individual is tolerating the medications and is able to swallow the medications. However, some individuals choose not to continue futile medical therapies, even if it results in shortening lifespan. The decision belongs to the individual, provided that it is made with adequate knowledge of the consequences and the symptoms that may develop if medications are not taken.

EXPECTED OUTCOMES

Expected outcomes for the individual with end-stage cardiovascular disorders should be tailored for the individual. It is not acceptable to develop a curative outcome. Measurable expectations may need to be adjusted every few days or weeks as condition deteriorates. For example, an expected out-come, "The individual will ambulate to the dining table for three meals each day," may need to be adjusted to "The individual will ambulate to the dining table for the evening meal with the family" and then to "The individual will consume one-half of the usual serving of food sitting in bed." This outcome refers to the declining ability to ambulate as well as the decreasing appetite and energy needed for consumption of food. The expected outcome in the fi-nal days may be modified to "The individual will drink one-half can of nutri-tional supplement twice a day."

SYMPTOM MANAGEMENT

Symptom management of end-stage cardiovascular disorders include contin-uation of medications until death approaches. Angiotensin-converting en-zyme (ACE) inhibitors with diuretics may be used to treat heart failure (Poole-Wilson 1999). Freudenberger, et al. (1999) described a four-part regimen for clinical heart failure consisting of diuretic, digoxin, ACE inhibitor, and beta blockers to help individuals feel better and live longer. This concept is im-portant given the prolonged nature of the illness. The individual is encour-aged to stay as active as possible for as long as possible.

Chest pain and general discomforts related to decreased tissue perfusion may be relieved with oxygen and short-acting nitrates (sublingual nitroglycer-ine). Occasionally the chest pain must be managed with low dose narcotics. Pulmonary and peripheral edema may be relieved with loop or thiazide di-uretics. Although vasopressor drugs may be used in acute exacerbations to in-crease blood pressure, they are generally not used in palliative care unless there is a specific need. Anemias may increase the fatigue, weakness, and dyspnea on exertion. If the individual wishes to improve activity tolerance for a special event, a blood transfusion may offer short-term relief of symptoms. Repeated transfusions, however, is not usually the treatment of choice as death nears.

The individual may complain of anorexia during the terminal phase of heart failure. Steroids or anabolic agents may be tried. Small frequent feedings, high-protein supplements, and preparing foods the individual wishes to eat may improve appetite. Usually, anorexia is a response to the progression of the disease and artificial or force feeding does not improve appetite or de-crease the cachexia which accompanies end-stage, long-term, chronic cardio-vascular disorders. The individual with end-stage heart failure may have in-tractable nausea without vomiting. Anti-emetics may be used to control nausea.

As death nears, this individual may become agitated, anxious, and restless. Having been near death before and having suffered through frightening episodes before, the individual may fear the dying process and the death event. It is natural to imagine the worst and to wish to escape that event. It is not uncommon for the level of consciousness to diminish as death approaches due to hypoxia and poor cerebral circulation. Until this occurs, anxiolytics such as lorazepam, diazepam, or haloperidol may be used for sedation, especially at night.

Oxygen demands may be increased by the restlessness which may exacerbate symptoms of breathlessness and chest pain, necessitating sedation. The experienced caregiver will develop skill in assessing the situation and responding accordingly. Sedation should not be used to mask spiritual distress or the emotional turmoil of unfinished business. These matters are better dealt with by talking, journaling, or consultation with psychologists or spiritual leaders. Individuals expressing a sense of hopelessness, guilt, and futility may be asking for help in accepting the inevitability of death. Listening to the individual and redirecting questions will allow resolution of distress and continuation of the grief work necessary for acceptance of the finality of death.

MANAGEMENT OF PHYSIOLOGIC CHANGES IN RESPIRATORY DISORDERS

Respiratory disorders, including chronic obstructive pulmonary disease and lung cancers, cause impaired gas exchange, alteration in breathing patterns, ineffective airway clearance. The symptoms of dyspnea, progressing from dyspnea on exertion to dyspnea at rest is frightening. Dyspnea causes the individual to either increase ventilatory effort or reduce activity (Kemp 1997). If the dyspnea is due to pneumonia, pleural effusion, ascites, or other treatable cause, and the individual is not actively dying, then treating the underlying causes will decrease the dyspnea for a time. Treatment of dyspnea include elevating the head of the bed or resting in a semi-reclining position and assuming a side-lying position (with the affected lung dependent) to improve movement of air to the unaffected side. Supportive treatment with positioning and oxygen may be necessary for symptoms related to weakness of the respiratory muscles. It is necessary to limit activity during exacerbations of dyspnea. Caregivers should space activities such as bathing, toileting, and medication administration to give the individual time to rest between exhausting activities. The room should be cool. A fan may be used to improve air flow near the individual's face. Mouth breathing may increase dryness of oral mucous membranes. Comfort measures such as sips of water and frequent mouth care is important.

Hypoxia causes agitation then sedation. Individuals experiencing dyspnea, agitation, and air hunger may benefit from oxygen administration, anxiolytics, and low dose narcotics, especially oral liquid morphine (Kemp 1997).

Nebulized morphine may also be used in palliative control of dyspnea in both heart and lung disorders. This treatment should be reserved for individuals who have already been treated with oral morphine. It is believed that this route has a local action on airway reflexes (Zeppetella 1997). Local anesthetics and steroids also have been given via nebulizer to reduce dyspnea. Other respiratory therapies and breathing exercises have been shown to relieve dyspnea. The ability of the individual to participate in the therapy may limit effectiveness as death nears.

Cough is another distressing symptom of respiratory problems. The individual complains of fatigue from not sleeping, rib and chest pain, sore throat, and headache. Providing increased humidity and removing irritants such as smoke and food odors may help. Although antitussives reduce coughing, they may lead to retained secretions, which could lead to infection. Most individuals should limit these medications to nighttime use. Opioids may be used to suppress cough alone or in combination with other medications. Hemoptysis generally occurs with cancer of the lung, but may occur during episodes of severe coughing. This is a distressing event and could precipitate the death event by hemorrhage.

Noisy breathing from retained secretions as death approaches—the "death rattle"—is distressing especially to the family since the individual may not be conscious. The use of an anticholinergic such as scopolamine transdermal patches may reduce secretions and decrease the noise. Suctioning does not usually decrease the secretions or the noise for any length of time.

Skilbeck, et al. (1998) studied the palliative care needs of the individual with chronic obstructive airway disease and noted inadequate continuity of care, including a plan of care, as they moved from curative to palliative to terminal care. Although most participants in the study believed that their physical care was adequate and that tasks were performed appropriately, emotional support for the chronic and debilitating illness was not adequate. The most common assistive devices provided were wheelchairs, walking aids, home alterations, nebulizers, and oxygen. Symptoms were evaluated in their study, and breathlessness was by far the most common and devastating. Other frequent symptoms were dry mouth, fatigue, and cough. Participants also reported distress with limitations in activities of daily living, citing going to the toilet as causing extreme dyspnea. It was very important to participants that quality of life had decreased. They verbalized concern related to role changes, sense of loss, depression, and worry. Individuals with chronic respiratory problems need continuous emotional and psychological counseling rather than crisis management. There was a high level of disability related to performance of activities of daily living, and these disabilities existed for a prolonged time before death occurred.

The term "terminal sedation"—referring to the deep sedation of terminally ill individuals to manage symptoms of dyspnea, pain, delirium, and vomiting—has been used in the literature for several years. Many of the individuals who require or request sedation also have unresolved psychological or spiritual problems as well as resistance to more commonly used palliative treatments of disturbing symptoms. When caregivers were asked to state reasons for terminal sedation, the major ones included intractable pain, anguish, respiratory distress and dyspnea, agitation and confusion, and severe anxiety (Chater et al., 1998).

SUMMARY

Chronic, debilitating diseases of the cardiovascular and pulmonary systems lead to end-stage disease and the terminal event. It is difficult to live with the knowledge of impending death. It is also difficult to predict with any certainty when or how the death will occur. Doka and Davidson (1997) describe the phases of illness as prediagnostic, acute, chronic, recovery, or terminal. It is the chronic phase that sets the stage for the terminal phase and death event. When the illness has a protracted course that consists of exacerbations, remissions, and gradual decline in health, individuals and families become immune to the expectation of death. The individual has survived so many near-death events that it seems death will not happen. When death finally occurs, it shocks the family and may precipitate a series of grief responses. The family has had to go on with their lives and may feel guilty at not having been there at the end. The caregivers verbalize physical and emotional fatigue. There are many unanswered questions related to why this crisis ended in death when the others didn't. "What went wrong?" they ask. It is important to provide supportive care to the individual and to the family, since your response to them during the terminal phase and the death event will impact their journey through grief.

Grief is an individual journey characterized by various steps toward integrating this devastating loss into one's life and being able to move on in spite of that loss. The journey through grief is different for each individual and each journey through grief is also different. Loss of a loved one brings with it the unfinished business of grieving previous losses. The family members may go back to resolve issues related to the time they first learned of their loved one's chronic illness and each succeeding crisis related to the illness. The caregiver must be willing to listen intently to what is being said and to the unspoken issues surrounding the death of a loved one.

REFERENCES

Chater, S. Viola, R., Paterson, J., & Jarvis, V. (1998). Sedation for intractable distress in the dying—A survey of experts. *Palliative Medicine*, 12(4), 255–270.

Doka, K., & Davidson, J. (Ed.). (1997). *Living with grief when illness is prolonged*. Washington, DC: Hospice Foundation of America.

Fristoe, B. (1998). Long-term cardiac and pulmonary complications in cancer care. *Nurse Practitioner Forum*, 9(3), 177–184.

Fruedenberger, R., Gottlieb, S., Robinson, S. and Fisher, M. (1999). A four-part regime for clinical heart failure. *Hospital Practice*, 34(9), 51–66.

Kaye, P. (1994). *Notes on symptom control in hospice and palliative care*. Essex: Hospice Education Institute.

Kemp, C. (1997). Palliative care for respiratory problems in terminal illness. *The American Journal of Hospice & Palliative Care*, 14(1), 26–30.

Poole-Wilson, P. (1999). Tailored treatment for heart failure: An emerging concept. *American Heart Journal,* 138(6), 1005–1006.

Porth, C. (1994). Alterations in oxygenation of tissues. In *Pathophysiology: Concepts of altered health states* (4th ed., pp. 321–588). Philadelphia, PA: J. B. Lippincott.

Skidmore-Roth, L., and McKenry, L. (1999). *Mosby's drug guide for nurses* (3rd ed). St. Louis, MO: Mosby.

Skilbeck, L., Mott, L., Page, H., Smith, D., Hjelmeland-Ahmedzai, S. & Clark, D. (1998). Palliative care in chronic obstructive airway disease: A needs assessment. *Palliative Medicine,* 12(4), 245–254.

Sommers, M., and Johnson, S. (1997). *Davis's manual of nursing therapeutics for diseases and disorders.* Philadelphia, PA: F. A. Davis.

Zeppetella, G. (1997). Nebulized morphine in the palliation of dyspnoea. *Palliative Medicine,* 11(4), 267–275.

CHAPTER 21

CARING FOR THE PATIENT DYING WITH A NEUROLOGICAL DISORDER

Susan Randol and Michelle Crain

When a relationship is lost—be it through separations, desertion, or death, but particularly through death—the emotional bonds that the surviving family members or friends had to the lost person must be slowly undone. This process, the inner psychological process of mourning and its accompanying emotions of grief, enables the relationship to be gradually relinquished in the face of the reality of its loss. The bereaved person eventually becomes able to renew old and establish new relationships, as the emotional focus moves again to life and, later, to the future.

Unlike the grief processes associated with these recognized losses, family members and friends of individuals who have experienced a severe brain injury related to trauma or a disease process experience the permanent loss of the loved one even though the body remains alive. The living body serves as an ongoing reminder of the enormity of the loss and serves as a significant barrier to grief. Additionally, the trajectory of neurological trauma and neurological disease processes proposes a future of limited functioning and decreasing capacities. This is in contrast to a predominate belief in Western culture that the future is full of promise and greater capabilities.

There are a variety of neurological conditions, disorders, and diseases that elicit these grief processes and produce end of life issues for both the patient and the family. Death may come very quickly and suddenly in some instances, and may be prolonged in others. Each neurological condition presents unique characteristics in relation to symptom onset, length of illness, treatment, and, finally, the dying process. For the purposes of this chapter, these neurological conditions will be grouped as traumatic injuries, neoplasms, strokes, and degenerative diseases and disorders. The authors will attempt to present the impact that these illnesses have on the patient and the patient's family. We will also discuss implications for the nurse providing care to this special patient population.

TRAUMATIC INJURIES

Both the brain and the spinal cord can be injured resulting in sudden death or a protracted and debilitating course leading, eventually, to death. Bergman (1999) identified that approximately 2 million people in the United States sustain some form of head injury each year, with about 80,000 resulting in long-term disability and 50,000 resulting in death. Spinal injury is included in this discussion of end of life issues because there are about 10,000 paralyzing spinal injuries in the United States each year, adding to already 200,000 to 500,000 individuals living with this life-altering injury (Hickey 1997).

Each head and spinal cord injury is different. The degree of loss or the probability of death depends on the location, type, and degree of primary injury and the presence of any secondary injury. The patient can be left with varying degrees of physical and psychological deficits involving movement, cognition, emotional stability, or vital functions such as breathing and body temperature control. Most traumatic injuries occur in individuals between 15 and 24 years old and are primarily a result of a motor vehicle accident. Such accidents are also the most frequent cause of spinal injuries, with the majority occurring in young people 16 to 30 years old (Hickey 1997). Other factors causing traumatic injuries include falls, especially in children and older adults, and penetrating injuries such as gunshots or knife wounds.

Head injury sequela can vary from minor to severe but the consequences of any head injury can be compounded due to secondary injuries caused by cerebral edema or increased intracranial pressure (IICP). Secondary injuries can occur immediately or can be insidious. A common initial symptom is a decrease in the level of consciousness. Later symptoms include an increase in systolic blood pressure without a corresponding rise in the diastolic blood pressure, a decrease in the pulse rate, and a decrease in respiratory drive. Unrelieved cerebral edema or increased intracranial pressure can lead to catastrophic deficits or death. Many patients who experience cerebral edema or increased intracranial pressure remain in coma or coma-like states for weeks or even years. These patients are then prone to multiple problems associated with immobility and often die of complications such as pneumonia or urosepsis.

Another complication leading to secondary injury in the head injury patient is the development of a hematoma, or blood clot. Cerebral hematomas can cause a rapid deterioration and death if not treated immediately. There are several types of cerebral hematomas. Epidural hematomas occur when there is bleeding into the space between the covering of the brain (dura mater) and the skull. Subdural hematomas, the most common type, are characterized by bleeding between the dura mater and the arachnoid space. This type of hematoma can occur within the first two days of injury (acute), within two to three weeks following the injury (subacute), or can even occur up to several weeks to months post injury (chronic) (Hickey 1997). Intracerebral hematomas generally have very dire outcomes and occur when there is bleeding into the brain tissue itself. Considered rare are the subarachnoid hemorrhages that occur between the arachnoid layers covering the brain and the pia mater or into the ventricles.

Head injuries are unpredictable and require intensive monitoring. This is very distressing to family members because the patient may be progressing satisfactorily and then suddenly be at the brink of death. The family begins to realize that they don't have this person as they used to be, but the body is still there, so many times, the family is simply unable to grieve their loss. Families may even lash out explosively, both verbally and physically, at anyone believed to be associated with the cause of the loss. Because they try to present the reality of the situation, nurses are frequently easy targets for the family frustration.

Spinal injuries can be fatal during the acute phase of the injury or as a result of complications years later. During the first year following the initial injury, death rates are the highest (National Spinal Cord Injury Statistical Center 1998). There are many different types of spinal injuries resulting in a variety of clinical problems. The spine is not always severed, but can be bruised, producing varying deficits and rehabilitation results. The initial injury is usually irreversible and can be extended with the development of swelling or hemorrhage in the spinal tissue (Hickey 1997). The location of the injury and the area or depth of the spinal cord damage determines the rehabilitation potential for the patient. Immediately following the initial injury, the patient goes into a spinal shock and will lose all muscle control, reflexes, and sensation below the level of the injury.

Cervical spine injuries are life threatening, as respiratory function is compromised. The patient may also go into a neurogenic spinal shock and develop problems maintaining adequate blood pressure, heart rate, and body temperature. These patients may also develop autonomic dysreflexia, characterized by sudden and severe blood pressure elevations and bradycardia. This condition is caused by common stimuli such as skin irritation from a wrinkled sheet, a full bladder, or fecal impaction. If not urgently treated, heart attack, stroke, or even death can occur.

Long term, the spine-injured patient may have complications involving any of the major organ systems due to the effects of immobility. For the spinal cord patient and the family, the losses to grieve are numerous. There is a loss of life as it was previously known. The patient will never be the same regardless of the level of recovery. There is also a reality that death can occur at any time and can be sudden, such as with autonomic dysreflexia, or can be slow and agonizing, as seen with sepsis and pneumonia.

When dealing with the family of a critically injured neurological patient, it is important to remember that waiting is one of the most difficult tasks. Every person handles crises in a different way; however, all families of neurologically injured patients experience uncertainty (Plowfield 1999). Many nurses are adept at managing the care of critically ill patients who have high technological and unstable physical needs. Time spent with the patient's family is often limited, and often the family member is viewed as an interruption to work. The nurse must realize that according to the family systems theory, there is never only one patient. Anything that affects one member affects the whole family. When a nurse cares for a patient, this care affects the whole family. By empowering families of critically injured neurological patients, there can be improved patient care and better overall outcomes for the patient.

CNS NEOPLASM

About 2% of all deaths attributed to cancer are a result of brain tumors (Curtis and Porth 1998). This chapter will briefly discuss the unique aspects of neoplasm or tumors located in the brain.

Malignant tumors encroach and destroy tissue, as well as take up cranial space meant for brain tissue. They can originate in the brain or grow as a result of metastasis. Symptoms occur and are more devastating when the tumor is fast growing. Tumors that are fast growing can cause cerebral edema and increased intracranial pressure. Slower-growing tumors allow adaptation and, therefore, symptoms are usually delayed or are not apparent until the tumor has reached a larger size. Even benign tumors or cysts on the brain can produce catastophic outcomes because of the enclosed environment of the cranium. The patient may have to endure multiple surgeries, often with only the hope of relieving symptoms. The surgery performed to remove the tumor may itself cause brain damage and loss of physical and psychological function.

The presentation of symptoms depends on where the tumor is located and the tumor size. The patient may demonstrate personality and behavioral changes or a deterioration in level of consciousness. Clumsiness or falls, gait disturbances, inability to walk straight, and dropping of objects are manifestations of motor disturbances that may present. For example, a family member may describe how the patient veers to the right when walking and cannot go left. Visual disturbances may be noted such as diplopia, or double vision, and hemianopia, blind areas in the visual fields that cause the patient to run into doorways or objects.

Often the behaviors described above may be thought to be of a psychological nature or may be attributed to "old age," thus delaying the diagnosis and treatment of the tumor. These generalizations may lead to feelings of guilt and anger for the patient and the patient's family.

Headaches are also a common symptom of brain tumors. The headache pain is related to compression within the skull or stretching of the brain tissues. These headaches initially occur primarily in the morning and may worsen with any type of straining or activity that increases intracranial pressure. As the tumor enlarges, the pain will worsen and may be continual. Nausea and vomiting are often symptoms related to the increased intracranial pressure and to the tumor compression of the vomiting center located within the medulla. If the medulla is compressed, vomiting may occur without the warning of nausea and is usually projectile. Seizure activity may also be a presenting symptom of a brain tumor, depending on what area of the brain is affected.

Brain tumor patients are unique. While this patient population resembles those of other neurodegenerative disorders, the nature of the illness can be progressive with a rapid cognitive and physical decline uncommon in other forms of malignancies and in most other neurodegenerative disorders. Frequently the diagnosis is made following a sudden emergent event, such as a seizure, and the patient never returns to normalcy in terms of physical function or cognitive abilities. The social stigma associated with cognitive and physical disabilities secondary to the brain tumor may cause more profound feelings of isolation and discrimination than other cancer patients' experiences.

Brain tumor patients may undergo treatments similar to those of other cancer patients such as surgery, radiation, and chemotherapy. Unfortunately, unlike many of the new treatments available for cancer patients, there has been limited progress in the development of highly effective therapies for brain tumors, specifically malignant brain tumors. The majority of therapies available for malignant brain tumors are palliative at best.

STROKE (BRAIN ATTACK)

Strokes, also referred to as cerebrovascular accidents (CVA), cerebrovascular infarcts, and more recently called brain attacks, are the third leading cause of death in the United States (Hickey 1997). An occluded, or blocked, artery secondary to a thrombus, embolus, or a spasm of the vessels can cause strokes. Brain attacks usually occur in older adults and may progress or evolve gradually. Brain attacks of an ischemic nature are not brought about by strenuous activity. Another type of brain attack occurs when there is bleeding into the brain; this type of stroke is referred to as hemorrhagic. Causes of hemorrhagic strokes include anything that causes bleeding such as trauma, drugs like coumadin or cocaine, hypertension, tumors, ruptured aneurysms or arteriovenous malformations, and blood clotting disorders. Hemorrhagic strokes are often associated with activity and straining, and although they account for only 15% to 20% of all strokes, they are the most fatal (Hickey 1997). Hemorrhagic strokes occur very suddenly with the patient complaining of the "worst headache of my life" then, almost immediately lapsing into unconsciousness or death.

Again symptoms depend on where the stroke occurs in the brain. General symptoms include decreased level of consciousness, sensory and motor impairments, difficulty speaking, and facial drooping. More specific symptoms are diagnostic of the location of the stroke. For example, a stroke located in the cerebellum will manifest with visual disturbances, dizziness, and dysphagia. A stroke in the frontal lobe of one side of the brain will manifest with impairments in the opposite extremities. This location will also cause problems with decision making, thought processes, and cognition.

DEGENERATIVE DISEASES

"The very nature of a degenerative disease indicates a process of loss" (Hickey 1997, 665). This process culminates eventually in death. The degenerative diseases that will be discussed in this section of this chapter include the dementias such as Alzheimer's disease, Parkinson's disease, amyotrophic lateral sclerosis (ALS), and multiple sclerosis.

Dementia

Most people with some form of dementia suffer for many years before dying. Because of the long-term nature of the dementias, it is not looked at as being terminal (Dunn 2000). It is a terminal disease, however, in which the patient dies of complications of the disease, much like many of the other neurologic problems discussed in this chapter. The patient loses functions, needs outside care, and eventually succumbs to problems like pneumonia.

Dementia is considered to be a syndrome of cognitive and intellectual impairments and is also called organic mental disorders (Hickey 1997). The course of dementia is usually gradual and sometimes goes unnoticed for years. Deterioration of the patient's memory, language, and concentration, as well as other aspects of their intellectual function slowly deteriorate. The patient eventually is unable to recognize family or even be aware of surroundings. This is especially distressing for family members.

One of the most common types of dementia is Alzheimer's disease. Onset is usually around 50 to 65 years of age, but can begin as early as age 40 (Thomas 1997). The cause is not completely understood, but changes in the brain include plaque deposits found in the frontal and temporal areas, atrophy of the cerebrum, and loss of neurons especially in areas related to thought and memory processes (Curtis and Porth 1998). One of the earliest symptoms is loss of memory, or forgetfulness, along with slight personality changes. The symptoms are progressive, and the patient may start to wander and lose orientation to place. The patient may also neglect personal hygiene, fail to follow instructions, become irritable and show obvious personality changes, and become socially isolated. Eventually the patient is unable to communicate or recognize family, is incontinent, and becomes bedridden and emaciated. Death often comes as a result of pneumonia or other complications related to immobility (Hickey 1997). The course of dying is usually 5 to 10 years.

Many other forms of dementia are similar in symptoms and may be differentiated by taking a complete history and physical. Diagnosis is confirmed with autopsy. Some other types of dementias include Huntington's disease, Creutzfeldt-Jakob's disease, Pick's disease, Acquired Immunodeficiency Disease (AIDS)–related dementias, and multi-infarct dementia. These differ from Alzheimer's in presentation, progression, and pathology.

Parkinson's Disease

Parkinson's disease is also degenerative and affects people during their middle to late years of life, usually after age 50 (Curtis and McDonald 1998). This disease can result from head injuries, brain tumors, strokes, or other degenerative conditions. The etiology is unknown but it is thought that the problem involves the basal ganglia (Hickey 1997). This area of the brain is involved with inhibiting tremors and controlling some voluntary movements (Thomas 1997).

The first symptom usually noted is resting tremors on one side. The most well known tremor is "pin-rolling" of the hand, but tremors may also be noted on the face and feet. These tremors progress to continual tremors bilaterally, along with progressive weakness, slow movement, and cogwheel rigidity (Curtis and McDonald 1998). The patient eventually has difficulty initiating movements such as walking and turning. Walking seems unusually slow and the gait has a shuffling quality. The posture and face of the Parkinson's patient is also easily identified, as their faces are expressionless with minimal blinking. Their posture tends to be stooped and they hold their arms in a semi-flexed position. The Parkinson's patient may eventually demonstrate cognitive changes much like dementia, and in 50% of these patients, serious depression ensues (Hickey 1997).

Because of the postural and gait changes, as well as difficulty with coordinated movements, the Parkinson's patient is at great risk for falls and injuries. As with most of the degenerative disorders, the patient will have increasing difficulty with swallowing and speaking, and are often immobile for long periods of a time. The patient will most likely become bedridden and die of complications.

Multiple Sclerosis

Multiple sclerosis (MS) is a chronic and progressive demyelinating disease that affects the central nervous system (Curtis and McDonald 1998). The disease usually strikes between 20 and 40 years of age, is more common in women, and seems to be more prevalent in cold climates (Hickey 1997). There are different classes of multiple sclerosis based on the course of the disease. Hickey notes the different types:

- Relapsing/remitting—acute onset in one-two weeks, with remissions and return to baseline in four-eight weeks; seen in 65% of patients. Pattern repeats with less and less improvements between exacerbations.
- Relapsing/progressive—similar to relapsing/remitting but does not return to baseline; occurs in 15% of cases.
- Chronic progressive disease—involves the cerebellum and spinal cord; relapsing/remitting can turn to this type; occurs in 20% of cases.
- Stable MS or benign—patients have long periods of only mild attacks or are symptom free for a year or more.

Symptoms of multiple sclerosis depend on where the individual patient's lesions are located, and a healthy person may suddenly develop symptoms of MS. Sensory symptoms are common and are manifested as numbness, or paresthesia, occurring on the face or extremities. Pain is usually felt as an electric shock type of pain upon flexion of the neck that radiates down the neck and arms. Spasticity may also produce pain symptoms in the MS patient. Other symptoms are visual such as diplopia, cloudy vision, visual loss, and pain with eye movement. Motor symptoms include weakness, usually starting in the lower extremities. Spasticity affecting the ability to walk and perform routine tasks is a usual symptom. Motor symptoms that worsen after a hot bath or shower are a diagnostic symptom of multiple sclerosis and are called Uhthoff's sign (Hickey 1997). Speech is also affected and may be slurred, very slow, staccato, and eventually indecipherable.

As with other degenerative and neurological diseases, death is due to complications such as pneumonia. Another problem facing the MS patient is depression, as the long-term and debilitating nature of the disease coupled with the young age of the patient wreak their devastation. Suicide is a possibility and the patient's mental outlook must be observed. Psychological changes may also include bipolar disease, dementia, emotional lability, and euphoria.

Amyotrophic Lateral Sclerosis

Amyotrophic lateral sclerosis (ALS) is also commonly known as Lou Gehrig's disease. This degenerative disease involves motor function and progresses very rapidly, with death ensuing within two to five years. There are about 5,000 cases of ALS in the United States each year primarily affecting men between the ages of 40 to 60 years (Curtis and McDonald 1998).

The disease involves upper and lower motor neurons, affecting cells in the cerebral cortex, the brain stem, the spinal cord, and the facial and hypoglossal cranial nerves (Hickey 1997). This results in decreased strength and spasticity, difficulty speaking, and dysphagia from the degeneration of upper motor neurons. Lower motor neurons contribute to the problems with muscle atrophy and flaccidity, fasciculations, loss of reflexes, and weakness (Curtis and McDonald 1998). One of the initial symptoms is muscle cramping and weakness in one of the extremities, usually one of the hands or arms. The symptoms will progress until the patient has serious difficulty with speech and swallowing along with difficulty breathing. A real concern is aspiration, especially in the presence of weak respiratory muscles. The patient may drool and demonstrate a very weak cough effort. These patients are extremely fearful of being unable to breathe; their minds are very clear to their physical weaknesses. The primary cause of death is from some form of respiratory difficulty or failure.

One of the unique aspects of ALS is that the patient's intellect is not affected. They are fully cognizant of their surroundings and are aware of their physical decline. This can be very frightening and distressing. Patients with

ALS, as with many of the neurological disorders, have difficulty expressing their thoughts, anxiety, pain, or other difficulties. These patients are prone to depression and anger and are very emotional (Kemp 1999). The sensory function also remains intact, therefore the patient may feel pain and be unable to call for assistance.

As nurses caring for this population, we must allow these patients to hold a sense of hope for the future. It is also important to allow these patients to communicate their lived experiences and understand that their coping strategies are accepted and encouraged.

Caring for the degenerative neurological patient at home places the caregiver in a double role: that of caregiver and that of family member (wife, husband, parent, child) (Habermann 1999). These individuals help their family members through very difficult times, support them financially and emotionally, and perform many of the everyday tasks of daily living. On the other hand, they also perform tasks that they are not prepared for—tasks that exceed what was inherent in the previous relationship. Through love for their family member, these caregivers may care too much and become so consumed in their responsibilities that they lose their sense of self. Many times they feel overburdened and unappreciated (Duijnstee and Borije 1998).

SUMMARY

Nurses and other health care professionals have a unique opportunity to make a difference in the lives of families and neurologically compromised individuals if they recognize that this population experiences chronic grief. Hansucker, Frank, and Flannery (1999), offered practice recommendations after studying how to meet the needs of families during critical illness. Their recommendations revolve around three common themes: individualize patient and family care, provide timely and frequent information, and empower the patient and the family to become active participants in care. The needs of these families and the patients will vary over the years as they encounter hurdles, obstacles, and difficult care decisions. It is essential that the nurse remain nonjudgmental about family or patient decisions and to support them through difficult times. Even though the patients are alive, they are not the people that they once were, and the grief continues.

REFERENCES

Bergman, A. (1999). *Testimony on children's health: Protecting our most precious resource in support of reauthorization of the Traumatic Brain Injury Act of 1996.* (On-line). http://www.biausa.org/childrens_health_testimony.htm.

Curtis, R., & McDonald, S. (1998). Alterations in motor function. In C. Porth (Ed.), *Pathophysiology: concepts of altered health states* (pp. 921–957). New York: Lippincott.

Curtis R., & Porth, C. (1998). Disorders of brain function. In C. Porth (Ed.), *Pathophysiology: Concepts of altered health states* (pp. 879–919). New York: Lippincott.

Dunn, H. (2000). *End of life decisions and the dementia patient.* Available at: http://www.nerds.net/aapublushers/dementia.html.

Duijnstee, M., & Borije, H. (1998). Homecare by and for relatives of MS patients. *The Journal of Neuroscience Nursing, 31*(4), 356–360.

Habermann, B. (1999). Continuity challenges of Parkinson's disease in middle life. *The Journal of Neuroscience Nursing, 31*(4), 200–207.

Hickey, J. (1997). *The clinical practice of neurological and neurosurgical nursing.* New York: Lippincott.

Hunsucker, S., Frank, D., & Flannery, J. (1999). Meeting the needs of rural families during critical illness: The APN's role. *Dimensions of Critical Care, 18*(30), 24–31.

Kemp, C. (1999). *Terminal illness: A guide to nursing care.* New York: Lippincott.

National Spinal Cord Injury Statistical Center. (1998). *National Spinal Cord Injury Association Resource Center Factsheet #2: Spinal cord injury statistics.* Birmingham, AL: University of Birmingham. Available at: http://www.eskimo.com/~jlubin/disabled/nscia/fact02.html.

Plowfield, L. (1999). Living a nightmare: Family experiences of waiting following neurological crises. *The Journal of Neuroscience Nursing, 31*(4), 231–238.

Thomas, C. (Ed.). (1997). *Tabor's cyclopedic medical dictionary* edition 18. Philadelphia, PA: F.A. Davis.

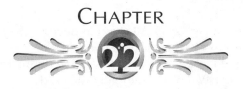

END OF LIFE EXPERIENCE AND CARE FOR THE AIDS PATIENT

Dr. Demetrius J. Porche

Human immunodeficiency virus (HIV) infection has culminated in an unprecedented amount of morbidity and mortality among productive men and women in the United States. As of June 1999, a cumulative total of 711,344 acquired immune deficiency syndrome (AIDS) cases had occurred in the United States (Centers for Disease Control and Prevention 1999). Of these, 420,201 individuals died as a result of complications from HIV disease; the greatest majority, 300,088, were 25 to 44 years old, very productive years of life (Centers for Disease Control and Prevention 1999). The amount of AIDS-related death remains alarming and imposes a burden on individuals, families, communities, and ultimately on various systems within society, especially the health care system.

Researchers and health care professionals have achieved multiple advances in the treatment of HIV disease. Recent advances in antiretroviral therapy continue to change the clinical spectrum of HIV disease and the resulting consequences of HIV infection. The natural history of HIV disease has evolved from that of an acute disease with a rapid and progressive advancement to death, to a chronic disease with a protracted and productive transition to death. This chapter will focus on the end of life experience and care for an AIDS patient from the paradigm of chronic illness.

THE NATURAL HISTORY OF HIV DISEASE EVOLVES TO A CHRONIC ILLNESS MODEL

Frequently in the early 1980s, the first presentation of HIV infection was symptoms of an opportunistic infection that eventually culminated in the person's death. By the 1990s, the HIV epidemic was growing exponentially with increasing numbers of AIDS-related deaths occurring after a longer period of illness. Medical therapy was limited at that time (Lashley 2000). In 1992, data predicted that by the year 2000, AIDS would become the number one cause of death for men 24 to 44 years of age (Puentes 1998).

Advances in the management of HIV infection during the 1990s, began to change the course of HIV disease. Currently, these advances in antiretroviral—especially protease inhibitors, introduced in 1995—and antimicrobial therapy for the various opportunistic pathogens are correlated with a decrease in the death rates resulting from AIDS. Better therapeutic management of HIV disease, better diagnostic and prognostic screening test, greater access to health care, and a redefinition of AIDS diagnosis has aided in the lowering of the AIDS-related mortality rates. The natural history of HIV disease has evolved from one of acute illness with rapid death to one of chronic illness with a protracted state of HIV disease (Lashley 2000, Puentes 1998).

Ferri (2000) reports that AIDS-related deaths have not occurred in their clinical practice within the past two years as a result of these advances in HIV disease management. Additionally, Ferri reports that causative factors associated with AIDS deaths have changed from acute opportunistic infections to death resulting from co-infections (hepatitis B or C, tuberculosis) or long-term complications of HIV disease management. AIDS-related deaths are occurring under the guise of liver dysfunction from pharmacological treatment or co-infections and cardiac disease attributable to long-term complications of metabolic abnormalities. Changes in the natural history of HIV disease has impacted the AIDS patient's emotional response to living and dying with HIV disease.

EXISTENTIAL EMOTIONAL ISSUES

The AIDS patient experiences personal grief that is manifested through various emotional states during the end of life experience. Some of these emotional states may be a coping measure and at other times it may be a hindrance to effective coping. These emotions may also be experienced by family members and significant others. The significant other of the AIDS patient may be HIV positive and view the partner's progression to illness and death as a reminder of their own mortality. In contrast, the significant other of the AIDS patient may not be HIV positive but feels a sense of overwhelming guilt for not being infected, which may compound the patient's coping with the end of life experience.

These existential emotional issues that confront persons infected with HIV may also affect the caring profession. Existential issues of medicalized care, social support, acceptance, repression, grieving, stigmatization, contagion, untimely death, and protracted end of life will be explored as emotional issues encountered during the end of life care for an AIDS patient. (Jones 1989, Worden 1991).

Medical Curative Care.   The medical profession in Western society focuses on the cure of illness at the avoidance of focusing on end of life experiences.

This medicalized approach consumes a considerable amount of energy by the medical profession and the patient in an attempt to deny the eventual consequence of chronic illness, death. However, discovering that one is HIV positive forces the patient to be confronted with the temporality of one's existence and the finite nature of life. Health care providers should be aware that an excessive focus on medicalized care (i.e. cure) may hinder an AIDS patient's coping with end of life issues (Jones 1989).

Social Support.   The level of emotional support from family, friends, significant others, and health care professionals influences an AIDS patient's ability to cope with death. During the end of life experience, AIDS patients experience anxiety and denial. Anxiety is a state of tension that motivates a person to act, whereas denial is a defense against anxiety that forces the patient to avoid the reality of their experience. The provision of social support assists the AIDS patient to achieve a balance among these emotions in order to cope with their end of life experience.

A lack of social support can compound or legitimize their grief experience. Many AIDS patients have had nontraditional relationships, which may create a barrier to achieving an appropriate level of understanding and support from others. If a relationship is not recognized by family and friends or socially sanctioned, the AIDS patient may feel socially isolated during the end of life experience. An excellent means of providing emotional support in such cases is through counseling and support groups (Grimes and Grimes 1995, Worden 1991).

Acceptance.   Persons infected with HIV must move through various emotions regarding past behaviors that may have contributed to their present illness and to the reality of their death. Acceptance of end of life permits patients not to postpone the death experience but to act in a manner to give significance to their life. Impending death and its acceptance can alter the way a patient perceives and lives in the world during the final days of life. Frequently AIDS patients experience a period of personal and spiritual growth while vacillating through various emotional states.

In coping with these issues of acceptance, AIDS patients experience behaviors such as projection, fixation, regression, rationalization, sublimation, and displacement (Jones 1989). Projection is the attributing to another person traits that are unacceptable to one's own ego, such as blaming another person for one's own behavior. Fixation is becoming stagnant in one developmental phase as a result of anxiety, such as the patient who never cycles to a coping state. Regression is the retreat to an earlier stage of development where the demands were less and the AIDS patient felt safe and secure. Rationalization is the development of reasons to explain issues that are a problem to one's own ego, such as AIDS patients providing excuses for their noncompliance with antiretroviral therapy. Rationalization is a self-deceptive process that prevents the patient from encountering the issues of reality. Sublimation is the utilization of a socially acceptable outlet for impulses, such as an angry

AIDS patient channeling energy into volunteering for HIV-related services. Displacement is directing energy onto another person or object, such as an AIDS patient displacing anger onto the nursing personnel.

Repression.   Repression is a defense mechanism in which the patient suppresses unacceptable reality into the unconscious state. Repression occurs when the patient avoids confronting progression toward death and proceeds in life without making end of life plans, such as a living will and medical power of attorney. An opposite coping mechanism is reaction formation. AIDS patients who act directly opposite to their conscious feelings are exhibiting reaction formation—for example, patients who are angry and hostile regarding their HIV infection act as though it does not affect them.

Grieving.   A patient's grief response is influenced by the intensity and course of the illness, support system, history of losses, and personal ego integrity (Worden 1991). Grief can occur early in HIV disease or at the end of life state. Individuals frequently grieve the loss of roles such as being an employee. A lack of necessary support systems can lead to an attempt to cope with grief in a dysfunctional manner. Grief may be delayed, masked, remain absent, or cumulative. Cumulative grief occurs when a person continues to experience multiple losses without progressing through the various stages of grief and bereavement with each loss or death, resulting in a multiple loss syndrome. Multiple loss syndrome consists of grief, a post-traumatic stress response, and burnout that affects the individual's personal ability. Multiple loss is frequently characterized by feelings of numbness, an inability to emote or feel feelings, expression of feelings in a new manner, pessimism, cynicism, fatalism, or insecurity. The health care professional should be alert to the fact that these individuals may engage in irresponsible or self-destructive behavior during the experience of multiple loss. Multiple loss syndrome can become a form of pathological grief when it begins to affect the patient's personal health status. Symptoms of pathological grief include intensified feelings of guilt or rage, increased physical symptoms or illness, denial, delayed reaction, and acting out of self-destructive behaviors. Pathological grief is frequently an unconscious event.

Stigmatization.   Stigma is an identifying mark of shame or discredit placed on a person based on socially interpreted standards of behavior. Stigmatization may leave an AIDS patient feeling rejected, judged, or alone during the end of life experience. A stigmatized AIDS patient is disqualified from social acceptance at a period of time when emotional support is needed. It may lead an AIDS patient or the family to attribute the cause of death to cancer or some socially acceptable causes. Stigmatization creates a state of fear for the AIDS patient during the end of life experience due to the concern about others discovering the illness. Stigmatization can occur after the patient's death, with the family, friends, or significant other being labeled unjustly.

Contagion. Contagion creates intense feelings of fear regarding the possibility of HIV transmission. Family members, friends, or significant others may experience intense fear regarding their own health and safety. This fear may be acted through behaviors that offend the AIDS patient, such as providing the patient with a disposable paper or plastic cup from which to drink. Some people reject close relationships with AIDS patients due to fear of contagion at a time when emotional support is critical.

Untimely Death. The majority of individuals who die from AIDS are relatively young. Death of children generally violates the parental notion that children would outlive their parents. This creates a difficult adjustment for parents and may be compounded by other existential issues presented. Untimely death precludes those left behind from experiencing anticipatory grief and increases awareness of their own mortality. HIV-infected patients with acquaintances who experience death are continually reminded of their potential untimely death. This continual reminder invokes feelings of denial, anger, anxiety, and depression.

Protracted Illness. The chronic nature of HIV disease has positive and negative consequences, depending on the individual patients' response to their illness and psychological coping mechanisms. The chronic and protracted illness associated with HIV currently may provide patients with more time to progress through and cope with the end of life psychological responses. In contrast, other individuals may experience the protracted illness as a state of intense negative emotional feelings related to their end of life.

HIV DISEASE END OF LIFE PSYCHOLOGICAL RESPONSE STATES

In addition to existential issues, AIDS patients experience numerous psychological responses such as depression, anxiety, suicidal ideation, affective numbing, denial, guilt, anger, hypochrondria, fixation, and obsession with death (Grimes and Grimes 1995). These responses appear to occur unpredictably throughout the clinical course of HIV disease. Nichols's (1985) classic work on the psychological response to HIV disease provides the nurse with a conceptual framework from which to assist health care providers in being proactive in dealing with such psychological states. The psychological states are crisis, transitional, acceptance, and preparatory.

Crisis State. The crisis state is considered the first psychological response to HIV infection. During this period, the person discovers the HIV infection status. Feelings experienced are affective numbing and acute denial, alternating with intense anxiety. The patient may experience the inability to understand instructions, with altered recall ability and memory failure due to preoccupation with the diagnosis (Grimes and Grimes 1995, Nichols 1985).

Transitional State.   This is the period in which patients realize their HIV infection status and begin integrating this into their self-image. During this realization, patients may experience physical suffering, social stigma, disfigurement, loss of sex life, and conflict associated with their choices. This is a
period of time with some negative alternating feelings of anger, guilt, self-pity,
anxiety, and denial. Feelings of regret and despondency may also occur, along
with suicidal ideation. Some patients may utilize the anxiety felt during this
period to mobilize their lives into a future orientation (Grimes and Grimes
1995, Nichols 1985).

Acceptance State.   Nichols (1985) correlates the acceptance state with a significant clinical event such as developing an opportunistic infection or beginning antiretroviral therapy. This state is frequently characterized as a very autonomous state in which the patient has a "take charge" attitude. Major
lifestyle changes may occur during this period in order to take charge of their
illness (Grimes and Grimes 1995).

Preparatory State.   The patient begins to be concerned with preparing for
death, with concerns regarding physical and emotional dependency. Reconciliation with family, friends, and significant others may occur during this state.
Typically the fear of dependence and loss of control is greater than the fear of
death. This fear may lead the patient to ponder suicidal ideation. Health care
professionals, as a coping mechanism, frequently deny patients' impending
death during this state by not permitting them to discuss their impending
death (Grimes and Grimes 1995, Nichols 1985).

Carter and Mc Goldrick (1989) provide an alternative framework from which
the health care provider can plan the AIDS patient's end of life care. The three
main phases create a general timeline associated with the natural history of
HIV disease: crisis, chronic, and terminal. During each phase, the patient is
faced with certain fairly predictable tasks that must be accomplished.

The crisis phase extends from the period prior to the diagnosis of HIV infection (including the contemplation of HIV testing) to the initial adjustment
to this diagnosis. The period of time from the crisis state (diagnosis) to the terminal phase is the chronic phase. During the terminal phase, the patient realizes that death is inevitable and the thought of death dominates the patient's life. The patient experiences intense feelings of mourning in the
terminal phase. Table 22–1 provides a description of the patient's task that
must be accomplished during each phase with some nursing actions.

END OF LIFE NURSING CARE
FOR AIDS PATIENT

Patients should receive compassionate and supportive care from nurses during their end of life experience with HIV disease. During this period, AIDS pa-

TABLE 22-1   TASK AND NURSING ACTIONS

PHASE	TASK	NURSING ACTIONS
Crisis	• Cope with diagnosis • Cope with symptoms • Seek health care • Cope with grief and loss	• Develop relationship with patient • Discuss feelings regarding health status • Refer for counseling • Refer to support groups
Chronic	• Cope with having a chronic illness • Attempt to live a "normal" life with a high quality of life	• Provide autonomy • Educate patient regarding disease process and current health status
Terminal	• Anticipatory grief • Cope with impending death • Resolve emotional issues	• Refer for grief counseling • Assist with end of life plans • Educate on end of life choices

tients experience physical, emotional and spiritual distress, and psychological pain and grief associated with their disease process and impending death. It is important that nurses support AIDS patients and promote their autonomy during the tenacious and cycling experience with the continuum of HIV disease (Bloomer 1998).

Nurses can provide compassionate and supportive palliative care to promote the AIDS patient's quality of life until death occurs. Palliative care is described as a specialty devoted to a patient-family center approach of anticipation, prevention, and treatment of suffering throughout the disease process. The nurse's focus on palliative care should be to promote comfort and function in order to maintain an acceptable quality of life for the patient (Bloomer 1998).

The nurse can initiate proactive care through the anticipation of the patient's psychological response states as described by Grimes and Grimes (1995) and Nichols (1985). Table 22-2 provides recommended nursing actions that correlate with each psychological response state.

SUMMARY

HIV disease has evolved from an acute illness with imminent death to a chronic illness with a protracted period of time that can be accompanied by a

TABLE 22–2   Psychological Response State: Nursing Actions

Psychological Response State	Nursing Actions
Crisis	• Ongoing assessment and early detection of psychological and neurological compromise • Written instructions to patient and significant other(s) • Remind patient of appointment via telephone calls • Consult with physician or nurse practitioner regarding anti-anxiety medicine • Consider psychotherapy
Transitional	• Active listening probing for suicidal ideation • Establish rules of conduct and courtesy • Use case management services and support groups • Provide positive reinforcement regarding healthy behaviors • Rapid referral for suicidal ideation
Acceptance	• Provide positive reinforcement of healthy behaviors • Continue to provide factual information • Refer for group or professional counseling as needed • Nonjudgmental regarding the seeking of multiple health care providers
Preparatory	• Discuss the patient's impending death; do not avoid the subject • Refer for legal consultation regarding living will and power of attorney • Explain options for end of life care • Provide reassurance that health care professional will not abandon patient • Provide information on home care and hospice services • Discuss funeral arrangements

high quality of life. The challenge of living with the HIV disease is that patients are plagued with numerous existential emotional issues prior to their end of life experience. Health care providers can provide quality health care through the anticipation of these emotional experiences.

REFERENCES

Bloomer, S. (1998). Palliative care. *Journal of the Association of Nurses in* AIDS *Care*, 9(2), 45–47.

Carter, B., & McGoldrick. (1989). *The changing family lifecycle:* A *framework for family therapy* Boston: Allyn & Bacon.

Centers for Disease Control and Prevention. (1999). HIV/AIDS *surveillance report*, 11(1), 1–42.

Ferri, R. (2000). Editorial. HIV *Frontline*, 39, 1–2.

Grimes, R., & Grimes, D. (1995). Psychological states in HIV disease and the nursing response. *Journal of the Association of Nurses in* AIDS *Care*, 6(2), 25–32.

Jones, A. (1989). AIDS and death: Some important considerations. *Senior Nurse*, 9(4), 14–17.

Lashley, F. (2000). The etiology, epidemiology, transmission, and natural history of HIV infection and AIDS. In J. Durham & F. Lashley, *The person with* HIV/AIDS: *Nursing perspective* (pp. 1–74). New York: Springer Publishing Company.

Nichols, S. (1985). Psychosocial reactions of persons with the acquired immunodeficiency syndrome. *Annals of Internal Medicine*, 103, 765–767.

Puentes, S. (1998). AIDS and death. *Annals of Long-Term Care*, 6(11), 358–360.

Worden, J. (1996). Grieving and a loss from AIDS. In AIDS *and The Hospice Community*, Madalon O'Rawe Amenta and Claire Tehan, eds. (pp. 143–150). Binghamton, New York: Haworth Press, Inc.

World Health Organization. (1990). *Cancer pain relief and palliative care*. (Technical Report Series 804.) Geneva, Switzerland: World Health Organization.

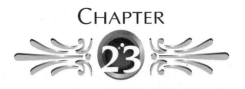

CHAPTER 23

EUTHANASIA, SUICIDE, AND THE TERMINALLY ILL

Dr. Regina Payne

INTRODUCTION

Kemp (1999b) stated that facing death may be life's greatest challenge but that most individuals meet death with equanimity. For some, however, the process of dying from a terminal illness with all its imagined and realized consequences presents an insurmountable obstacle from which suicide seems the only escape. Nurses can assume that individuals who are terminally ill think about suicide at some time during their illness.

The concept of suicide has nuances of meaning. Traditionally, suicide (from Latin *sui*, of oneself, and *cidum*, from *caedere*, to kill) is the act of intentionally destroying one's own life by one's own hand—what Wrobleski (1999, 206) calls "real suicide." Successful suicide is a serious, maladaptive, self-destructive behavior whose consequences have a ripple effect like a pebble thrown into a pond—except in suicide, the pebble takes on boulderlike proportions.

Most persons who contemplate or commit suicide are thought to be mentally ill, depressed, and acting irrationally. A subtle shift in thinking about suicide has occurred in the United States over the last few years. In certain circumstances, suicide is considered a rational act. This change is partly the result of the ability of medical science to prolong life.

While Americans live longer and more productive lives, there is an excessive use of technology to prolong dying, with scant regard for our obligation to relieve pain and suffering, promote a dignified and peaceful death, and respect the patient's right to refuse life-sustaining treatments (SUPPORT 1995). An avalanche of debate has ensued the last 10 years centered on physician-assisted suicide and euthanasia—issues about quality of life, sanctity of life, and patient self-determination. The 1997 U.S. Supreme Court decision affirming the right of Oregon to legalize physician-assisted suicide (Oregon Death with Dignity Act, 1994) has taken the national debate to new dimensions. The legal and ethical ramifications of these debates affect each individual nurse.

KEY TERMS

To facilitate participation in these debates, knowledge of key terms related to suicide and euthanasia is important, since misunderstandings ensue when meanings are unclear and confused. The following definitions are presented to clarify discussion:

- **Suicide:** The act of intentionally taking one's own life (Bongar 1991); death-resulting injury, poisoning, or suffocation with explicit or implicit evidence that the injury was self-inflicted and intended to result in death (O'Carroll, et al. 1996); synonymous with completed suicide.
- **Suicidal ideation:** Thoughts of or wishes to be dead and the active consideration of the pros and cons of taking one's own life (Shea 1999).
- **Suicide threat:** Verbal or nonverbal behavior that indicates the person is thinking about suicide, ranging from vague, veiled comments ("Things will be better soon") and behaviors (making a will, giving away possessions) to direct statements of immediate intent to kill oneself ("I have a gun and am going to use it") (Stuart 1998); behavior suggests that a suicidal act may occur in the near future (O'Carroll, et al. 1996).
- **Suicide attempt:** Potentially self-injurious act that would lead to death if not interrupted or if a more lethal means had been used (Stuart 1998). There is evidence that the person intended to kill himself or herself (O'Carroll, et al. 1996).
- **Lethality of suicide attempt:** The potential for death associated with the selected method (Moscicki 1999).
- **Intent of suicide attempt:** The individual's desire to die or expect to die as a result of his or her action (Moscicki 1999).
- **Completed suicide:** A self-injurious act that ends in the person's death (Stuart 1998).
- **Parasuicide:** A self-inflicted, injurious suicide-like act with low lethality (Bongar 1991) usually referred to as a "suicide gesture."
- **Euthanasia:** The act of bringing about the death of a terminally ill person usually through injection of a lethal medication (Back, et al. 1996; Hendin 1999). In euthanasia, the physician performs the intervention (American Medical Association 1999).
- **Voluntary active euthanasia:** The act of intervening "to cause the patient's death at the patient's explicit request and with full informed consent" (Emanuel 1994, 1891); also termed *physician assisted death* (PAD); euthanasia performed on a competent person at the person's request; the physician administers the lethal medication (Kemp 1999a).
- **Nonvoluntary active euthanasia:** Euthanasia performed on an incompetent person who is incapable of explicitly requesting a hastened death (Emanuel 1994).

- **Involuntary euthanasia:** Euthanasia performed on a competent person without that person's consent (Kemp 1999a, Waisel and Truog 1997).
- **Assisted suicide:** Providing an individual with the means to end his or her own life usually by deliberately prescribing large doses of medication which are likely to produce death when taken by the patient (physician-assisted suicide) or administered by the physician (physician-assisted death) (National League for Nursing 1997).
- **Physician-assisted suicide (PAS):** The patient self-administers a lethal medication which has been prescribed by a physician who understands that the person intends to use it to end his or her life (Emanuel 1994, Hendin 1999). In the United States, the only state in which physician-assisted suicide is legal within prescribed safeguards is Oregon (Oregon Death with Dignity Act 1994).
- **Rational Suicide:** Suicide in which the individual reaches a decision to end his or her life within the following parameters outlined by Werth (1996), the leading proponent of rational suicide:
  1. The person has an unremitting, hopeless condition, including but not limited to terminal illness, severe physical or psychological pain, physically or mentally debilitating or deteriorating conditions, or the quality of life is unacceptable to the person
  2. The person makes the decision freely without pressure from others
  3. The person has discussed the decision objectively with significant others
  4. The person is judged competent, nonimpulsive, and acting within his or her values to engage in a sound decision-making process
  5. The person has considered the impact of suicide on others
  Rational suicide includes: voluntary euthanasia or PAD; assisted suicide; physician-assisted suicide; and some instances of suicide by one's own hand without assistance from another person.
- **Palliative Care:** The comprehensive management of the physical, psychological, social, spiritual, and existential needs of individuals with incurable, progressive illness. The goal of palliative care is to achieve the best quality of life through relief of suffering, control of symptoms, and restoration of functional capacity (Last Acts Palliative Care Task Force 1997).

EUTHANASIA AND ASSISTED SUICIDE

Euthanasia (from Greek *eu*, good or noble, and *thanatos*, death) was used in the 17th century by Francis Bacon to mean an easy, painless death (Hendin 1999). Euthanasia connotes "mercy killing" or the active causation of a patient's death usually from lethal injection by a physician. While euthanasia is illegal in the United States, the Netherlands and the Northern Territory of

Australia have legalized voluntary euthanasia or physician-assisted death (PAD). Physician-assisted suicide (PAS) is legal in the United States only in the state of Oregon, and it differs from PAD. In PAD the physician administers the lethal medication, while in PAS, the physician prescribes the lethal medication but the patient must be able to take the medication without assistance.

Key Historical Events Related to End of Life Issues

In the last two decades, primarily because of advanced medical knowledge, technology to prolong the life of critically ill persons, and increased societal concerns about quality of life and rights of self-determination, the debate over end of life issues has intensified. The legalization of assisted suicide as a means to end suffering contradicts nursing ethics and will have a profound effect on nurses and nursing practice.

Professional organizations within health care have taken a variety of positions on assisted suicide. The American Society of Clinical Oncology (ASCO) position is to "neither condone nor condemn" assisted suicide (ASCO 1998, 1987). The American Nurses' Association (ANA) Code for Professional Nurses is more restrictive: "The nurse does not act deliberately to terminate life of any person" (ANA, 1991, 3). This position was reconfirmed in the ANA position statements (1992). The America Academy of Hospice and Palliative Medicine oppose the legalization of euthanasia and assisted suicide (American Academy of Hospice and Palliative Medicine 1997). Key historical events that have brought the debate over euthanasia and assisted suicide to its current status are summarized in Table 23–1.

Assisted Suicide in the Netherlands and United States

Physician-assisted death is legal in the Netherlands but is subject to criminal law. The Dutch recognize no ethical difference between PAD or voluntary euthanasia and physician-assisted suicide (PAS), so a large percentage of PAD consists of euthanasia (Waisel and Truog 1997). To safeguard against abuses, a notification procedure for PAD is used in which physicians report each PAD to the coroner who notifies the public prosecutor. An Assembly of Prosecutors General decides whether or not to prosecute. Of the 6,324 cases reported between 1991 and 1995, only 13 physicians were prosecuted, the outcomes of which were light: One case was dismissed, three were acquitted, three were found guilty without punishment, and three received suspended sentences (van der Wal, et al. 1996). The researchers also found that only 41% of all cases of euthanasia and physician-assisted suicide were reported in 1995, up from 18% in 1991. Many procedural requirements were not met in the unreported cases, such as securing a written request from the patient for PAS, consultation with another physician, and filing a written report. Other problems with the

TABLE 23–1 KEY HISTORICAL EVENTS RELATED TO END OF LIFE ISSUES

DATE AND EVENT	DESCRIPTION OF EVENT
1968 Brain Death	Withdrawal of life support from a living person, considered unethical behavior for physicians (Ad Hoc Committee of the Harvard Medical School to Examine the Definition of Brain Death 1968).
1974 CPR	The American Medical Association endorsed a policy confirming that cardiopulmonary resuscitation (CPR) is not appropriate in cases of terminal irreversible illness where death is expected (Waisel and Truog 1997).
1976 DNR Policies published	Boston's Beth Israel Hospital and Massachusetts General Hospital published the first do not resuscitate policies in the *New England Journal of Medicine* (Waisel and Truog 1997).
1976 Quinlan Decision "Right to Die"	Karen Ann Quinlan became comatose in 1976 as a result of alcohol and drug ingestion. Her parents fought successfully to have mechanical life support withdrawn, and Karen Ann lived nine more years in a permanent vegetative state following this action. Courts upheld the legality of discontinuing life support from a patient in a permanent vegetative state and dependent on a ventilator; surrogate had right to decline medical treatment for incompetent patient based on surrogate's intimate knowledge of the patient (substituted judgment standard) (In the Matter of Karen Ann Quinlan, 1976).
1980 Hemlock Society	Derek Humphry established the Hemlock Society, an organization for those who support the rights of terminally ill to choose death with dignity and to exercise personal autonomy over end of life decisions. Members believe that laws should allow a terminally ill person the choice of medical assistance to hasten their death.
1988 "It's over, Debbie"	An anonymous essay was published in JAMA by a resident physician describing his giving a lethal dose of medication to end the suffering of a 20-year-old woman dying from ovarian cancer (It's over, Debbie, 1988). Responses ranged from horror to sympathetic understanding.
July 1990 to Present "Doctor Death"	Jack Kevorkian, MD, used his "suicide machine" to euthanize at least 21 patients suffering from physical and mental disorders. In late 1998, Dr. Kevorkian was charged with murder after videotaping himself euthanizing a patient.
1990 Cruzan Decision	Nancy Cruzan was in a persistent vegetative state following a car accident in 1990. At the request of her parents and on the basis of testimony of two friends, her feeding tube was removed and she died. Basing treatment on previously stated preferences for end of life care is called "subjective standard" and is grounded on direct knowledge of the patient's wishes while competent (Waisel and Truog 1997). The United States Supreme Court upheld the legality of discontinuing medical care when a once-competent patient

TABLE 23–1 CONTINUED

	makes formal statements regarding end of life care and not wanting to live in diminished capacity. In addition, the Supreme Court's ruling significantly extended the Quinlan decision by including artificial nutrition and hydration (tube feeding) as medical treatment which may be refused or discontinued by a competent patient or surrogate (*Cruzan v. Director* 1990). The decision also upheld the rights of states to determine evidentiary standards and held that states may require "clear and convincing" evidence that an incompetent patient would prefer to have care limited.
1991 Assisted Suicide	Dr. Timothy Quill published a signed article in the *New England Journal of Medicine* describing his relationship with and actions to assist a young woman dying of leukemia, and his helping her to commit suicide by referring her to the Hemlock Society and prescribing barbiturates (Quill 1991).
1991 *Final Exit*	Derek Humphry published *Final Exit: The Practicalities of Self-Deliverance and Assisted Suicide for the Dying*, a do-it-yourself guide to suicide.

1991
Patient Self-
Determination Act
(PSDA)
	The federal PSDA was enacted to ensure an active role and voice for patients in the health care system. Officially ended medical paternalism by requiring all agencies to do the following:
	• Inform all patients of their right to refuse any treatment
	• Provide information about advance directives
	• Facilitate the execution of advance directive if patient so chooses
	• Patients must be given information about the following (Waisel and Truog 1997):
	  • Advance Directive: A legal document which provides information about the patients' treatment preferences should they no longer be competent to communicate their wishes.
	  • Living Will: An advance directive in which patients state in writing (and witnessed) their desire to avoid extraordinary care should they become hopelessly ill.
	  • Health care Proxy: Durable power of attorney for health care decisions; identifies a person to speak for a patient should that patient become incompetent to make health care decisions.

1994 Oregon Death with Dignity Act and Reaffirmed in 1997	The U.S. Supreme Court ruled that there is no constitutional right to assistance in committing suicide; this allowed states to make laws permitting or prohibiting assisted suicide (Oregon Death with Dignity Act 1994). The law permits terminally ill adult residents of Oregon to obtain, under strict conditions, a physician-prescribed lethal dose of medication to end their own life.

TABLE 23–1 CONTINUED	
1995 SUPPORT Study	The Study to Understand Prognoses and Preferences for Outcomes and Risks of Treatment (SUPPORT 1995) found that, even with increased information about patient prognosis and patient-surrogate preferences, patients and families were rarely consulted about 1) treatment decisions; 2) pain management was largely absent; and 3) dying and suffering were prolonged. Also, tenants of informed consent, the Patient Self-Determination Act, and the WHO guidelines on pain management were absent in medical practice with critically ill and dying patients.
1996 Patient Self- Determination	Competent patients have unlimited right to refuse any medical treatment, including life-saving treatments such as mechanical ventilation (AMA 1999).

Dutch system have been uncovered, the most serious of which are cases in which patients who had not given consent had their lives ended by the physician: The number of such cases was 4,813 in 1990 (3.7% of all deaths), increasing to 6,368 in 1995 (4.7% of all deaths) (Hendin 1999).

Kelly, Mufson, and Rogers (1999, 509) acknowledge that assisted suicide in all its forms is a "highly public and controversial issue." In the United States, public support for physician-assisted suicide became evident with the passage of the 1994 Death with Dignity Act in Oregon and its reaffirmation by voters in 1997. The law legalizes physician-assisted suicide within these highly controlled conditions (Official 1994 General Election Voter's Pamphlet, 1994):

- Patient must be a competent adult resident of Oregon.
- Patient must have a terminal illness (incurable, irreversible disease producing death within six months) confirmed by attending and consulting physicians.
- Patient must provide two oral and one written request for medication to end life in humane and dignified manner.
- Oral requests must be no less than 15 days apart.
- No less than 48 hours may elapse between the written request and the prescription.
- The patient must be fully informed of the diagnosis, prognosis, lethal medication and its risks, expected result from taking the medication, and feasible alternatives, including comfort care, hospice care, and pain control.
- The patient may rescind the request at any time.
- The patient is requested to notify next of kin but may: Inform family and ask their opinions, decide not inform family, or have no family to inform.

- Two witnesses (not a relative or heir; not connected with patient's health care facility) are required to attest that the patient is acting voluntarily.
- The physician may refer the patient for counseling; if a psychiatric disorder or depression is present, life-ending medication may not be prescribed.
- Any health care provider or physician may decline to participate.
- Health professionals and family members who attend the suicide are immune from prosecution.

Fears that the law would be overused by the poor, underinsured, and terminally ill are unsupported. In 1999, 27 persons died by PAS in Oregon compared with 16 in 1988. Only one in six persons who requested PAS in Oregon received a prescription for lethal medication. This is due, in part, to counseling patients about the availability of palliative care. Oregon public health officials, who are closely monitoring the law, found that persons who died under the Death with Dignity Act were "educated, thoughtful people who reflect about the meaning of the life and death and how they want to die" (Erikson 2000, 13). The following summarizes data for 1999, the second year of implementation for the Oregon law (Sullivan, Hedberg, and Fleming 2000):

- 33 persons received prescriptions for the lethal medication permitted by the law, secobarbital 9 grams (9,000 mg) orally.
- Of the 33 persons receiving prescriptions for lethal medication, 26 died after taking the medication, 5 persons died from their illness, and 2 were alive at the end of 1999.
- 1 additional person received the medication in 1998 but died in 1999 after taking the lethal medication, bringing the total to 27 persons who died by physician-assisted suicide (PAS) in 1999.
- 21 out of 27 were receiving hospice care at the time of death.
- Median age was 71 years.
- 16 out of 27 were male.
- 26 out of 27 were Caucasian.
- 12 out of 27 were married.
- Diagnoses: End-stage cancer (largest number lung cancer) 17 out of 27; 4 out of 27 amytrophic lateral sclerosis; 4 out of 27 chronic obstructive pulmonary disease; 1 out of 27 AIDS; 1 out of 27 multiple organ failure.
- 27 out of 27 persons had health insurance.
- 13 out of 27 were college graduates.

ASSISTED SUICIDE AND THE TERMINALLY ILL

Many terminally ill persons who request assisted suicide are motivated not by current pain and suffering, but by dread of what lies ahead as their illness progresses. They fear pain, loss of control, indignity, being a burden, and death itself. Clinically depressed terminally ill persons are four to five times more likely to consider physician-assisted suicide and harbor wishes for an early death than other terminally ill. The desire for death among terminally ill patients with cancer is correlated most strongly with depression, followed by physical pain, isolation, and lack of social support. More than 8% of patients who were terminally ill with cancer expressed a pervasive wish for death to come quickly (Chochinov, et al. 1995). The first step in treating depression in terminally ill patients is to control pain (Block 2000).

Pain
While pain is the most common symptom in dying patients, terminally ill patients across all settings rarely experience adequate pain management and relief (Foley 1997). This situation is intolerable since oral medications can effectively manage pain without severe side effects in 70% to 95% of terminally ill patients when given following World Health Organization (WHO) guidelines for managing cancer pain (Jadad and Browman 1995). Opponents to the Oregon Death with Dignity Act assert that patients who chose PAS are not receiving good palliative care and experience unrelieved suffering. With palliative care, pain and other symptoms can be controlled to the degree that the desire of terminally ill patients for physician-assisted suicide would be relieved (AMA, EPEC Project, 1999).

Depression
The diagnosis of depression is difficult in terminally ill patients since the vegetative symptoms of depression (changes in appetite, sleep, energy level, libido) frequently occur as a result of the terminal illness, and the usual DSM IV criteria for depression do not apply to patients with terminal illness. Asking the patient, "Are you depressed?" will open the door for exploration of this important risk factor for suicide. A person who answers positively to this question must be further assessed for the presence of the following indices of depression in terminally ill persons (Block 2000):

Psychological Symptoms:
- Dysphoria
- Depressed mood
- Sadness
- Tearfulness
- Lack of pleasure (anhedonia)
- Hopelessness
- Helplessness
- Worthlessness
- Social withdrawal
- Guilt
- Suicidal ideation

Other Symptoms:
- Intractable pain and other symptoms
- Excessive somatic preoccupation
- Disproportionate disability
- Poor cooperation and refusal of treatment
- Hopelessness, aversion, and lack of interest on part of nurse
- Treatment with Interferon and/or corticosteriods

History-Related Indicators:
- Personal or family substance abuse, depression, or bipolar disorder
- Pancreatic cancer

Common Fears

Persons dying from a terminal illness are challenged not only to cope with current realities but also with future ambiguities. Dying persons worry about many things: worsening of pain, loss of control over activities ranging from familiar routines to bodily functions, being a burden to families, dying an undignified death, and being emotionally or physically abandoned by friends, family, and caretakers. These common fears may lead a terminally ill person to attempt suicide or to request assistance with a hastened death. Common fears associated with living with a terminal illness are presented in Table 23–2, along with measures for preventing or reducing their effects (AMA 1999).

National Initiatives

Concerns about the quality of care provided to persons near the end of life has spurred several national initiatives: The Project on Death in America (PDIA) and Last Acts. The mission of the Project on Death in America is to broaden understanding and transform the culture and experience of dying and bereavement through initiatives in research, scholarship, the arts, and humanities and to foster innovations in the care of dying individuals through public education, professional education, and public policy. More information about the Project on Death in America can be found at its web site http://www.soros.org/death/.

Last Acts is a national coalition to improve care of the dying and to share issues and ideas at the national, state, and local levels. Last Acts members believe in palliative care as the best approach for care of individuals with incurable, progressive illnesses (see Appendix A). Access to information and membership in Last Acts is found on its home page at http://www.lastacts.org. Additional palliative care and assisted suicide web sites are listed in Appendix B.

TABLE 23–2   COMMON FEARS PREDISPOSING TO SUICIDE IN THE TERMINALLY ILL AND MEASURES FOR PREVENTING OR REDUCING EFFECTS

COMMON FEARS	MEASURES FOR PREVENTING OR REDUCING EFFECTS
Fear of Pain and Other Symptoms	Teach about: • Control of pain • Control of other symptoms • Sedation for intractable pain Display professional commitment to manage symptoms
Fear of Loss of Control and Autonomy	Explore specific important issues over which each person seeks control: • Daily activities, routines, and schedules • Medical care and treatment decisions Educate about right to determine own medical care and assist patient in decision making: • Right to refuse any treatment • Right to intensive symptom management • Right to refuse artificial nutrition, hydration, antibiotics, mechanical ventilation Encourage patient to prepare living will and select health care proxy Assist patient to plan for death Make personal commitment to help patient maintain as much control as possible
Fear of Being a Burden	Explore meaning of "being a burden" with patient Assess caregiving capacity of family: • Family willing and able to assume care • Arrange backup alternate and respite care settings Discuss financial concerns: • Help patient and family find community resources and services Elicit assistance from social worker and nurses for connecting to community resources and teaching care to family
Fear of Indignity	Explore meaning of "indignity" and "dignity" with patient Explore approaches to care and resources to support dignity Address issues of control: • Everyone has permission for their roles and responsibilities • Affirm patient's right to participate in decisions Reassure patient that he or she has dignity
Fear of Abandonment and Being Alone	Explore details and how realistic patient's fears are Discuss how well family, caregivers, and health care professionals are coping with patient's illness Offer respite care or care in alternate setting Increase hospice and palliative care involvement, if needed

NURSING RESPONSES TO REQUESTS FOR HASTENED DEATH

Nurses caring for terminally ill patients receive direct and indirect requests for hastened death and must be prepared to respond to this difficult request in a way that is ethical, legal, and compassionate. Any request for PAS must be taken seriously (AMA 1999). Patient requests for assistance in dying engenders anxiety and dissonant emotions in nurses (NLN 1997). Nurses may understand why a patient would make such a request but be strongly opposed to PAS and euthanasia. Arguments supporting and opposing legalization of physician-assisted suicide are presented in Table 23–3.

Pierce (1999, 621) found that oncology nurses were vehemently against actively intervening to bring about death even to relieve suffering. There was an "ethical uncertainty" about the correctness of assisting a patient to die. This did not mean that caretakers would initiate vigorous treatment. Nurses wanted a dignified, nontechnical death for terminally ill cancer patients. No practitioner accepted hastened death as an explicit goal of pain management.

Clarifying Personal Values

While PAS is legal only in Oregon at this time, the Death with Dignity movement is likely to be taken up in other states. Nurses experience first hand the depth of physical, psychosocial, and spiritual suffering endured by terminally ill patients who die not only in institutions but also at home. Honest self-exploration of one's own values about euthanasia and physician-assisted suicide is essential for nurses to fully enact their roles as advocate, caregiver, comforter, teacher, communicator, and confidant. A National League for Nursing task force (1997) examined the moral, ethical, and legal dimensions of the nurse's role in caring for patients who request assisted suicide. The following questions were proffered to help guide nurses:

- What are my values and beliefs about assisted suicide?
- What is the position of the state board of nursing?
- What are the values and beliefs of the community?
- What is the legal status of physician-assisted suicide in my state?
- Am I willing to take a stand on the issue of physician-assisted suicide?
- Am I willing to take a public stand in some way as a panel member, social activist, or leader in my place of employment?
- What are the choices that patients have when making end of life decisions?
- What is my professional responsibility depending on the position I take?
- If assisted suicide were legal in my state, what care would I be willing to provide?
- If I am not opposed to PAS, what exactly am I willing to do?
- Do I have access to an ethics review board from whom I can seek information?

TABLE 23–3   ARGUMENTS SUPPORTING AND OPPOSING LEGALIZATION OF PHYSICIAN-ASSISTED SUICIDE

ARGUMENTS SUPPORTING PHYSICIAN-ASSISTED SUICIDE	ARGUMENTS OPPOSING PHYSICIAN-ASSISTED SUICIDE
Autonomy/Self-Determination • Freedom to control one's own body • Since the definition of a "good death" is personal, individuals should be allowed to control the circumstances of death	**Autonomy/Self-Determination** • Inadequate patient and physician education about pain management, comfort measures, and treatment of depression lead to uninformed choice • Patient may be depressed, feel like a burden and not make choice freely
Beneficence • Well-being and compassion dictate that dying patients should not suffer unduly • If the burdens of being alive outweigh the benefits, physicians are obligated to perform assisted suicide	**Beneficence** • Medicine can do better job of pain control with less loss of dignity **Nonmalfeasance** • Ethical principle of do no harm forbids any deliberate act to cause death
Legalization • Distinction between withholding or withdrawing treatments in terminal situations versus directly ending a life is artificial • Legalization of PAS will increase public accountability of the practice • Legalization of PAS will ensure medical safeguards and prevent abuses • Patients will feel supported by physicians during their death	**Legalization** • Permitting PAS gravely harms image of the physician as healer • Concerns about caregiver's motives for offering euthanasia: elderly, infirm, or indigent may be subjected to subtle pressure to die to reduce social, emotional, economic burden • Permitting PAS will discourage physicians from seeking solutions to end of life problems • PAS diverts attention away from the need to optimize palliative care • PAS may have long-lasting negative effects on family who may or may not have role in decision • PAS devalues the sanctity of life and predicts a slippery slope to nonvoluntary euthanasia for patients who may or may not be terminally ill • Euthanasia circumvents the normal grief process

Note. Adapted from D. B. Waisel and R. D. Truog. "The End-of-Life Sequence," Anesthesiology 87 (1997): 676–686; National League for Nursing, "Life-Terminating Choices: A Framework for Nursing Decision Making," Nursing and Health Care Perspectives 18 (1997): 198–204; V. P. Tilden and M. A. Lee, "Oregon's Physician-Assisted Suicide Legislation: Troubling Issues for Families," Journal of Family Nursing 3 (1997): 120–128.

Choosing Palliative Care

A request for PAS may be a sign that the terminally ill patient is experiencing a crisis resulting from the overwhelming presence of unmet needs. Palliative care proponents argue that PAS is morally wrong and propose that withholding and withholding unnecessary treatments, aggressively treating pain, depression, and suffering, and educating physicians and nurses in the care of the dying will preclude the need for PAS.

Withholding and Withdrawing Life-Sustaining Treatment.   In the setting of terminal illness, withholding and withdrawing life-sustaining therapies are ethically and medically sound (AMA 1999). There is no legal or ethical difference between *withholding* and *withdrawing* certain treatments. Nurses, because of their intimate involvement with patients and families, play an essential role in the decision-making process. Understanding the terminally ill patient's goals for care and facilitating the best decision to withhold or withdraw therapy require skill. There is a wide variety of treatments that might be considered by the patient and family. These include cardiopulmonary resuscitation (CPR), elective intubation and ventilator support, surgery, dialysis, blood transfusions or blood products, oxygen, intravenous fluids, tube feedings, diagnostic tests, antibiotics, and future hospitalization (AMA 1999).

Principle of Double Effect.   Providing palliative care that may have fatal side effects—called the principle of double effect—is ethically appropriate. The ANA (1991, 2) states, "The increased titration of medication to achieve adequate symptom control, even at the expense of maintaining life or hastening death secondarily, is ethically justified." The principle of double effect is most often used in terminal pain relief but may also be used to justify the use of opiates to relieve cough and breathlessness (Pace 1996).

Palliative Care Protocol.   Emanuel (1998, 644) outlined an eight-step clinical protocol for professional response to requests for PAS (see Figure 23–1). Her recommendations are based upon two widely held ethical principles of palliative care: autonomy, the patient's right to be free of unwanted interventions, including withholding and withdrawing life-sustaining treatment; and non-malfeasance, the health professional's obligation to respect human dignity and provide comfort and relief from pain and other illness-related suffering. Emanuel's approach necessitates a team approach, with clearly stated values about end of life care that embrace hospice philosophy and palliative care.

Choosing Physician-Assisted Suicide

Kemp (1999b) asserted that lack of clarity, misunderstandings, and continual anxiety are hallmarks of end of life decision making. A typical sequence of events in the process of terminal illness illustrates this point:

- The person first notices an "ominous symptom" (p. 18) bringing on feelings of fear, anxiety, and denial.

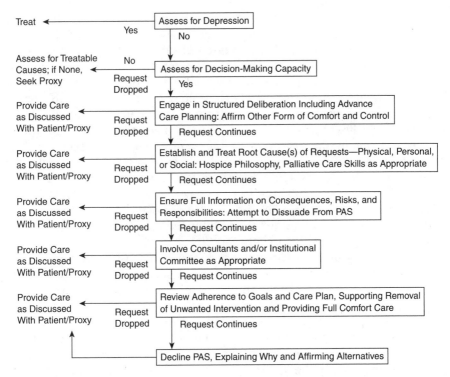

Figure 23–1 Approach to the Patient Who Requests Physician-Assisted Suicide (PAS) (Emanuel, 1998, p. 644).

- Help is sought which boosts hope, but hope is clouded by fear, anxiety, and denial.
- A diagnosis is made. The prognosis and treatment options are discussed. The illusion of "living forever" is shattered, and the individual and family feel overwhelmed, confused, fearful of the future, and abandoned.
- Treatment is begun. The intensity of the side effects and suffering surprise the individual and family.
- The suffering may be endured or may be overwhelming, which prompts requests to discontinue therapies. Individual and family worry if the right choice was made.
- The outcome of treatment is ambiguous, and the individual and family wait and hope for a remission in the illness.
- Symptoms recur and hope falls; suffering and mortality become realities.
- As the disease progresses, the individual and family experience emotional and physical exhaustion. They are tired of hoping and failing, tired of sickness, and tired of worry.
- When death comes, there is a "deep weariness that surpasses all previous experience" (p. 19).

Studies show that the physical, emotional, social, and spiritual needs of critically and terminally ill persons are unmet even following efforts to improve care. The SUPPORT (1995) study—a well-controlled, prospective, multisite study of 9,105 critically ill patients to improve end of life decision making and reduce the incidence of mechanically supported, painful, and protracted dying—found that efforts to prolong life only prolonged death, even following an intervention to improve physician-patient communication. Approximately 40% of patients spent at least 10 days in intensive care where invasive treatments and isolation were the norm. At least half of patients able to communicate reported having serious pain in their final days. Physicians were unaware of patients' resuscitation preferences, and do not resuscitate (DNR) orders were written in the last two days of the patient's life. Families were economically devastated by the care. In spite of these shortcomings with end of life care, both control (68%) and intervention (69%) patients or surrogates rated care as excellent to very good.

The public is painfully aware of the crisis atmosphere that surrounds the final hours of dying with a terminal illness in any setting. This causes dying to be worse than it should be and predisposes terminally ill persons to consider "real suicide" or to request physician-assisted suicide. When a patient requests physician-assisted suicide, the nurse's personal values may conflict with the patient's decision to terminate life. In this case, the nurse has the right to withdraw from further participation in patient care after conscientiously informing the patient and family of the ethical dilemma, formally referring the patient to another health care provider, or transferring care to another nurse (NLN 1997). When nursing values are congruent with a patient's request for PAS and nursing participation in PAS is within the legal scope of nursing practice, as in Oregon, the following nursing interventions guide practice with patients who determine that PAS is the correct choice (AMA 1999, Block 2000, NLN 1997):

- Provide care and comfort to relieve pain and suffering:
    Assess for and work collaboratively for control or reduction of pain, breathlessness, weakness, fatigue, anorexia, depression, anxiety, delirium, and other illness-related symptoms.
    Assess for troubling side effects from medications.
- Assess quality of patient coping with issues of loss of control, dependency, uncertainty, and grief:
    Are fears about the dying process contributing to the desire to die?
- Explore the reasons for the patient's request for PAS by asking:
    What makes you ask for PAS at this time?
    What will your death accomplish for you? For others?
- Evaluate rationality of patient's choice:
    Do hopelessness and depression distort the patient's judgment?
    Are there cognitive deficits?
    Does the patient understand the condition, its course?

- Inform the patient of all available legal options including living will, advance directives, durable power of attorney, palliative care, withholding and withdrawing treatments, and PAS.
- Encourage the patient to communicate openly with family and significant others about plans and wishes:
  - Explore the question, How do you think your death will affect others?
- Facilitate discussion between the patient and physician about end of life preferences.
- Inform the patient about available community resources, such as hospice care, respite care, home health, complementary therapies, spiritual support.
- Expand and involve the patient's social and familial network:
  - Has there been a recent loss, conflict, or rejection?
  - Are there fears about abandonment, rejection, or financial burden?
  - With whom has the patient spoken about PAS plans?
  - How do these individuals feel about the patient's wishes?
  - Are interpersonal tensions contributing to psychosocial suffering?
- Explore religious, spiritual, and existential concerns:
  - Are there unresolved or distressing questions or concerns?
- Maintain confidentiality about the patient's decisions, except in the case of imminent suicide.
- Assist the patient in meeting prescribed legal safeguards in PAS protocol.
- Determine from the patient the time, circumstances, involvement of others, and amount of assistance desired during the final hours.
- Assist the patient in obtaining prescribed drugs for PAS.
- Be present during the patient's self-administration of lethal medication, during death, and afterwards to console significant others who may be present.
- Assist the family and significant others to arrange long-term bereavement support.
- Provide care to a patient admitted to the emergency room after a failed assisted suicide attempt.
- Be involved in policy development at local health care facility, community agency, or local and state legislative level.

SUMMARY: EUTHANASIA AND ASSISTED SUICIDE

End of life decisions are among the most difficult and confusing for patients, families, and health care providers. Although there has been significant improvements in the care of terminally ill persons, the dying experience has not been similarly improved. There is agreement that it is ethical and legal to withhold and withdraw medical treatments and to relieve physical suffering even if the patient's life is shortened. However, whether the ethical arguments of autonomy and beneficence justify active voluntary euthanasia or physician-assisted suicide remain controversial (Emanuel 1994). With the passage of the 1994 Oregon Death with Dignity Act and its reaffirmation in 1997, the consequences of permitting physician-assisted suicide in the United States will be evaluated. Nurses are challenged to clarify their values and beliefs about requests for hastened death from terminally ill patients. The accountability of nurses to counsel patients and families about end of life choices is more complex today than ever before.

ASSESSING RISK OF SUICIDE IN TERMINALLY ILL PATIENTS

Suicide is difficult to predict. Even in high risk groups, suicide is infrequent and the rate in the general population is low (Plutchik, et al. 1996). Shea (1999) asserts that the decision to kill oneself is an internal, secretive process, made after a complex and stressful process of weighing the pros and cons. The importance of determining the presence or absence of risk factors cannot be overemphasized. The focus of suicide prevention rests on recognizing circumstances and symptoms that indicate the individual is at risk for suicide and intervening appropriately. Suicide risk assessment must be as thorough as possible even in persons with advanced disease and known to be terminally ill.

Risk factors for suicide are measurable personal characteristics, aspects of one's lifestyle, or environmental hazards that are statistically associated with and increase the likelihood of completed suicide and precede the suicide in time (Last, 1995; Kraemer, et al. 1997). The greater the number of risk factors present, the greater the degree of risk. Nurses are cautioned that one single risk factor rarely precipitates suicide, but the cumulative, interactive, and additive effects of coexisting risk factors create an increased risk. Suicide risk should always be assessed and documented at these times (Moscicki 1999):

- upon first admission or initial psychiatric evaluation
- occurrence of any suicidal ideation or behavior
- significant clinical change in depression, either improvement or worsening
- prior to increasing privileges or granting passes
- prior to discharge from agency

Several authors (Moscicki 1999, Shea 1999) recommend organizing suicide risk factors into categories that distinguish between distal and proximal risk factors. Distal risk factors are longstanding characteristics which predispose the individual to increased risk and are statistically related to suicide. Distal risk factors are unreliable in assessing the immediate risk but are key in framing an overall judgment of risk. Assessing the presence of distal risk factors and gauging the degree of risk alerts the nurse not that the patient is at higher risk, but that the patient may be at higher risk. Distal predisposing risk factors include demographic and epidemiological factors, psychopathological factors, historical, familial, social support, and neurobiological factors.

Proximal risk factors are characteristics of a specific living person that may act as "triggers" to precipitate an immediate suicide (Shea 1999). Both proximal and distal risk factors must be assessed for safe, effective practice. The primary goal of suicide risk assessment is not to predict suicide but to place an individual along a continuum of risk, to understand the forces driving the individual, and to determine appropriate interventions (Jacobs, Brewer, and Klein-Benheim 1999). Proximal risk factors include access to lethal means of suicide, recent severe stressful life events, and social isolation.

DISTAL PREDISPOSING RISK FACTORS FOR SUICIDE

Demographic and Epidemiologic Risk Factors

Suicide is a persistent, worldwide public health problem. In the United States, approximately 75 persons kill themselves daily, and one suicide occurs every 20 minutes (Roy 2000). The overall age-adjusted suicide rate is 11.4 per 100,000, unchanged since 1994 and much lower than the rate for cardiovascular disease, the leading cause of death, at 271.6 per 100,000 (National Center for Health Statistics 1999). The main source of data on suicide mortality in the U.S. is death certificate information reported to the National Center for Health Statistics (NCHS). Suicide mortality is underreported in official data due to the social stigma associated with suicide but Moscicki (1999) believes the undercount is low.

Age and Gender. Suicide is the eighth leading cause of death in the United States, resulting in 30,535 deaths in 1997 (NCHS 1999). Suicide rates vary by age, gender, marital status, socioeconomic status, and ethnicity. The suicide rate for 15-24 year olds has more than tripled over the last 30 years (Aguilera 1998) and is currently the third leading cause of death in this age group at 11.4 per 100,000 population (NCHS 1999). Rates increase with age, with the highest rates among elderly white men. Although individuals age 65 and over comprise 26% of the population, they account for 40% of suicide deaths (Stuart 1998). The U.S. Centers for Disease Control reports that the number of suicides among Americans age 65 and older has risen 36% since 1980, with rates of 40 per 100,000 population in men 65 years and over (Roy 2000) and 63.1 per 100,000 men age 85 and older (Moscicki 1999). In women, suicide rates increase until midlife, when rates plateau.

Men consistently have higher suicide rates than women. White males account for 73% and white females for 18% of all suicide deaths (Firestone 1997). Men commit suicide more than four times more frequently than women, but women attempt suicide three times more often than men. This difference in completed suicides relates to men selecting more lethal means such as firearms, while women overdose on medications. The age-adjusted suicide rate for men is 18.7 per 100,000 (NCHS 1999), while that for women is 4.1 per 100,000 (Moscicki 1999).

Marital Status, Socioeconomic Status, and Occupation. The suicide rate for single persons is twice that for married persons, and single, divorced, and widowed persons have suicide rates four to five times greater than married persons (Roy 2000). Individuals in the highest and lowest social classes have higher rates than those in middle classes (Kaplan and Sadock 1998). During economic recessions, depressions, and times of high unemployment, the suicide rate increases; in times of high employment and during wars, the rate decreases (Roy 2000). Suicide rates are higher among physicians, musicians, dentists, police officers, lawyers, and insurance agents than they are in the general population (Stuart 1998).

Ethnicity. Sociocultural factors contribute to suicidality. Suicide rates for African Americans are lower than for whites, although there has been a recent increase in suicide among young black men ages 15-19 which corresponds with the increase in homicides in this group (Shaffer, Gould, and Hicks 1994). Mortality data show that the age-adjusted suicide rate among African Americans of both sexes rose more than 36% between 1960 and 1985, and the rate among black males rose 45% (Burr, Hartman, and Matteson 1999). Gender differences are similar by race (NCHS 2000):

- Age-adjusted suicide rate for black men—12.4 per 100,000
- Age-adjusted suicide rate for white men—19.7 per 100,000
- Age-adjusted suicide rate for black women—2.0 per 100,000
- Age-adjusted suicide rate for white women—4.4 per 100,000

PSYCHOPATHOLOGICAL RISK FACTORS

Psychiatric and Addictive Disorders

The strongest and most frequently occurring risk factor for completed and attempted suicide is having a recent major mental illness (Moscicki 1999). The three most common DSM IV Axis I diagnoses associated with attempted and completed suicide are: mood disorders (major depression and bipolar illness); alcohol and substance abuse or dependence; and schizophrenia (Fawcett, Clark, and Busch 1993). The DSM IV Axis II diagnoses of borderline personality and antisocial personality disorder follow the above Axis I diagnoses in importance as clinical risk factors for suicide (Jacobs, Brewer, and Klein-Benheim 1999).

Mood Disorders.   Individuals with mood disorders are far more likely to commit suicide than persons with any other psychiatric diagnosis. More than 90% of all persons who commit suicide have a diagnosed psychiatric illness, and depressive disorders account for nearly 60% of this figure. The annual suicide rate for persons with major depression is eight times that found in the general population. Mood disorders are more frequently associated with completed suicide in older adults and women, while substance abuse and personality disorders are most often associated with suicide in adolescents and young adults (Henriksson, et al. 1993 and 1995; Lesage, et al. 1994). Characteristics associated with high risk of imminent suicide are (Fawcett, et al. 1990):

* severe anxiety
* panic attacks
* severe anhedonia
* global insomnia
* difficulty concentrating
* abuse of alcohol

Although depression contributes greatly to disease morbidity in the United States, depression frequently goes underdiagnosed and undertreated (Block 2000, AMA 1999). Depression is one of the 10 most costly illnesses in the United States at approximately $43 billion per year (Hirschfeld, et al. 1997). The vast majority of individuals treated with antidepressants are not treated with an adequate dose nor for a long enough period. Roy (2000) reported that most depressed suicide victims had received inadequate or no treatment for depression prior to their death. Therefore, early diagnosis and treatment of depression and bipolar disorders are important first-line steps in preventing suicide.

Block (2000) strongly urges nurses that major depression is a treatable condition in the terminally ill and recommends antidepressants, supportive psychotherapy, and family and patient education. Block also recommends using psychostimulants such as dextroamphetamine, methylphenidate, and pemoline in terminally ill patients who are debilitated and fatigued. The dose is tapered after one or two weeks while therapeutic levels of antidepressant medications are reached.

Depression should be treated in the terminally ill. Depression interferes with the dying process in the following ways: the patient's capacity for pleasure, meaning, and connection is impaired; pain and other symptoms are made worse; quality of life suffers; the patient's separation process is made more difficult; family members and others worry; and depression increases risk for suicide and requests for physician-assisted suicide. The comparison of normal grief with depression in terminally ill patients in Table 23–4 will assist nurses in recognizing depression in patients with advanced disease (Block 2000).

Substance Abuse.   Substance abuse, especially alcohol addiction, is associated with a greater frequency of attempts, more lethal attempts, more serious

TABLE 23–4   GRIEF COMPARED WITH DEPRESSION IN TERMINALLY ILL PATIENTS

CHARACTERISTICS OF GRIEF	CHARACTERISTICS OF DEPRESSION
Patients experience feelings, emotions, and behaviors that result from a specific loss.	Patients experience feelings, emotions, behaviors that fulfill criteria for a major psychiatric disorder; distress is usually generalized to all facets of life.
Almost all terminally ill patients experience grief, but only a few develop clinical depression requiring treatment.	Major depression occurs in 7%-53% of terminally ill patients.
Patients usually cope with distress on their own.	Medical or psychiatric intervention is usually necessary.
Patients experience somatic distress, loss of usual patterns of behavior, agitation, sleep and appetite disturbances, decreased concentration, social withdrawal.	Patients experience similar symptoms plus hopelessness, helplessness, worthlessness, guilt, and suicidal ideation.
Grief is associated with disease progression.	Depression has an increased prevalence in patients with advanced disease; pain is a major risk factor.
Patients retain the capacity for pleasure.	Patients enjoy nothing.
Grief comes in waves.	Depression is constant and unremitting.
Patients express passive wishes for death to come quickly.	Patients express intense and persistent suicidal ideation.
Patients are able to look forward to the future.	Patients have no sense of a positive future.

intent, and higher levels of suicide ideation (Lewinsohn, Rohde, and Seeley 1996). Alcohol abuse is a factor in approximately 23% of suicides (Murphy, et al. 1992). Drug and alcohol abuse are significant risk factors because these agents decrease impulse control, contribute to psychotic thinking, and impair memory. When the addicted person stops drinking, the risk of suicide escalates. For some, alcohol abuse enables individuals to cope with otherwise intolerable levels of anxiety and stress. Due to the long-term consequences of alcohol abuse, alcoholic persons usually commit suicide following years of drinking (Roy 2000). Other factors linked to suicide in alcoholism are continued drinking, lack of support systems, serious medical illness, unemployment, loss of close relationships, isolation, living alone, and communicating suicidal intent.

Schizophrenia. Schizophrenia accounts for 10%-15% of all suicides, and persons with schizophrenia have a 10% lifetime risk of suicide (Murphy 1986a). Since rational thought often acts as the last barrier to suicide, every psychotic illness or episode warrants a thorough assessment for suicide risk. Shea (1999) identified three patterns of psychotic thinking that are especially dangerous in persons with psychosis: command hallucinations, feelings of alien control, and religious preoccupation. Most persons with schizophrenia who commit suicide do so during the first few years of their illness (Roy 2000).

Persons with paranoid schizophrenia are at greatest risk for suicide due to the predominance of positive symptoms (hallucinations, delusions, disorganized speech, catatonia) over negative symptoms (affective flattening, alogia, avolition, anhedonia). The "healthier" the person with schizophrenia, the more likely he or she is to attempt suicide (Fenton, et al. 1997), since these individuals are painfully aware of the seriousness of their illness. The risk factors associated with suicide in persons with psychotic illness such as schizophrenia or manic depressive illness are listed below (Jacobs, Brewer, and Klein-Benheim 1999):

* young age
* early stage of illness
* good premorbid history (school or work progress)
* good intellectual functioning
* frequent exacerbations and remissions
* painful awareness of the discrepancies between the "normal" future once envisioned and the likely degree of chronic disability in the future
* periods of clinical improvement following relapse
* presence of a depressive episode and increased hopelessness
* communication of suicidal intent

The more severe the psychiatric illness, the greater the suicide risk. Comorbidity has been identified in 70%-80% of all completed suicides (Henriksson, et al. 1993) and in a large number of attempted suicides (Lewinsohn, et al. 1996; Moscicki 1995). Mood and addictive disorders, and mood and personality disorders appear to be deadly combinations.

Personality Disorders. Individuals with borderline personality disorders and antisocial personality disorders are at highest risk for suicide (Roy 2000). The three aspects of personality most clearly associated with suicide are hostility, impulsivity, and depression (Stuart 1998). In young men completing suicide, the combination of borderline personality disorder, depression, and untreated alcoholism is an especially lethal combination (Lesage, et al. 1994).

HISTORICAL AND FAMILIAL RISK FACTORS

Previous Suicide Attempt

A history of suicide attempt is an important risk factor for completed suicide. There is no reliable source of data on suicide attempts since there is no standard definition for attempted suicide (Moscicki 1997). However, estimates of lifetime prevalence of attempted suicide among adults range from 1.1 to 4.3 per 100 (Moscicki 1997). Higher rates are reported for older adolescents at 7.1 per 100 overall—10.1 per 100 for females, and 3.8 per 100 for males (Andrews and Lewinsohn 1992). Women report more suicide attempts than men. The suicide rate among persons who have previously attempted suicide is five to six times greater than for the general population. Between 18% and 38% of persons who commit suicide had at least one previous attempt (Clark and Fawcett 1992b). However, the majority of persons who have completed suicide had never made a prior attempt (Jacobs, Brewer, and Klein-Benheim 1999).

Especially vulnerable are older adult men, since this population has lower ratios of attempts to completions resulting from more lethal means. Therefore, older males presenting with a history of attempted suicide are at great risk for suicide and require immediate intervention and determination if hopelessness is present (Szanto, et al. 1998).

Approximately 40% of attemptors have made a previous attempt, and 1% of those who attempt suicide will commit suicide within one year (Roy 2000); therefore, identifying persons at risk for repeated suicide may prevent unnecessary death. The following are important factors for identifying persons at risk (Roy 2000):

- problems with alcohol
- antisocial personality disorder
- impulsivity
- previous inpatient treatment of a psychiatric disorder
- previous outpatient treatment of a psychiatric disorder
- previous suicide attempt(s) leading to inpatient treatment
- living alone

Family History

Higher risk for suicide is associated with a family history of suicide, especially in a same-sex parent; mental illness; or substance abuse (Lesage, et al. 1994; Moscicki 1997; Townsend 2000). Family lifestyles disrupted by divorce, separation, or widowhood can contribute to suicidal behavior (Wagner 1997). These families are characterized by family conflicts, stress, legal troubles, and separation of children from parents. Physical and sexual abuse are associated with adolescent suicide attempts and completed suicide (Brent, et al. 1996).

Nurses are cautioned that while positive family history increases risk, the absence of family history does not decrease risk.

Family members must understand the seriousness of the threat or attempt and that the patient is not to be left alone (Shea 1999). It is considered safe and appropriate to discuss the patient's suicide risk with the family openly and frankly. The family should be encouraged to talk openly about their concerns and role in the safety plan.

Social Supports

A strong interpersonal support system may be the suicidal individual's primary lifeline. Significant others, including family and relatives, can be helpful, distant, injurious, or toxic. A hostile interpersonal environment increases suicide risk. Family, relatives, and friends can consciously or unconsciously undermine any plans for safety (Shea 1999). Others may deny the suicidal behavior and withdraw emotionally and physically. The nurse must determine who can support the person during crisis: family, relatives, friends, clergy, physician, therapist, or employer. Aguilera (1998) recommends that the responsibility for a suicidal person be shared among as many people as possible.

In addition to fulfilling caring and caregiving roles, family members, close friends, and relatives can be a valuable source for corroborating the patient's history, gauging lethality, and determining if the patient meets criteria for involuntary admission. Shea (1999) suggests the following questions may be useful:

- Have you seen [patient] do or say anything that indicates he/she is thinking about killing himself or herself?
- Has [patient] made any comments about "being better off dead?"
- Has [patient] joked about killing himself or herself?
- Has [patient] made statements about "things will be better soon"?
- Does [patient] have potential weapons available such as guns or knives?
- Has [patient] ever tried to hurt himself or herself, even in seemingly harmless ways such as "scraping" wrists or taking a few too many pills?
- Has [patient] appeared sad, depressed, despondent, tearful?
- Is [patient] isolating himself or herself or spending more time than usual alone?

Neurochemical Imbalances

Decreased brain stem levels of the brain neurotransmitter serotonin (5HT) or its principle cerebral spinal fluid metabolite (CSF 5HIAA) have been consistently found in postmortem studies of those who completed suicide (Mann, et al. 1995). Abnormal serotonin transmission is related to the etiology of depression and schizophrenia. Antidepressant drugs increase the amount and efficiency of 5HT. Mann and Arango (1992) found deficiencies in 5HT and 5HIAA and an increase in one of the 5HT postsynaptic receptors ($5HT_{2A}$) in suicidal persons. People hospitalized for violent suicide attempts with low CSF 5HIAA are 10 times more likely to commit suicide within one year. Although there is no biological test to differentiate suicide risk, there is a great deal of interest in identifying a biological marker for suicide (Stuart 1998).

PROXIMAL PRECIPITATING RISK FACTORS

Access to Lethal Means of Suicide

The most common method of suicide in the United States in all age groups in both genders is by firearms (Moscicki 1995), followed by hanging for men and poisoning for women (Moscicki 1999). A firearm in the home is a potent proximal risk factor, with approximately 60% of all suicides in the United States involving firearms (Sloan, et al. 1990). An especially dangerous combination is having an emotional illness or substance abuse disorder, being intoxicated, and having a firearm (Brent, Perper, and Allman 1987).

Recent, Severe Stressful Life Events

Stressful life events precipitate suicide attempts. Often the number of stressors rather than a specific type of stressor may lead to suicide. Suicide may result from any stress that the individual feels is overwhelming (Stuart 1998). The nurse must determine which stressful events have precipitated the current crisis. The most common proximal stressors are losses: loss of a loved one through death, divorce, or separation; loss of job, money, prestige, or status; loss of health; loss of esteem following prosecution or criminal involvement.

In a study of 50 alcoholic suicides, Murphy (1986b) found that in only one of the victims could no precipitating event be identified. The most important precipitating events were:

- loss of a close relationship through divorce, separation, or family conflict
- job trouble
- financial trouble
- trouble with the law
- depression
- disgrace
- fear of rehospitalization
- inability to control drinking

Stressors frequently associated with completed suicide in adolescents and young adults are interpersonal loss or conflict, separation or rejection, legal problems (arrest, imprisonment), and humiliating events (financial ruin, scandal, lost job) (Brent, et al. 1993; Lesage, et al. 1994; Rich, et al. 1991). Economic problems (job loss) are important stressors in midlife and may precipitate suicide during that period.

Physical Illness

Physical illness is the dominant stressor in older adult suicides (Rich, et al. 1991): 50% of persons who die by suicide have been seen by a physician within one month of their death (Fawcett, Clark, and Busch 1993). Conwell and Caine (1991) found that 75% of older adults who commit suicide had seen a physician within one month of the suicide. Because of the potential increased risk for suicide associated with comorbid depression and physical illness, a diagnosis of a terminal illness, especially in an elderly person, is an important indicator of increased suicide risk. Late-life suicide is highly associated with the following circumstances: physical illness, especially painful illness, sensory losses, cognitive decline, mental illness, retirement, death of spouse, threat of dependency or institutionalization, drug and alcohol use, and combinations of these (Roy 2000).

Until recently, HIV-positive status was strongly associated with increased suicide risk. Current research shows that individuals at risk for HIV are also at risk for other factors associated with suicide and HIV infection such as drug abuse (Marzuk, et al. 1997).

A severe, debilitating, or terminal illness associated with pain, disfigurement, restricted function, and fear of dependence and exacerbation or precipitation of depression or delirium were associated with increased risk of suicide (Mackenzie and Popkin 1990, Blumenthal 1990). Harris and Barraclough (1994) identified the following diagnoses with an increased risk for suicide: Huntington's disease, malignant neoplasias, multiple sclerosis, peptic ulcer, kidney disease, spinal cord injuries, and systemic lupus erythematosis. Epilepsy is associated with the increased incidence of suicide in children and adolescents (Brent, et al. 1990).

Terminal Illness

The suicide rate among terminally ill patients is unknown, but several studies support the notion that suicide is rare in this population. Ripamonti, et al. (1999) reported only five deaths (0.027%) occurred by suicide in a population of 17,964 terminally ill patients with cancer being cared for at home by palliative care teams in Italy between 1985 and 1997. In a five-year study of palliative care units in the United Kingdom, Grzybowska and Finlay (1997) found 14 suicides (0.019%) among 72,633 terminally ill cancer patients receiving palliative care. Holland (1997) speculated that the suicide rate among terminally ill cancer patients is somewhat higher than in the general population and is likely underreported.

Patients with cancer who are most at risk for suicide have gastrointestinal, head or neck, or metastasized cancer (Finkleman 1997). Risk factors associated with suicide in patients with cancer are (Valente and Saunders 1989):

- prior suicide attempt(s)
- substance abuse
- single marital status
- severe emotional distress
- exhausted social resources
- conflict with family or significant others
- poor prognosis
- pain, nausea, or other side effects of treatment or the illness

Additional risk factors for suicide in terminally ill patients include advanced age, male gender, diagnosis of cancer or AIDS, depression, hopelessness, delirium, exhaustion, pain, preexisting psychiatric illness, and personal or family history of suicide (Block 2000).

Social Isolation

While 41% of individuals who committed suicide in Finland had contact with a health care professional up to 28 days before their deaths, in only 22% was suicide discussed during the final visit (Isometsa, et al.). In a study comparing 67 male alcoholic suicide victims with 106 male alcoholics in the community, Murphy, et al. (1992) found that every suicide victim had at least one of six suicide risk factors:

- major depression
- suicidal thoughts
- poor social support
- living alone
- unemployment
- inability to control drinking

ASSESSING SUICIDAL THOUGHTS, INTENTIONS, AND BEHAVIORS

Because suicide is considered by the individual to be the only solution to an unbearable problem, initiating a suicide risk assessment requires much skill on the part of the nurse. Suicidality is the result of a complex interaction among environmental stressors, coping mechanisms, presence (or lack) of a supportive network, accurate perception or distorted perception of stressors, and biochemical influences. There is wide variability in the circumstances surrounding each individual instance of completed suicide. In the nursing assessment, approach each patient without preconceptions. Actively listen to each patient's unique story. Do not worry that directly asking, "Are you thinking about killing yourself?" will cause an individual to commit suicide. Be assertive and direct in questions about suicide risks, thoughts, plans, and behaviors.

Determining Presence of Suicidal Thoughts

Evaluation of suicide risk begins by asking patients if they are thinking about suicide. Contrary to common belief, directly questioning the patient about suicidal intent will not cause the person to commit suicide. It is estimated that more than 5 million people in the U.S. think about killing themselves each year (Moscicki, et al. 1989), yet only about 30,000 actually die by suicide (NCHS 1999).

Suicidal Ideation.   These are an individual's thoughts of death and the active consideration of the pros and cons of suicide. The individual may or may not begin to formulate suicide plans at this stage. Suicide ideation is not a "robust indicator" of imminent suicide but psychological autopsy studies reveal that 70% of suicide victims communicated their intent shortly before death (Jacobs, Brewer, and Klein-Benheim 1999).

The purpose of exploring a patient's suicidal thoughts is to gauge the severity or seriousness of the ideation and assess the quality and quantity of thought. The following questions are suggested to uncover suicidal thinking:

- Are you having thoughts about killing yourself?
- What are your thoughts?
- When did these thoughts begin?
- How frequently do you think about suicide?
- How persistent are these thoughts?
- Can you control these thoughts?
- Can you get these thoughts out of your mind?
- Are these thoughts active or passive?
- Do you hear voices telling you to kill or harm yourself (command hallucinations)?

If the patient relates having thoughts of suicide, the degree of risk is determined by assessing ambivalence, feelings of hopelessness, and specifics of the plan: method, time, place, and availability of method.

Ambivalence.   Once the nurse has determined that suicidal ideations are present, the actual content of the thoughts is explored. Ideation usually contains emotional conflicts between a wish to live or be rescued and a wish to die. Ambivalence is almost always present in suicidal persons (Shneidman 1989). Ambivalence is not uncertainty or doubt, it is psychic energy generated by two opposing forces (Jacobs, Brewer, and Klein-Benheim 1999)—in this case, the desire to live and the desire to die. Ambivalence associated with suicide increases anxiety and agitation that may increase suicide risk. Conversely, if the patient's anxiety, dysphoria, and agitation suddenly decrease, the patient may have resolved to die. A key question to assess reasons for not following through with suicidal ideations is to ask, "What stopped you from acting on your thoughts to kill yourself?" The therapist should listen carefully to the answers patients give to this question. The following are frequently given reasons for not killing oneself (Clark and Fawcett 1992a):

- responsibility for dependent children, especially under 18 years old
- fear of pain and self injury
- reluctance to expose family to stigma
- wish to be present at future events
- religious beliefs

Psychological Pain and Despair.   According to Shneidman (1999, 83), "The psychological dimensions . . . of committed suicide . . . can be understood in terms of intensely felt psychological pain (called psychache), coupled with the idea of death . . . as the best solution to the problem of unremitting and intolerable psychache." The psychological pain is related to frustrated or blocked psychological needs. Assessing the patient's psychological pain may be helpful in determining risk (Jacobs, Brewer, and Klein-Benheim 1999):

- Do you feel disconnected, empty, uninvolved, and worthless?
- Are you at the point where you cannot tolerate any more emotional pain?

Hopelessness.   Hopelessness is defined as the degree to which the individual holds negative expectations about the future (Beck, et al. 1993). Hopelessness was found to be better than depression in predicting suicide ideation in clinically depressed adults and suicide attempts in older adults who had recovered from depression (Szanto, et al. 1998). Fawcett (1988) found high levels of hopelessness and anhedonia in patients who committed suicide within one year following their initial assessment. Among older adults, hopelessness may be a persistent trait that predisposes to suicide attempts even in the absence of depression. The following questions will help uncover feelings of hopelessness in suicidal patients:

- Do you feel hopeless now?
- Do things seem so hopeless that you wish you were dead?
- Have you been discouraged or felt hopeless?
- What kind of future do you see for yourself?
- Can you see yourself or your situation getting better?
- Do you believe you have lost your main reason for living?
- Have you had any thoughts that life isn't worth living either recently or in the past?

Determining Suicidal Intent or Lethality
Nurses must be comfortable and skilled with asking explicit questions aimed at uncovering the seriousness or intensity of a patient's secret wish to be

dead. The process and techniques for forming a therapeutic alliance, creating a safe environment for dialog about suicide, and exploring the hidden meanings behind words are beyond the scope of this text, but the reader is referred to Shea's text (1999) for a discussion of "the practical art of suicide assessment." For Shea, no detail of an individual's suicide plan is insignificant. As the individual talks about thoughts of suicide, the depth of the person's suffering emerges and this exploration becomes part of the therapeutic process for healing. Making an accurate determination of the seriousness of the patient's desire to die is crucial since treatment decisions rest most heavily on this aspect of the patient's behavior. The following questions will help reveal the seriousness of the person's suicidal thinking:

- How intense is the wish to die?
- How long have you been thinking about dying or harboring a wish to die?
- To what degree does the wish to die outweigh the wish to live?
- At what point are you in your wish to die—a vague wish to die or a concrete plan to kill yourself?
- What form does the wish to die take?
- What is the motive behind the wish to die? To hurt someone else? To punish oneself? To escape? To end suffering? To not be a burden?
- What does the suicide mean to the patient?
- Is there a wish for rebirth or reunion?
- Have there been past suicide attempts? How many? Lethality?
- Does the person have the energy to act on his or her plan?
- Is the person using drugs or alcohol?
- Is there identification with a significant other?
- What is the person's view of death?
- Does death have a positive meaning for the person?
- Does the person believe, think, or feel that others would be better off if he or she died?

Identifying Suicide Method or Plan

After learning the patient has suicidal ideas and the degree of intent has been estimated, the nurse should thoroughly assess the plan. The more detail to the plan, the more serious the risk. Pay close attention to violent, nonreversible methods such as shooting, jumping, car wrecks, and carbon monoxide. The following questions will uncover details of the patient's plan:

- What is the plan?
- When will the plan be carried out?
- Is there a specific method, place, and time?
- Is the plan specific?
- Can the patient say exactly when the plans are to be carried out?
- Does the patient have the means available?

- Has the patient rehearsed the plan?
- Has the person been hoarding pills?
- Are there plans to leave a suicide note? Has the note been written?
- Is there someone the person can call before acting on the plans?
- Have there been final acts of pre-preparation: Writing a will, giving away possessions?
- Are there elements of deception built into the plan?
- Has the patient spent time planning a funeral, leaving instructions?
- How long has the patient spent planning the suicide?
- What is the goal: death or self injury?

If the patient denies he has a specific suicide plan, nurses should ask if the patient intends to follow through with suicide ideations in the future.

Assessing Recent Immediate Suicide Event

An attempted suicide is a psychiatric emergency. Following an actual suicide attempt, the nurse focuses on understanding the seriousness and severity of the event (Shea 1999). A serious attempt usually results in hospitalization. Shea presents the following schema for "entering the patient's world at the time of the suicide attempt" to understand how the patient feels about not dying:

- Explore how the patient tried to commit suicide. What method was used?
- How serious was the action taken with the stated method? What pills were taken? How many?
- Did the patient realize the medication was not lethal?
- To what extent did the patient intend to die?
- Did the patient tell anyone beforehand? Afterward?
- Did the patient select an isolated spot or main area where rescue was likely?
- Did the patient leave a will or suicide note, confirm insurance status, or tell significant others goodbye beforehand?
- How does the patient feel about the fact the event was not successful?
- What are the patient's thoughts about the fact the patient is still alive?
- Was the event well planned and executed as planned or was the attempt more impulsive?
- Did alcohol or drugs play a role?
- Were there interpersonal issues at play such as fear of failure?
- What role did stressor(s) play? Number? Length of time present?
- How hopeless did the patient feel at the time?

Assessing Coping Potential

As a psychological process, coping is perceiving, appraising, and contending with a threat. Coping involves the interaction between the resources and capacities of the individual to resist the stressor. The individual can focus on the actual problem to directly solve it or can focus on the emotional aspects of the stress by managing one's own emotional responses to the threat. The following questions can be used to assess the ability of the patient to work with caregivers in mobilizing coping resources needed to meet the challenges of dying from a terminal illness:

- Are there recent stressors in the patient's life?
  Is the patient facing real or perceived loss, disappointment, humiliation, or failure?
- What is the patient's potential for autonomy?
  Does the patient have a history of regressive, compulsive, or aggressive behavior?
  Does the patient need or use his or her support system to bolster self-esteem?
- Is the patient able to participate in treatment?
  Did the patient verbalize willingness to comply with treatment?
  Does the patient have the capacity to form a therapeutic alliance?

A person's overall usual pattern of coping is determined by one's genetic makeup, temperament, and past experiences. Although there is a wide range of individual differences in response to stress, the responses are somewhat predictable in individuals. A typology of coping strategies and related behaviors is presented in Table 23–5.

TABLE 23–5 COPING STRATEGIES AND RELATED COPING BEHAVIORS

COPING STRATEGY	COPING BEHAVIOR
Initial immobilization or delay	• The individual reduces the initial shock of the situation (accidents, ICU, terminal diagnosis). • Behaviors include temporarily postponing confronting the stressor (not entering ICU or funeral home until able to confront the situation) or taking a time-out to gain emotional control. • The time frame is not specific but is individualized.
Visual survey	• The patient or family concentrate on aspects of environment or situation (noise, odors, bedrails) rather than on immediate problem (wound, dressings, ostomy, confusion, pain, death). • Nurses may need to wait until the family/parent/patient are able to concentrate before asking not-so-immediate questions. • Patient and family questions may seem irrelevant and critical of care but must be answered patiently and honestly.
Selective inattention or restructuring (Wilson and Kneisl 1996)	• The individual controls or filters out noxious or stressful sensory stimuli. • Behaviors include focusing on a part of a crisis or problem such as tape, hair, or linens. • Selective inattention is used to control moderate to severe anxiety.

TABLE 23–5   CONTINUED

COPING STRATEGY	COPING BEHAVIOR

Withdrawal (Stuart and Laraia 1998)	• The individual withdraws; withdrawal is within a variable time frame and can be physical and/or emotional.
	• Examples of withdrawal behavior are as follows:
	    Destructive withdrawal behaviors–apathy, lower aspirations, admit defeat, isolate self; do not ask questions; do not talk about fears, problems, situation; sleeping; daydreaming; fatigue.
	    Constructive withdrawal behaviors–withdrawal from biological stressors such as dust, smoke, radiation.
	    Active withdrawal behaviors–physically leave the stressful situation (leaving hospital against medical advice).
	    Passive withdrawal behaviors–patient does not ask questions or talk about problems.
	    Interpersonal withdrawal behaviors–superficiality, clichés, limited self-disclosure, poor eye contact; verbal hesitation, blocking, vacillation.

Planning ahead	• Planning ahead is future oriented and is generally a positive, active coping strategy. • The individual decides where he or she is in time and what future goals and options might be. • Behaviors include analyzing risks, organizing the environment, arranging transportation, taking a leave of absence from work, keeping an appointment calendar, or planning one's funeral.
Setting limits	• The individual limits time, effort, resources, or money expended in coping with stressors. • Behaviors include limiting the number of visitors, or limiting time spent on certain activities.
Modifying situational goals, priorities, expectations (Aguilera 1998)	• The individual decides he or she can be happy with less, especially when situational constraints are outside one's control. • The individual makes compromises and redirects or rechannels energies toward more realistic and attainable goals. • Behaviors include substituting one goal with another, for example, using a wheelchair rather than walking.
Diversion/Distraction	• The individual refocuses his or her attention on a nonthreatening situation to reduce anxiety and/or pain. • Behaviors include music, reading, exercise, television, eating, or talking.
Intellectualization (Stuart and Laraia 1998)	• The individual deals with stressful situations on a cognitive level rather than an emotional level. • Intellectualization is adaptive in the early phase of a health crisis. • Behaviors include detailed interest in equipment, blood work, medications, or vital signs. • Approach families patiently and answer each question since questions mask real concerns about terminal illness of family member.

TABLE 23–5   CONTINUED

COPING STRATEGY	COPING BEHAVIOR

Confront the problem (Stuart and Laraia 1998)	• The individual faces the stressful situation indirectly or directly.
	• Examples of confronting the problem indirectly and directly are as follows:
	    Indirect action–Tends to be destructive in nature and includes angry, hostile, blaming, or intimidating behavior.
	    Direct action–Tends to be constructive in nature and includes problem-solving; self-assertiveness; review of crisis event; seeking information; making plans; learning new tasks and self-care skills (medications, wound care, exercise, rest, meal preparation), setting goals; rehearsing alternate solutions/outcomes.

Turning to comforting person (Wilson and Kneisl 1966)	• The individual seeks help from another person. • Turning to a comforting person can be adaptive or maladaptive if the individual becomes too dependent on another person. • Coping behaviors include touching, rocking, stroking, patting, soothing words, singing to, feeding, or verbal reassurances.
Relying of self-discipline (Wilson and Kneisl 1996)	• The individual uses self-control/stoicism with self-admonitions to keep a "stiff upper lip" or "bite the bullet." • Individuals who rely on self-discipline view "turning to a comforting person" and dependency as weak.
Privately thinking it through (Wilson and Kneisl 1996)	• The individual uses introspection or reflection to think about a problem. • The individual may state, "I have to think about this" and withdraw to think through the problem.
Intense expression of feelings (Wilson and Kneisl 1996)	• The individual expresses strong emotions such as joy, anger, anxiety, and fear. • Behaviors include swearing, shouting, laughing, striking out, or crying. • Intensely expressing feelings may have calming effect.
Talking it out (Wilson and Kneisl 1996)	• The individual uses communication to cope with stressful situations. • Behaviors include telling stories, rehearsing solutions, projecting "what if," and discussing ways to cope with stressors. • New ideas and solutions may emerge when talking about problems.
Working it off (Wilson and Kneisl 1996)	• The individual relieves tensions through both pointless, non-goal directed behaviors (finger tapping, pacing floor, smoking) or through using energy constructively (playing tennis, washing walls, scrubbing floors).

TABLE 23–5 CONTINUED

COPING STRATEGY	COPING BEHAVIOR
Using symbolic substitutes (Wilson and Kneisl 1996)	• The individual gives symbolic value to acts or objects in order to manage tension. • Behaviors include internal comforting measures such as meditation, prayer, or confession; buying symbols of power/prosperity such as cars, clothes, or vacations. • Meanings beyond usual/obvious ones are attached to objects, experiences, and people.
Minimizing the Situation/Selective Reappraisal	• The individual reinterprets the situation as less threatening by relabeling the stressor. • Behaviors include comparing problem with others with more problems ("She lost both her husband and son in the same year. I just lost my husband.").
Somatizing (Wilson and Kneisl 1996)	• The individual communicates tensions through "organ language" with behaviors such as blushing, stuttering, yawning, sweating, or palpitations.
Reminiscing	• The individual recalls past, pleasant events when self-worth and capabilities were higher. • Reminiscing may decrease negative, painful aspects of losses.

SUMMARY: ASSESSING RISK OF SUICIDE IN TERMINALLY ILL PATIENTS

While the risk of suicide among terminally ill patients is low, the presence of risk factors that predispose and precipitate suicide is high. Nursing vigilance is needed to prevent suicide among this population of patients. A terminally ill person may have a history of suicide attempts, be abandoned by friends and family, be clinically depressed, and use drugs and alcohol to control pain and other distressing symptoms. This person is at high risk for suicide, and nursing assessment of the risk and the person's coping potential is essential to prevent suicide.

REFERENCES

Ad Hoc Committee of the Harvard Medical School to Examine the Definition of Brain Death. (1968). The definition of irreversible coma: Report of the ad hoc committee of the Harvard Medical School to examine the definition of brain death. *Journal of the American Medical Association, 205,* 337–340.

Aguilera, D. C. (1998). *Crisis intervention: Theory and methodology* (8th ed.). St. Louis, MO: Mosby.

American Academy of Hospice and Palliative Medicine. (1997). Position statement on comprehensive end-of-life care and physician-assisted suicide. [On-line]. Available: *http://www.aahpm.org/pas/htm*

American Medical Association. (1999). Module 5: Physician-assisted suicide. In American Medical Association, *Education for physicians on end-of-life care* (EPEC): *Trainer's guide* (pp. 1–27). Washington, DC: Author.

American Nurses Association (1992). *Compendium of position statements on the nurse's role in end-of-life decisions.* Washington, DC: American Nurses Association.

American Nurses Association (1991). *Code for professional nurses with interpretive statements.* Washington, DC: American Nurses Association.

American Society of Clinical Oncology (1998). Cancer care during the last phase of life. *Journal of Clinical Oncology*, 16, 1986–1996.

Andrews, J. A., & Lewinsohn, P. M. (1992). Suicidal attempts among older adolescents: Prevalence and co-occurrence with psychiatric disorders. *Journal of the Academy of Child and Adolescent Psychiatry*, 31, 655–662.

Back, A. L., Wallace, J. I., Starks, H. E., & Pearlman, R. A. (1996). Physician-assisted suicide and euthanasia in Washington state: Patient requests and physician responses. *Journal of the American Medical Association*, 275, 919–925.

Beck, A. T., Steer, R., Beck, J. S., & Newman, C. F. (1993). Hopelessness, depression, suicidal ideation, and clinical diagnosis of depression. *Suicide and Life Threatening Behavior*, 23, 139–145.

Block, S. D. (2000). Assessing and managing depression in the terminally ill patient. *Annals of Internal Medicine*, 132, 209–218.

Blumenthal, S. J. (1990). An overview and synopsis of risk factors, assessment, and treatment of suicidal patients over the life cycle. In S. J. Blumenthal & D. J. Kupfer (Eds.), *Suicide over the life cycle: Risk factors, assessment, and treatment of suicidal patients* (pp. 685–733). Washington, DC: American Psychiatric Press.

Bongar, B. (1991). *The suicidal patient: Clinical and legal standards of care.* Washington, DC: American Psychiatric Association.

Brent, D. A., Bridge, J., Johnson, B. A., & Connolly, J. (1996). Suicidal behavior runs in families. *Archives of General Psychiatry*, 53, 1145–1152.

Brent, D. A., Kolko, D. J., Allen, M. J., & Brown, R. V. (1990). Suicidality in affectively disordered adolescent inpatients. *Journal of the American Academy of Child and Adolescent Psychiatry*, 29, 586–593.

Brent, D. A., Perper, J. A., & Allman, C. J. (1987). Alcohol, firearms, and suicide among youth. *Journal of the American Medical Association*, 257, 3369–3372.

Brent, D. A., Perper, J. A., Moritz, G. M., Baugher, M., Roth, C., Balach, L., & Schweers, J. (1993). Stressful life events, psychopathology, and adolescent suicide: A case-control study. *Suicide and Life-Threatening Behavior*, 23, 179–187.

Burr, J. A., Hartman, J. T., & Matteson, D. W. (1999). Black suicide in U.S. metropolitan areas: An examination of the racial inequality and social integration-regulation hypotheses. *Social Forces*, 77, 1049–1080.

Chochinov, H. M., Wilson, K. G., Enns, M., Mowchun, N., Lander, S., Levitt, M., & Clinch, J. J. (1995). Desire for death in the terminally ill. *American Journal of Psychiatry*, 152, 1185–1191.

Clark, D. C., & Fawcett, J. A. (1992a). An empirically based model of suicide risk assessment for patients with affective disorders. In D. G. Jacobs (Ed.), *Suicide and clinical practice* (pp. 55–73). Washington, DC: American Psychiatric Press.

Clark, D. C., & Fawcett, J. A. (1992b). Reviews of empirical risk factors for evaluation of the suicidal patient. In B. Bongar (Ed.), *Suicide: Guidelines for assessment, management, and treatment* (pp. 16–48). New York: Oxford University Press.

Conwell, Y., & Caine, E. D. (1991). Suicide in the elderly chronic population. In E. Light & B. D. Lebowitz (Eds.), *The elderly with chronic mental illness* (pp. 31–52). New York: Springer Publisher.

Cruzan v. Director, Missouri Department of Health, 497 U.S. 261 (1990).

Emanuel, E. J. (1994). Euthanasia: Historical, ethical, and empiric perspectives. *Archives of Internal Medicine*, 154, 1890–1901.

Emanuel, L. L. (1998). Facing requests for physician-assisted suicide: Toward a practical and principled clinical skill set. *Journal of the American Medical Association*, 280, 643–647.

Erikson, J. (2000). Year 2 of Death with Dignity Act find Oregon law working as expected. *Oncology Times*, 22(4), 1, 13–15.

Fawcett, J. (1988). Predictors of early suicide: Identification and appropriate intervention. *Journal of Clinical Psychiatry*, 49 (Suppl. 10), 7–8.

Fawcett, J., Clark, D. C., & Busch, K. A. (1993). Assessing and treating the patient at risk for suicide. *Psychiatric Annals*, 23, 244–255.

Fawcett, J., Schefter, W. A., Fogg, L., Clark, D. C., Young, M. A., Hedeker, D., & Gibbons, R. (1990). Time-related predictors of suicide in major affective disorder. *American Journal of Psychiatry*, 147, 1189–1194.

Fenton, W. S., McGlashan, T. H., Victor, B. J., & Blyler, C. R. (1997). Symptoms, subtype, and suicidality in patients with schizophrenia spectrum disorders. *American Journal of Psychiatry*, 154, 199–204.

Finkelman, A. W. (1997). *Psychiatric home care*. Gaithersburg, MD: Aspen Publishing.

Firestone, R. W. (1997). *Suicide and the inner voice: Risk management, treatment, and case management*. Thousands Oaks, CA: SAGE Publications.

Foley, K. M. (1997). Competent care of the dying instead of physician-assisted suicide. *New England Journal of Medicine*, 336, 54–58.

Grzybowska, P., & Finlay, I. (1997). The incidence of suicide in palliative care patients. *Palliative Medicine*, 11, 313–316.

Harris, E. C., & Barraclough, B. M. (1994). Suicide as an outcome for medical disorders. *Medicine*, 73, 281–296.

Hendin, H. (1999). Suicide, assisted suicide, and euthanasia. In D. G. Jacobs (Ed.), *The Harvard Medical School guide to suicide assessment and intervention* (pp. 540–560). San Francisco: Jossey-Bass Publishers.

Henriksson, M. M., Aro, H. M., Marttunen, M. J., Heikkinen, M. E., Isometsa, E. T., Kuoppasalmi, K. I., & Lonnqvist, J. K. (1993). Mental disorders and comorbidity in suicide. *American Journal of Psychiatry*, 150, 935–940.

Henriksson, M. M., Marttunen, M. J., Isometsa, E. T., Heikkinen, M. E., Aro, H. M., Kuoppasalmi, K. I., & Lonnqvist, J. K. (1995). Mental disorders in elderly suicide. *International Psychogeriatrics*, 7, 275–286.

Hirschfield, R. M. A., Keller, M. B., Panico, S., Arons, B. S., Barlow, D., Davidoff, F., Endicott, J., Froom, J., Goldstein, M., Gorman, J. M., Guthrie, D., Marek, R. G., Mauren, T. A., Meyer, R., Phillips, K., Ross, J., Schwenk, T. L., Sharfstein, S. S., Thase, M. E., & Wyatt, R. J. (1997). The national depressive and manic-depressive association consensus statement on the undertreatment of depression. *Journal of the American Medical Association, 277*, 333–340.

Holland, J. C. (1997). Principles of psycho-oncology. In J. F. Holland, R. C. Bast, D. L. Morton, E. Frei, D. W. Kufe, & R. W. Weischselbaum (Eds.), *Cancer medicine* (4th ed., pp. 1327–1343). Baltimore: Williams & Wilkins.

Humphry, D. (1991). *Final exit: The practicalities of self-deliverance and assisted suicide for the dying.* Eugene, OR: Hemlock Society.

In the Matter of Karen Ann Quinlan. 70 N. J. 10, 335 A.2d 647, Cert. Denied, 429 U.S. 922, (1976).

Isometsa, E. T., Heikkinen, M. E., Marttunen, M. J., & Henriksson, M. M. (1995). The last appointment before suicide: Is suicide intent communicated? *The American Journal of Psychiatry, 152*, 919–921.

It's over, Debbie. (1988). *Journal of the American Medical Association, 759*, 272.

Jacobs, D. G., Brewer, M., & Klein-Benheim, M. (1999). Suicide assessment: An overview and recommended protocol. In D. G. Jacobs (Ed.), *The Harvard Medical School guide to suicide assessment and intervention* (pp. 3–39). San Francisco: Jossey-Bass Publishers.

Jadad, A. R., & Browman, G. P. (1997). The WHO analgesic ladder for cancer pain management: Stepping up the quality of its evaluation. *Journal of the American Medical Association, 274*, 1870–1873.

Kaplan, H. I., & Sadock, B. J. (1998). *Synopsis of psychiatry: Behavioral science/chemical psychiatry* (8th ed.). Baltimore, MD: Williams & Wilkins.

Kelly, M. J., Mufson, M. J., & Rogers, M. P. (1999). Medical settings and suicide. In D. G. Jacobs (Ed.), *The Harvard Medical School guide to suicide assessment and intervention* (pp. 491–519). San Francisco: Jossey-Bass Publishers.

Kemp, C. (1999a). Ethics. In C. Kemp, *Terminal illness: A guide to nursing care* (2nd ed., pp. 87–94). Philadelphia: J. B. Lippincott.

Kemp, C. (1999b). Psychosocial needs, problems, and interventions: The individual. In C. Kemp, *Terminal illness: A guide to nursing care* (2nd ed., pp. 17–33). Philadelphia, PA: J. B. Lippincott.

Kraemer, H. C., Kazdin, A. E., Offord, D. R., Kessler, R. C., Jensen, P. S., & Kupfer, D. J. (1977). Coming to terms with the terms of risk. *Archives of General Psychiatry, 54*, 337–343.

Last Acts Palliative Care Task Force. (1997). Precepts of palliative care. *Electronic Newsletter of Last Acts Campaign.* [On-line]. Available: *http://www.lastacts.org*

Last, J. M. (1995). *A dictionary of epidemiology* (3rd ed.). New York: Oxford University Press.

Lesage, A. D., Boyer, R., Grunberg, F., Vanier, C., Morissette, R., Menard-Buteau, C., & Loyer, M. (1994). Suicide and mental disorders: A case-control study of young men. *American Journal of Psychiatry, 151*, 1063–1068.

Lewinsohn, P. M., Rohde, P., & Seeley, J. R. (1996). Adolescent suicidal ideation and attempts: Prevalence, risk factors, and clinical implications. *Clinical Psychology: Science and Practice, 3*, 25–46.

Mackenzie, T. B. & Popkin, M. K. (1990). Medical illness and suicide. In S. J. Blumenthal & D. J. Kupfer (Eds.). *Suicide over the life cycle: Risk factors, assessment, and treatment of suicidal patients* (pp. 205–232). Washington, DC: American Psychiatric Press.

Mann, J., & Arango, V. (1992). Integration of neurobiology and psychopathology in a unified model of suicidal behavior. *Journal of Clinical Psychopharmacology, 12* (2, Suppl): 2S–7S.

Mann, J. J., McBride, P. A., Malone, K. M., DeMeo, M., & Keilp, J. (1995). Blunted serotonergic responsivity in depressed patients. *Neuropsychopharmacology, 13,* 53–64.

Marzuk, P. M., Tardiff, K., Leon, A. C., Hirsch, C. S., Hartwell, N., Portera, L. & Iqbal, M. I. (1997). HIV seroprevalence among suicide victims in New York City, 1991–1993. *American Journal of Psychiatry, 154,* 1720–1725.

Moscicki, E. K. (1995). Epidemiology of suicidal behavior. *Suicide & Life-Threatening Behavior, 25,* 22–34.

Moscicki, E. K. (1997). Identification of suicide risk factors using epidemiological studies. *Psychiatric Clinics of North America, 20,* 499–517.

Moscicki, E. K. (1999). Epidemiology of suicide. In D. G. Jacobs (Ed.), *The Harvard Medical School guide to suicide assessment and intervention* (pp. 40–51). San Francisco: Jossey-Bass Publishers.

Moscicki, E. K., O'Carroll, P., Lock, B. Z., Rae, D. S., Roy, A., & Regier, D. A. (1989). Suicidal ideation and attempts: The epidemiologic catchment area study. In U.S. Department of Health and Human Services; Alcohol, Drug Abuse, and Mental Health Administration, K. Bale (Ed.), *Report of the Secretary's Task Force on Youth Suicide: Vol. 4. Strategies for the prevention of youth suicide.* (DHHS Publication No. ADM 89-1624) (pp. 115–128). Washington, DC: U.S. Government Printing Office.

Moskowitz, E. H., & Nelson, L. L. (1995). The best laid plans. *Hastings Center Report, 25* (6, Suppl.), 3–6.

Murphy, G. E. (1986a). Suicide and attempted suicide. In G. Winokur & P. Clayton (Eds.), *The medical basis of psychiatry* (pp. 562–579). Philadelphia, PA: W. B. Saunders Co.

Murphy, G. E. (1986b). Suicide in alcoholism. In A. Roy (Ed.), *Suicide.* Baltimore, MD: Williams & Wilkins.

Murphy, G. E., Wetzel, R. D., Robins, E., & McEnvoy, L. (1992). Multiple risk factors predict suicide in alcoholism. *Archives of General Psychiatry, 49,* 459–463.

National Center for Health Statistics (2000, June 8). FASTATS A to Z [On-line]. Available: *http://www.cdc.gov/nchs/suicide.htm*

National Center for Health Statistics (1999, June 30). *National Vital Statistics Reports, Vol. 47, No. 19* [On-line]. Available: *http://www.cdc.gov/nchswww/data/nvs47_19.pdf*

National League for Nursing (1997). Life-terminating choices: A framework for nursing decision making. *Nursing & Health Care, 18,* 198–204.

O'Carroll, P. W., Berman, A. L., Maris, R. W., Moscicki, E. K., Tanney, B. L., & Silverman, M. M. (1996). Beyond the tower of babel: A nomenclature for suicidology. *Suicide & Life-Threatening Behavior, 26,* 237–252.

Official 1994 General Election Voter's Pamphlet—Statewide Measures, Measure No. 16, Nov 8, 1994. Oregon, state of.

Death with Dignity Act. Oregon Revised Statute 1953. ORS ch. 13 Sections 127.800–127.995 (1994).

Pace, N. (1996). Withholding and withdrawing medical treatment. In N. Pace & S. A. M. McLean (Eds.), *Ethics and the law in intensive care* (pp. 48–65). New York: Oxford University Press.

Pierce, S. F. (1999). Allowing and assisting patients to die: The perspectives of oncology practitioners. *Journal of Advanced Nursing*, 30, 616–622.

Plutchik, R., Botsis, A. J., Weiner, M. B., & Kennedy, G. J. (1996). Clinical measurement of suicidality and coping in late life: A theory of countervailing forces. In G. J. Kennedy (Ed.), *Suicide and depression in late life: Critical issues in treatment, research, and public policy* (pp. 83–102). New York: John Wiley & Sons, Inc.

Quill, T. (1991). Death and dignity—a case of individualized decision making. *New England Journal of Medicine*, 324(10), 691.

Rich, C. L., Warsradt, G. M., Nemiroff, R. A., Fowler, R. C., & Young, D. (1991). Suicide, stressors and the life cycle. *American Journal of Psychiatry*, 148, 524–527.

Ripamonti, C., Filiberti, A., Totis, A., DeConno, F., & Tamburini, M. (1999). Suicide among patients with cancer cared for at home by palliative care teams. *Lancet*, 354, 1877–1878.

Roy, A. (2000). Psychiatric emergencies: Suicide. In B. J. Sadock & V. Sadock (Eds.), *Kaplan & Sadock's comprehensive textbook of psychiatry: Vol. 2* (7th ed., pp. 2031–2040). Philadelphia, PA: Lippincott, Williams & Wilkins.

Shaffer, D. A., Gould, M. S., & Hicks, R. C. (1994). Worsening suicide rate in black teenagers. *American Journal of Psychiatry*, 151, 1810–1812.

Shea, S. C. (1999). *The practical art of suicide assessment: A guide for mental health professionals and substance abuse counselors.* New York: John Wiley & Sons, Inc.

Shneidman, E. S. (1989). Overview: A multidimensional approach to suicide. In D. G. Jacobs & H. N. Brown (Eds.), *Suicide: Understanding and responding* (pp. 1–30). Madison, CT: International Universities Press.

Shneidman, E. S. (1999). Perturbation and lethality: A psychological approach to assessment and intervention. In D. G. Jacobs (Ed.), *The Harvard Medical School guide to suicide assessment and intervention* (pp. 83–97). San Francisco: Jossey-Bass Publishers.

Sloan, J. H., Rivara, F. P., Reay, D. T., Ferris, A. J., Path, M. R. C., & Kellermann, A. L. (1990). Firearm regulations and rates of suicide: A comparison of two metropolitan areas. *New England Journal of Medicine*, 322, 368–373.

Stuart, G. (1998). Self-protective responses and suicidal behavior. In G. W. Stuart & M. T. Laraia (Eds.). *Stuart & Sundeen's principles and practice of psychiatric nursing* (6th ed., pp. 385–404). St. Louis: Mosby.

Sullivan, A. D., Hedberg, K., & Fleming, D. W. (2000). Legalized physician-assisted suicide in Oregon—the second year. *New England Journal of Medicine*, 342, 598–604.

SUPPORT Principle Investigators. (1995). A controlled trial to improve care for seriously ill hospitalized patients: The study to understand prognoses and preferences for outcomes and risks of treatments (SUPPORT). *Journal of the American Medical Association*, 274, 1591–1598.

Szanto, K., Reynolds, C. F., Conwell, Y., Begley, A. E., & Houck, P. (1998). High levels of hopelessness persist in geriatric patients with remitted depression and a history of attempted suicide. *Journal of the American Geriatrics Society, 46,* 1401–1406.

Tilden, V. P., & Lee, M. A. (1997). Oregon's physician-assisted suicide legislation: Troubling issues for families. *Journal of Family Nursing, 3,* 120–127.

Townsend, M. C. (2000). The suicidal client. In M. C. Townsend, *Psychiatric mental health nursing: Concepts of care* (pp. 225–234). Philadelphia, PA: F. A. Davis Company.

Valente, S., & Saunders, J. (1989). Dealing with serious depression in cancer patients. *Nursing 89,(2),* 44–47.

van der Wal, G., van der Maas, P. J., Bosma, J. M., Onwuteaka-Philipsen, B. D., Willems, D. L., Haverkate, I., & Kostense, P. J. (1996). Evaluation of the notification procedure for physician-assisted death in the Netherlands, *New England Journal of Medicine, 335,* 1706–1711.

Wagner, B. M. (1997). Family risk factors for child and adolescent suicidal behavior. *Psychological Bulletin, 121,* 246–298.

Waisel, D. B., & Truog, R. D. (1997). The end-of-life sequence. *Anesthesiology, 87,* 676–686.

Werth, J. L. (1996). *Rational suicide? Implications for mental health professions.* Washington, DC: Taylor & Francis.

Wilson, A. S., & Kneisl, C. R. (1996). *Psychiatric nursing* (5th ed.). Menlo Park, CA: Addison-Wesley.

Wrobleski, A. (1999). Rational suicide: A contradiction of terms. In J. L. Werth (Ed.), *Contemporary perspectives on rational suicide* (pp. 206–211). Philadelphia, PA: Brunner/Mazel.

APPENDIX A

LAST ACTS

A National Coalition to Improve Care and Caring at the End of Life

Palliative Care Task Force

December 1997

Palliative care refers to the comprehensive management of the physical, psychological, social, spiritual, and existential needs of patients. It is especially suited to the care of people with incurable, progressive illnesses.

Palliative care affirms life and regards dying as a natural process that is a profoundly personal experience for the individual and family. The goal of palliative care is to achieve the best possible quality of life through relief of suffering, control of symptoms, and restoration of functional capacity while remaining sensitive to personal, cultural, and religious values, beliefs, and practices.

Palliative care can be complementary to other therapies that are available and appropriate to the identified goals of care. The intensity and range of palliative interventions may increase as illness progresses and the complexity of care and needs of the patients and their families increase. The priority of care frequently shifts during this time to focus on the dying process, with an emphasis on end of life decision making and care that supports physical comfort and a death that is consistent with the values and expressed desires of the patient. Palliative care guides patients and families as they make the transition through the changing goals of care, and helps the dying patient who wishes to address issues of life completion and life closure.

Palliative care has become an area of special expertise within medicine, nursing, social work, pharmacy, chaplaincy, and other disciplines. However, advances in palliative care have not yet been integrated effectively into standard clinical practice. The fundamental precepts of palliation should be a basic component of the attitudes, knowledge base, and practice skills of all nurses.

The Last Acts Palliative Care Task Force believes that acknowledgment and incorporation of the following core precepts into all end of life care can serve as a starting point for needed reform.

Precepts of Palliative Care

Respecting Patient Goals, Preferences, and Choices
Palliative Care:

- Is an approach to care that is foremost patient centered and addresses patient needs within the context of family and community.
- Recognizes that the family constellation is defined by the patient and encourages family involvement in planning and providing care to the extent the patient desires.
- Identifies and honors the preferences of the patient and family through careful attention to their values, goals, and priorities, as well as their cultural and spiritual perspectives.
- Assists patients in establishing goals of care by facilitating their understanding of their diagnosis and prognosis, clarifying priorities, promoting informed choices, and providing an opportunity for negotiating a care plan with providers.
- Strives to meet patients' preferences about care settings, living situations, and services, recognizing the uniqueness of these preferences and the barriers to accomplishing them.
- Encourages advance care planning, including advance directives, through ongoing dialogue among providers, patient, and family.
- Recognizes the potential for conflicts among patient, family, providers, and payors, and develops processes to work toward resolution.

Comprehensive Caring
Palliative Care:

- Appreciates that dying, while a normal process, is a critical period in the life of the patient and family, and responds aggressively to the associated human suffering while acknowledging the potential for personal growth.
- Places a high priority on physical comfort and functional capacity, including, but not limited to: expert management of pain and other symptoms, diagnosis and treatment of psychological distress, and assistance in remaining as independent as possible or desired.
- Provides physical, psychological, social, and spiritual support to help the patient and family adapt to the anticipated decline associated with advanced, progressive, incurable disease.
- Alleviates isolation through a commitment to nonabandonment, ongoing communication, and sustaining relationships.
- Assists with issues of life review, life completion, and life closure.
- Extends support beyond the lifespan of the patient to assist the family in their bereavement.

Utilizing the Strengths of Interdisciplinary Resources

Palliative Care:

- Requires an interdisciplinary approach drawing on the expertise of, among others, physicians, nurses, psychologists, pharmacists, pastoral caregivers, social workers, ancillary staff, volunteers, and family members to address the multidimensional aspects of care.
- Includes a clearly identified, accessible, and accountable individual or team responsible for coordinating care to assure that changing needs and goals are met and to facilitate communication and continuity of care.
- Incorporates the full array of inter-institutional and community resources (hospitals, home care, hospice, long-term care, adult day services) and promotes a seamless transition between institutions/settings and services.
- Requires knowledgeable, skilled, and experienced nurses, who are provided the opportunity for ongoing education, professional support, and development.

Acknowledging and Addressing Caregiver Concerns

Palliative Care:

- Appreciates the substantial physical, emotional, and economic demands placed on families caring for someone at home, as they attempt to fulfill caregiving responsibilities and meet their own personal needs.
- Provides concrete supportive services to caregivers such as respite, round-the-clock availability of expert advice and support by telephone, grief counseling, personal care assistance, and referral to community resources.
- Anticipates that some family caregivers may be at high risk for fatigue, physical illness, and emotional distress, and considers the special needs of these caregivers in planning and delivering services.
- Recognizes and addresses the economic costs of caregiving, including loss of income and nonreimbursable expenses.

Building Systems and Mechanisms of Support

Palliative Care:

- Requires an environment that supports innovation, research, education, and dissemination of best practices and models of care.
- Needs an infrastructure that promotes the philosophy and practice of palliative care.
- Relies on the formulation of responsible policies and regulations by institutions and by state and federal governments.

- Promotes equitable and timely access to the full array of interdisciplinary services necessary to meet the multidimensional needs of patients and caregivers.
- Demands ongoing evaluation, including the development of research-based standards, guidelines, and outcome measures.
- Assures that mechanisms are in place at all levels (e.g., systems, direct care services) to guarantee accountability in provision of care.
- Requires appropriate financing, including the development of new methods of reimbursement within the context of a changing health care financing system.

APPENDIX B

WEB SITES RELATED TO EUTHANASIA, ASSISTED SUICIDE, AND TERMINAL ILLNESS

American Academy of Hospice and Palliative Medicine
The AAHPM is an organization of physicians who embrace and/or practice palliative or hospice care.
http://www.aahpm.org

Americans for Better Care of the Dying
ABCD is a nonprofit coalition of lay persons and professions working together to influence public policy for the betterment of individuals and families coping with a terminal illness.
http://www.abcd-caring.com

American Pain Society
APS is a nonprofit multidisciplinary educational and professional organization providing education, research, and treatment for persons with pain.
http://www.ampainsoc.org

American Society for the Advancement of Palliative Care
ASAP Care is a personal effort to help reform health care practice in terminal illness.
http://www.asap-care.com

American Society for Bioethics and Humanities
ASBH is a professional organization interested in bioethics and humanities.
http://www.asbh.org

American Society of Law, Medicine, and Ethics
ASLME provides opportunities for debate, scholarship, and critical thinking on issues crossing law, medicine, and ethics.
http://www.aslme.org

Approaching Death: Improving Care at the End of Life
A report from the Institute of Medicine calls for pervasive changes to improve end of life care.
http://www2.nas.edu/hcs/21da.html

Better Health
Better Health is an on-line interactive forum to air medical concerns and conditions.
http://www.BetterHealth.com/

Center for Medical Ethics and Mediation
CMEM is an educational association dedicated to providing training, research, consultation, and mediation for health care professionals.
http://www.wh.com/cmem

Center for Improving Care of the Dying
CICD is an interdisciplinary team of individuals working to improve the care of the dying through research, advocacy, and education. CICD is located at the RAND Institute.
http://www.medicaring.org

Choice in Dying
Choice in Dying is a nonprofit organization that provides advance directives, counseling, training, advocacy, and public information about dying.
http://www.echonyc.com/~choice/

Death, Dying, and Grief Resources
This web site provides a holistic collection of Internet resources on death and dying.
http://www.katsden.com/webster/index.html

Dying Well
Resources for patients and families facing terminal illness.
http://www.dyingwell.com/

Education for Physicians on End-of-Life Care (EPEC)
EPEC is a comprehensive education program about palliative care to improve physicians' knowledge and skill with terminally ill patients.
http://www.epec.net

Growthhouse
This web site is an international gateway to resources for life-threatening illness and end of life issues.
http://www.growthhouse.org/

Hemlock Society USA and PRO-USA
An organization for individuals who support rational suicide and believe laws should permit euthanasia.
http://www.hemlock.org/hemlock/index.html

Last Acts
Last Acts is a call-to-action campaign dedicated to improving end of life care.
http://www.lastacts.org

Medical College of Wisconsin Palliative Care Program
This program is committed to improving palliative care through innovative education and clinical care programs.
http://www.mcw.edu/pallmed/

Oregon Health Sciences University Center for Ethics in Health Care
The Center for Ethics combines opinions of health care professionals, patients, and families to improve teaching, research, and practice about ethical issues in patient care and health policy.
http://www.ohsu.edu/ethics/

Oversight Hearing: "Assisted Suicide in the United States"
This web site keeps others informed about actions of the Judiciary Committee.
http://www.house.gov/judiciary/2.htm

Project on Death in America
The Project on Death in America aims to transform the culture and experience of dying and bereavement and to foster innovations in care, public education, professional education, and public policy.
http://www.soros.org/death/

University of Buffalo Center for Clinical Ethics and Humanities in Health Care
This is an interdisciplinary academic center using the knowledge of a wide range of individuals.
http://wings.buffalo.edu/faculty/research/bioethics/index.html

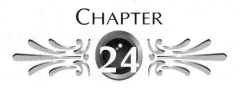

END OF LIFE CARE FOR ALCOHOLIC PATIENTS

Patricia LaBrosse
Dr. Sudah Patel

INTRODUCTION

Alcoholism is a widespread biophysiological and psychological problem in the United States. It carries serious implications for the alcoholic's physical health, economical well-being, psychological equilibrium, and family and social relationships. In addition, it offers unique challenges for those providing nursing care to alcoholics and their families during the end of life stage.

STATISTICS AND EPIDEMIOLOGY

It is estimated there are 10 million to 13 million alcoholics in the United States, and there are 19,576 alcohol-induced deaths each year, not including motor vehicle fatalities (CDC 1997). The prevalence of alcoholism places family members at risk for highly dysfunctional patterns, a variety of dependencies, and emotional illness (Louie 1991).

Alcoholism is estimated to affect 14% of adults at some time in their lives. Nearly identical rates of alcoholism are found in Caucasians as in African Americans. Those at higher risk for alcoholism than the general populations are Native Americans, African American women, and Eskimos. The reasons for this vulnerability are unknown. This disease is present in upper socioeconomic classes, affects five times as many men as women, and has been found to have a high prevalence in certain occupational groups such as nurses and physicians (Pies 1994; American Psychiatric Association, Diagnostic and Statistical Manual of Mental Disorders, 1994). Approximately 21% of all intensive care unit admissions are directly alcohol related (Marik and Mohedin 1996), and 20% to 40% of all persons admitted to general hospitals have alcohol-linked problems and are often undiagnosed alcoholics being treated for the consequences of their drinking.

PATHOPHYSIOLOGICAL COMPLICATIONS

Historically, the health care professions debated the question of alcoholism as a disease rather than a moral and spiritual weakness. Current thinking includes alcoholism as a disease because it meets the following criteria: It can be diagnosed, it is a primary disorder, it is the cause of other medical and psychiatric disorders, it is predictable and progressive in its course, and it is treatable. Alcoholism affects every system of the body. The most severe functional and structural alterations occur in the liver leading to cirrhosis. Chronic liver disease and cirrhosis are the 10th leading causes of death in the United States, accounting for 25,175 deaths annually (CDC 1997). Specifically, 11,000 Americans die each year from alcoholic cirrhosis of the liver (CDC 1999). This multisystem disease can manifest itself in many ways and usually begins to impact the body five years after heavy drinking begins. Table 24–1 shows some of the systemic complications related to alcoholism.

TABLE 24–1   SYSTEMATIC COMPLICATIONS RELATED TO ALCOHOLISM

Cardiopulmonary System	Hypertension
	Tachycardia
	Dysrhythmia
	Cardiomegaly
	Edema
	Acute respiratory distress syndrome
Hepatic System	Hepatomegaly
	Edema
	Ascites
	Cirrhosis
	Fatty liver
	Alcoholic hepatitis
	Pancreatitis
Gastrointestinal System	Gastritis
	Esophagitis
	Duodenal ulcers
	Gastric ulcers
	Nausea
	Malabsorption syndrome
	Colitis
	Cancer of GI system
	Alcoholic pancreatitis

TABLE 24–1 CONTINUED

Neurological System	Fatigue
	Unsteady gait
	Depression
	Irritability
	Memory and learning deficits
	Severe head trauma from falls
	Tremors
	Polyneuropathy (typically begins in the feet)
	Cerebellum degeneration
	Wernicke-Korsakoff Syndrome
Reproductive System	Decreased testosterone levels
	Erectile dysfunction
Immune System	Immune impairment and infection
Hematopoietic System	Toxic effect on bone marrow and blood cells
	Megaloblastic anemia related to folate deficiency
	Thrombocytopenia
	Anemia
Musculoskeletal System	Bone demineralization results in easier fractures
	Acute myopathy (muscular swelling and pain)
	Chronic myopathy (proximal muscle wasting)
Integumentary System	Facial edema
	Rosacea
	Rhinophyma
	Psoriasis
	Discoid eczema
	Erythema
	Bullous lesions

END OF LIFE CARE

Historically the health care profession has viewed end of life as the time when all treatment options have been exhausted. This view can result in feelings of guilt and helplessness among nurses. Those feelings form the perception that "there is nothing left to offer" and may lead to avoidance of the patient and family. In turn, the patient and family perceive the nurse's behavior as abandonment. The current approach embraces a positive, proactive perspective, which regards end of life as the final phase of life. This implies that a cure is no longer possible, and the patient, family, and health professionals turn their focus toward care. By doing so, fears of abandonment carried by both patients and families are significantly decreased. The nursing focus addresses symptom relief, comfort, the nurse's presence, time with family, and assisting both patient and family with the transition to the final phase of life.

With proactive efforts, the focus naturally moves to how death is approached. This approach enhances achievement of patient goals, desires, and wishes, thereby assisting with personal growth and enriched relationships at the end of life. What is the nurse's role in end of life care? To comfort when there is no cure; to honor patient instructions; to effectively manage symptoms; to engage in therapeutic use of self; to coordinate needed resources (i.e. spiritual advisor, family, friends, hospice); and to actively engage in this final phase of life so no patient faces death alone.

ROLE OF THE NURSE

Much has changed about how people come to the end of their lives. No more than a century ago, dying afflicted every age group. With advances in medicine and technology, people are living longer, and they are living longer with terminal illnesses. How society arranges services to support end of life care has profound effects on the quality of life. Current societal issues revolve around how to assure that terminally ill persons can live well despite living for a long time, and find peace and comfort during the end of life phase. "Nursing, like other professions, is an essential part of the society of out which it grew and with which it has been evolving. Nursing can be said to be owned by society, in the sense that nursing's professional interest must be perceived as serving the interests of the larger whole of which it is a part" (American Nurses Association 1980, 3). Alcoholism and the comorbid disease processes require that the nursing profession examine its crucial role in end of life care.

Nursing has been defined as "the diagnosis and treatment of human responses to actual or potential health problems" (ANA 1980, 9). When cure or prolongation of the alcoholic's life is no longer possible, nursing care must focus on the individual's response to dying.

The provision of nursing care requires a holistic approach to patient needs by addressing the physical, psychological, emotional, and spiritual dimensions. In many instances, care provided to the terminally ill alcoholic patient will focus primarily on those symptoms which arise from multisystem failures. While the management of symptoms such as pain, anorexia, dehydration, nausea and vomiting, dyspnea, fatigue, cachexia, and confusion will provide physical comfort, it is paramount that care for the dying alcoholic patient includes nursing interventions related to psychosocial and spiritual needs. Most patients with terminal illness say they are more concerned about the process of dying than with death itself. They may be fearful of pain, abandonment, loss of identity, worthlessness, meaninglessness, and dying alone (Herbst, et al. 1995; Shives 1998). A nursing process framework presents specific strategies for providing comfort measures associated with symptoms arising from the physical, emotional, and spiritual needs of the dying alcoholic patient.

Physical Comfort

While alcoholism produces multiple systems problems, the predominant effect is on the liver. Liver damage may occur in three irreversible stages: fatty liver, alcoholic hepatitis, and cirrhosis. Symptoms of liver disease include the following: severe fatigue, weakness, and exhaustion; abdominal pain and swelling; jaundice; fever; nausea and vomiting; swelling of the legs; easy bruising and bleeding; itching; gallstones; personality change; bleeding problems in the upper stomach and esophagus; sexual problems; and trembling hands.

Terminally ill patients experience many of the same symptoms and syndromes regardless of their underlying medical conditions. Therefore, nursing assessment in the physical domain for the alcoholic patient must include systemwide data such as pain, elimination, nausea and vomiting, fatigue, muscle wasting, dyspnea, respiratory distress, anorexia, dysphagia, skin integrity, dehydration, and oral hygiene, to name a few.

Pertinent nursing diagnoses might include chronic pain, activity intolerance, ineffective breathing pattern, altered elimination patterns, fluid volume deficit, altered nutrition, alteration in oral mucous membranes, impaired physical mobility, self-care deficits related to activities of daily living, impaired skin integrity, and impaired swallowing.

Nursing care planning goals must focus on the maintenance of physical comfort for the dying alcoholic patient. As with other disease processes, it is imperative to include the patient, family members, and significant others when the nurse plans care.

Nursing interventions to provide general supportive measures are essential in the end of life care of the alcoholic patient. Prioritizing the multiple presenting symptoms will facilitate symptom control and identification of appropriate interventions. The use of therapeutic communication with patients and family provides the crucial framework for all other nursing interventions.

Emotional Comfort

Assessing the emotional needs of a dying alcoholic patient is not unlike other terminally ill patients. The two major emotions the nurse will need to assess are grief and fear. Grief is the reaction to numerous losses that are likely to occur during the course of illness that is approaching a fatal outcome. Some of the perceived losses include loss of security, loss of physical functions, loss of body image, loss of strength, loss of independence, loss of self-esteem, loss of respect of others, and loss of the future. Grieving is a natural response, which needs to be acknowledged and expressed. Movement through the five stages of grief (Kubler-Ross 1969) will require support and therapeutic communication.

Fear is a psychological reaction to danger. While fear in the dying alcoholic patient may be obvious, nurses should not assume to know what the fear is. Some causes of fear include: separation from loved objects; becoming a burden to others; dying; losing control; inability to meet life responsibilities; unmet goals; exacerbation of the illness; and reflected fears of family, friends, and significant others.

Pertinent nursing diagnoses might include fear, anxiety, defensive coping, body image disturbance, self-esteem disturbance, powerlessness, hopelessness, anticipatory grieving, impaired verbal communication, and altered role performance.

Nursing interventions designed to meet emotional comfort needs must extend from a therapeutic communication base. Specific techniques include:

- engage, but don't enmesh—in other words, provide an empathetic environment for patients to process feelings without emotional interference from the nurse;
- maintain adult-to-adult communication patterns;
- do not personalize the patient's anger;
- facilitate the patient's life review and determine how you can best act within that value system;
- help the patient to deal with guilt feelings by identifying the source of guilt, correcting cognitive distortions, encouraging making amends if possible, and encouraging forgiveness so that peace and acceptance can occur;
- assist with exploration of each stage of grief;
- review the family system for dysfunctional patterns; and
- facilitate appropriate responses and behaviors whenever possible.

As patients successfully prepare for death, they may want to talk about life, death, and life after death. All they may need is someone to listen, to touch, or to hold a hand. It is important to reassure them that you will do everything possible to ensure that they remain comfortable.

Successful interventions will provide the patient with the ability to identify factors that may hinder the grieving process, communicate openly, express feelings, process through the stages of grief, and verbalize the acceptance of death.

Spiritual Comfort

The *Code for Nurses* adopted by the International Council of Nurses in 1973 requires the nurse to provide an environment of care that includes the patient's values, customs, and spiritual beliefs. An essential component in nursing care for the dying alcoholic is the aspect of spirituality. The term *spirituality* can have varying definitions and encompass several concepts. For this discussion, spirituality is defined as "whatever provides meaning in an individual's life." It is broader than "religion"—it is the need to feel connected to God or a Higher Power. Other elements of spirituality include interactions with others or nature, prayer, and meditation. The exploration, identification, and utilization of spiritual supports enables the terminally ill patient to carry a sense of meaning and purpose in life.

Recent data reveal that nursing care does not always address the spiritual needs of the patient (Brant 1998). In a study of 12 hospice nurses, 25% of the sample never initiated discussions around spirituality. Responses indicated that they felt their patients did not want to enter into spiritual discussions, and the nurses themselves were uncomfortable with the issue (Grey 1994). The importance of spirituality as part of a dying person's developmental task of transcendence is cited by Mudd (1992) who indicates the need for nurses to recognize and facilitate achievement of this task. In order to properly care for the alcoholic patient, it is important for nurses to assess, reassess, and self-intervene, when necessary, regarding their own beliefs, attitudes, and values related to spirituality. It is also crucial that the nurse caring for a dying alcoholic patient re-examine personal attitudes, values, and beliefs related to this disease.

Nursing assessment of spiritual needs may include the alcoholic patient, the family, and significant others. Dr. Christina Puchalski (1999) developed a spiritual assessment tool, which is useful to nurses as they plan care for their dying alcoholic patients. The four components (F.I.C.A.) of the assessment include: faith or beliefs; importance or influence of those spiritual beliefs; community; and application. Examples of assessment questions include:

- **F**—What things do you believe in that give meaning to your life?
- **I**—How have your beliefs influenced your behavior during this illness?
- **C**—Is there a person or group of people you really love who are really important to you?
- **A**—How would you like me to incorporate these issues in your nursing care?

The dying alcoholic patient may currently be active in Alcoholics Anonymous (AA) or may have at some previous time been affiliated with that program. One of the central tenets to an alcoholic's continued sobriety and recovery is the inclusion of a spiritual relationship with self, others, and a Higher Power. Nursing assessment related to the spiritual needs of end of life care for the alcoholic must include data related to the patient's level of involvement with AA.

Nursing diagnoses to address the spiritual needs of the alcoholic patient facing death might include spiritual distress, potential for enhanced spiritual well-being, powerlessness, hopelessness, and social isolation, to name a few. Once again, nursing care planning must include the patient, patient's family, and significant others. Remain sensitive to and respectful of values, beliefs, and practices, which may be different from your own.

Nursing interventions related to spirituality may include:

* active listening to facilitate harmony and connectedness of body, mind, and spirit;
* helping patient and family to connect with appropriate spiritual leaders if so desired;
* supporting the patient's spiritual practices such as prayer and cultural healing ceremonies;
* remaining open to participating in the patient's spiritual activities;
* facilitating accessibility to religious services;
* encouraging displays of religious and spiritual symbols;
* promoting use of preferred music;
* assisting the patient in incorporating principles from AA;
* facilitating the patient's connection with the sponsor and other members of the AA community; and
* promoting use of the Serenity Prayer if the patient so chooses (be willing to the recite prayer along with the patient).

Spirituality should be regarded as an integration rather than a separate part of nursing care.

Evaluation of nursing interventions related to the dying alcoholic will focus on the patient's resolution of ambivalent feelings regarding past behaviors. As patients move from spiritual distress to that desired connectedness of mind, body, and spirit, they will be able to verbally and nonverbally demonstrate physical, emotional, and spiritual peace. Indicators of peacefulness might include: reduced physical discomfort; reduced anxiety related to the dying process; achievement or near-achievement of the developmental task related to death (transcendence); the ability to find a purpose in the suffering and see beyond it; the ability to describe what enhances a sense of personal value; and the ability to express spirituality through prayer, writing, reflection, art, reading, guided imagery, rituals, and connection to others and God or a Higher Power.

FAMILY ISSUES

Alcoholism is a disease that affects more than just the alcoholic. It involves family members, the spouse, the children, and the parents. Talbott and Cooney (1982, 97–98) cite studies at the University of Indiana which reveal that

* if a patient had severe heart disease, usually one member of the family was discernibly affected, either emotionally or psychologically;
* if the patient had cancer, two members of the family were involved, either psychologically, situationally, or emotionally;
* if, however, the patient had alcoholism or drug addiction, that figure rose to anywhere from three to five members of the family being measurably affected.

The end stages of alcoholism may bring multiple emotional responses from family members and significant others in relationship to past behaviors of the patient. Many of these responses—fear, anxiety, anger, loneliness, and guilt—may be observed in varying degrees, and must be included in any nursing assessment of end of life care for the alcoholic patient.

Chronic alcoholism impacts on multiple body systems. However, the alcoholic's family has been dealing with the emotional, social, and spiritual aspects of this disease for many years prior to the terminal phase. Throughout the course of the illness, the alcoholic has suffered disintegration in many facets of life—health, work, family, friendship, self-image, and community. Many similar losses are also experienced by family and significant others.

Talbott and Cooney (1982) identified the "spousolic" behaviors and phases that spouses or significant others move through during their relationship with the alcoholic. These phases impact on past and current relationships within the family. The first phase includes silence and solicitous caretaking, which manifests as denial, rationalization, and defensiveness on the part of the spouse or significant other. He or she makes excuses; becomes protective; and hides liquor, car keys, and guns. Progression through phase one results in guilt and fear, but without confrontation of the alcoholic behaviors. Reality of the potential losses associated with this disease start to impact the spousolic, and he or she begins to give up the protective role. At this time, the emotions of hopelessness and despair emerge.

During phase two, the spouse or significant other mimics the alcoholic's isolative behavior, becoming unreliable to self by breaking appointments, sleeping more, arriving late to work, neglecting personal hygiene, and neglecting other relationships. He or she also develops many somatic complaints. Toward the end of this phase, the spousolic evolves as the arrogant controller who now has the dominant role in the relationship and family. At this point many family fights occur; the spousolic becomes a workaholic and will now do anything to avoid personal and emotional contact. Anxiety and anger mount, and the spouse develops his or her own form of the disease.

Now comes the third and final phase. The spousolic begins to experience true grief similar to Kubler-Ross's (1969) stages of loss. For all intents and purposes, the alcoholic is considered dead. The body is still there and active in the disease of alcoholism, but there is no communication, physical contact, or sexual relationship. At this time, the spousolic experiences an increase in somatic complaints, trips to the doctor, and quantity of medications taken. Loneliness is exacerbated by guilt, anger, fear, and depression, and the spousolic reaches out for love. He or she may become involved in an extramarital affair. Often the relationship experiences geographical or legal separation. Deterioration has reached the point that the family no longer exists.

Children in alcoholic families pay a huge emotional price at the expense of the disease. The past will certainly impact how they may involve themselves at the end stage of the alcoholic's life. Living in a family with an alcoholic and a spousolic results in certain predictable behaviors related to the children.

Wegscheider (1981) identifies four roles which might be adopted by children of alcoholics. They include Hero, Scapegoat, Mascot, and Lost Child. Usually one set of characteristics is predominant, but the nurse may find multiple characteristics from each role present in one child. Following are some identifying characteristics and behaviors for each role (Wegscheider, 1981):

1. Hero children are motivated by inadequacy and guilt, and become overachievers in order to compensate for these underlying feelings and to deflect the focus from the alcoholic and the spousolic. Secondary gain at a personal level is positive attention from family, peers, and community. The family's secondary gain is that of self-worth which reflects the Hero's achievements. A high price paid by the Hero is that of operating from compulsive drives in order to maintain the appearance of success and achievement.
2. Scapegoat children are motivated by hurt which they are often unable to identify. A function of their role is to divert attention away from the alcoholic by acting out family anger. Delinquency is often a characteristic, along with hazardous exploits and promiscuity. The price associated with this role can include addiction and self-destruction.
3. Lost Children are motivated by loneliness. They try not to attract attention, withdraw from the family, and lose themselves in solitary activities. Escape is the secondary gain for this role, and the payoff for the family is relief at not having to address the needs of the Lost Child. Social isolation in both childhood and adulthood is the price reflected in this role.
4. Mascot children are motivated by fear. They are hyperactive clowns. Their function is to decrease family stress by providing comic relief. Secondary gain for the Mascot is amused attention from those present, and the family's gain is engaging in the fun provided by this child. Immaturity and emotional illness are prices attached to the Mascot role.

Nurses working with dying alcoholics and their families may also be working with old, unresolved family issues. It is important to have an understanding of the dynamics associated with family processes related to alcoholism. Nursing assessment for end of life care is incomplete if family function is omitted.

Assessment data related to alcoholic family function will include feelings, behaviors, roles, and relationships. Some pertinent areas for examination of feelings will be powerlessness, anger, repressed emotions, lingering resentment, shame, and embarrassment. Behavioral examination should include communication patterns, inappropriate expressions of anger, manipulation, defense mechanisms used by family members, criticism and blaming, poor problem-solving skills, inability to meet emotional needs of members, history of broken promises, and an inadequate understanding of the disease, to name a few.

Data provided by assessment of roles and relationships should include ability of family members to relate to one another, level of cohesiveness, disrupted family rituals, lack of respect for individual members and their autonomy, history of economic problems and neglected obligations, lack of relationship skills, history of inability to meet security needs of family members, and a history of the inability of family members to relate to each other for mutual growth and maturation. Additionally, nursing assessment of family member needs should include data regarding current or past participation in Al-Anon or other recovery groups.

Nursing diagnoses related to family function for the dying alcoholic can include: altered family processes, altered role performance, anticipatory grieving, caregiver role strain, impaired social interactions, impaired verbal communication, social isolation, ineffective family coping, anxiety, and altered parenting. While these and other nursing diagnoses might be applicable to the dying alcoholic patient, family, spouse, or significant others, it is critical that priority is given to those upon which the nurse can successfully intervene. Many of the family issues are a product of years of dysfunction, and the nurse may be unable to address all these issues during end of life care. Nursing care should remain within the legal scope of practice, and some family issues may require referral to other resources, such as advanced practice psychiatric or mental health clinical nurse specialists.

A comprehensive goal in planning care for the dying alcoholic would be to assist the family in progressing through stages of adaptation to impending death and resolving those feelings that may prevent expressions of timely grieving. However, while planning care for the dying alcoholic and the family, the nurse must be continually aware of the degree of dysfunction present within the family unit. Nursing interventions may require some level of modification, depending on the emotional presentation of the patient, family members, and significant other.

Of primary importance is the establishment of a trusting relationship which mandates the therapeutic use of self. Other interventions include, but are not limited to:

- continually encourage ventilation of feelings regarding patient's condition;
- assess congruency of information given to patient and family;
- clarify information where needed;
- refer to other members of the health care team as appropriate;
- monitor family members for destructive or inappropriate behaviors caused by anxiety, tension, or fear related to the impending death;
- remain supportive and nonjudgmental of patient and family;
- monitor for pathological grieving responses;
- assist family members to deal with guilt feelings by identifying source of guilt, correct cognitive distortions, and encourage making amends if possible;

- facilitate discussions of final arrangements such as funeral services and burial wishes; and
- support progress as the family moves through each stage of grief (Reighley, 1988).

Evaluation of nursing interventions will measure the following: the family's ability to express thoughts and feelings related to losses as a consequence of the disease of alcoholism; the ability to verbalize a perception of the future without the alcoholic; cohesiveness among family members; effective coping under stress; increased knowledge base regarding community resources; and utilization of support systems to facilitate progression through the grieving process.

ETHICAL ISSUES

"The goal of nursing actions is to support and enhance the client's responsibility and self-determination to the greatest extent possible" (ANA 1985, ii). The American Nurses Association first formulated the Code for Nurses in 1950. Since that time, periodic revisions have been made to reflect ethical considerations for current nursing practice. It is from this ethical base that all nursing judgments and evaluations should flow. The ethical principles associated with nursing care include: respect, autonomy (self-determination), beneficence (doing good), nonmaleficence (avoiding harm), veracity (truth-telling), confidentiality (respecting privileged information), fidelity (keeping promises), and justice (fair treatment for all people). Each principle must be reflected in end of life nursing care for the dying alcoholic patient.

Close to 2.5 million Americans die annually from various causes (Cassel and Foley 1999). Technological advances have increased longevity even in the face of varied terminal disease processes, and issues around dying and end of life care have moved to the forefront of ethical questions for both providers and consumers of health care. While patients may die of different causes, it is important that the professionals delivering care agree on basic principles involved in roles and responsibilities surrounding end of life care.

In addition to clinical practice, health care organizations participating in the accreditation process are mandated to address end of life care in the form of policies and ethical decision-making processes. The Joint Commission on the Accreditation of Healthcare Organizations (JCAHO 1993) has specific standards related to care of the dying patient. These standards align with the core principles of end of life care designed by multiple medical specialties, along with JCAHO, to guide physicians with the care rather than the cure of patients (Cassel and Foley 1999).

Many boards of medicine are taking an active role in the development of guidelines related to palliative care and end of life treatment. However, there have been no initiatives by boards of nursing in addressing regulation of end of life care (ANA 1998). While the nursing profession as an entity has not yet articulated specific standards related to end of life care, the American Nurses Association (ANA 1994) adopted a position on end of life decisions. This position statement acknowledges that the role of the nurse is to promote, preserve, and protect human life. In that regard, nurses are obligated to provide comprehensive and compassionate care to the dying patient. End of life nursing care must reflect ethically driven decisions which include the promotion of comfort, the relief of pain, and, at times, forgoing life-sustaining treatments.

In January 1999, the Nursing Leadership Consortium on End of Life Care was developed to advance the nursing profession's commitment and efforts to improve care of the dying patient in the last stage of life. In June 1999, the consortium brought together 23 nursing specialty organizations, the National Institutes of Health, Project Death in America, the Robert Wood Johnson Foundation, and other institutions to address end of life nursing care. The overarching paradigm was the initiative coming from the Palliative Care Task Force of the Last Acts Campaign (1997), setting forth precepts of palliative care. These precepts include: respecting patient goals, preferences, and choices; comprehensive caring; utilizing the strengths of interdisciplinary resources; acknowledging and addressing caregiver concerns; and building systems and mechanisms of support.

The five precepts of palliative care reflect many of the ethical principles incorporated in the *Code for Nurses with Interpretive Statements* (ANA 1985), and they operationalize current goals for end of life nursing care. Fifteen action points were set forth in the report from the consortium, including that nursing organizations endorse the precepts of palliative care and that end of life care be included in each organization's strategic planning processes (American Association of Critical Care Nurses 1999). In light of the current momentum related to end of life issues, the profession should soon adopt a set of generic practice standards for nursing care of the dying patient. From there, each specialty can be expected to develop and adopt standards related to specific areas of nursing practice.

Nursing assessment focused on the ethical issues surrounding end of life care for the dying alcoholic patient should stem from the five precepts of palliative care as stated above and also include the following data:

- patient and family understanding of the course of the illness,
- available treatment options including associated risks and benefits,
- how informed the patient and family are regarding end of life decisions (alleviation of suffering; adequate pain control; do not resuscitate orders; and withdrawing/withholding artificially provided nutrition and hydration);
- communication and collaboration among those providing care; and
- designation of a health care agent to act on the patient's behalf in accordance with the patient's wishes.

In addition, the nurse caring for a dying alcoholic patient must assess quality of life. Erlen (1996) addresses quality of life as one of the seven components in end of life care. Others include pain management, double effect of medication, respect for autonomy, trust, nonabandonment, and suffering. The amount of suffering one endures sets the framework for quality of life, and Cassell (1991) identifies three key points associated with suffering:

- Individuals do experience suffering.
- Suffering is associated with severe distress and threats to a person's integrity.
- Suffering can be associated with any dimension of the individual.

Suffering is a unique biopsychosocial and spiritual phenomenon, and is truly known only to the dying individual. Assessment data related to suffering would include asking the patient the significance of the illness as it pertains to current reality, and how it influences perception of the future.

As stated earlier in this chapter, a valuable nursing tool related to care of the dying alcoholic is the nurse's self-assessment regarding attitudes, beliefs, and values pertaining to alcoholism. An honest appraisal of one's own perception of this disease and how it affects patients and their families will serve to identify issues of cognitive dissonance. These issues will need to be addressed and, hopefully, resolved. When therapeutic use of self cannot be achieved because of one's own issues, ethics require the nurse to use facility guidelines to be removed from delivering nursing care as soon as possible.

Identification and articulation of any ethical issues related to end of life care for an alcoholic patient will help the nurse to remain in keeping with the principles of respect as set out in the Code for Nurses (ANA 1985). Nurses are in a unique position to hear and understand the concerns of the patient, family, physician, and other members of the health care team. Acting in the advocacy role, the nurse can coordinate efforts to assure that end of life care issues are addressed from an ethical framework.

LEGAL ISSUES

The first ethical principle in the Code for Nurses addresses the professional obligation to render care that is respectful of human dignity and considers the uniqueness of each individual. This includes the right to make treatment choices based on accurate information and a clear understanding of the risks and benefits associated with each treatment option. Informed consent is the key element to any decisions made by patients.

It is important to assess the execution of informed consent as it relates to the dying alcoholic's treatment decisions. Assessment questions should provide data which answer the following:

- Are the patient's expressed treatment choices being honored?
- What are the patient's religious beliefs regarding treatment?

* How is the family impacted by treatment choices?
* What is the probability of adverse side effects?
* What is the prognosis with treatment?
* What is the prognosis without treatment?

Patient and family responses to these questions will guide the nurse in making decisions related to what, if any, additional actions must be taken to advocate for the dying alcoholic's right to informed consent (Feutz-Harter 1997).

Nurses have an obligation to be knowledgeable about the legal issues associated with the patient's right to make informed treatment choices. This right to accept or refuse treatment is mandated by the Patient Self-Determination Act of 1990, which became effective December 1, 1991. The premise of this legislation is to offer the patient information about advance directives. These documents, known as living wills and health care power of attorney, communicate choices regarding treatment options and the appointment of surrogates should the patient's decision-making capacity be lost.

Many factors influence patient decisions related to advance directives. These include diagnosis, age, gender, economic status, educational level, and values attached to culture and ethnicity. The dying alcoholic is no different from other patients facing death, and the nurse is responsible for advocating for the patient's right regarding advance directives and end of life treatment choices as they relate to cultural and ethnic values (DePalma 1996).

The Patient Self-Determination Act legislates that health care organizations provide advance directive information to all patients, and that there be mechanisms in place to allow for the execution of these documents. Organizations are assessed on their staff education, patient education, completion of advance directives, and appropriate documentation in the medical record (Parkman 1997). Some questions to ask would be:

* Do organizational policies exist that address advance directives?
* Has the staff been educated on the state's laws, state statutes, and organizational policies related to advance directives?
* Has the information regarding advance directives been included in the alcoholic's admission packet?
* Has the patient or family been educated about advance directives?
* Has the existence of a current advance directive been determined?
* Was the process for completing an advance directive facilitated by specially trained staff?
* Does the medical record indicate the presence or absence of an advance directive?
* Does the medical record reflect discussions with the patient regarding the intent of the advance directive?

Identification of potential legal problems regarding advance directives is a nursing responsibility and well within the professional scope of practice.

Properly executed advance directives clearly indicate the alcoholic patient's choices regarding treatment decisions and support patient autonomy. The absence of these documents lays the groundwork for unnecessary questions associated with the legality of end of life treatment choices.

Some nursing interventions associated with the legal aspects of advance directives and the dying alcoholic include:

- If a properly executed advance directive exists, it is placed in the medical record.
- If an advance directive does not exist, provide advance directive information to patient or family.
- Clarify questions related to advance directives.
- Support the patient's decision regarding acceptance or rejection of advance directives.
- Ensure compliance with organizational policy and procedure related to execution of advance directives.
- Review the medical record to assure documentation of the entire process related to advance directives and patient treatment choices.

Other end of life treatment issues which carry legal implications include do not resuscitate orders (DNR), withholding or withdrawing treatment, and artificial nutrition and hydration. The American Nurses Association (1992, 1994) developed position statements regarding nursing care as it relates to these issues. Once again, the Code for Nurses provides the ethics-driven framework for the statements, and it guides professional actions associated with end of life choices. These statements acknowledge the complexity of end of life issues, and regard the nurse's role as one of advocacy for patient rights and the legal implementation of those rights.

It is important for nurses to be familiar with, and follow, organizational policies and procedures associated with do not resuscitate orders. These orders must be clearly documented, reviewed, and updated periodically to reflect changes in the patient's condition (JCAHO 1993). Legal documentation in the medical record supporting a do not resuscitate order must include at least the following (Feutz-Harter 1997, 287):

- the process leading to the patient's current condition
- an estimation of the patient's prognosis and reversibility of the condition
- a summary of the discussions, identifying with whom they were held
- who authorized the do not resuscitate order

Patients must define what their needs are and how they are to be addressed, and nurses must act out of duty and compassion. If the dying alcoholic patient has the capacity to make health care decisions and requests that any treatment be withheld or withdrawn, there is no duty to contact or seek input of family members or next of kin. Professional duties and responsibilities that have both legal and moral implications related to withholding or withdrawing treatment should be considered. Failure to fulfill duties related to end of life treatment decisions could result in the risk for legal liability. Furthermore, actions to treat without consent or contrary to expressed wishes is considered battery (Feutz-Harter 1997).

Acceptance or refusal of artificial nutrition and hydration is the right of the competent dying alcoholic patient or the surrogate in the event the health care power of attorney is exercised. This parameter of end of life care evokes mixed emotions among nurses. In 1987, the ANA committee on ethics issued "Guidelines on Withdrawing Foods or Fluids," which indicate that "in most circumstances, it is not morally permissible to withhold or withdraw food and fluid. However, if it is clearly evident that more harm than benefit is present with the administration of food and fluids, then it is morally permissible to withhold" (Feutz-Harter 1997, 297). Many nurses find withdrawing treatment that has already begun more difficult than withholding a treatment that has not yet begun (Dalinis and Henkelman 1996). It is assumed that withdrawal of food and fluids would add to the discomfort of the dying alcoholic patient. Rousseau (1991) indicates the only commonly reported discomfort is a dry mouth (xerostomia) which can be alleviated by palliative mouth care. The benefits of withholding fluids include: reduction in edema and associated pressure points; reduction in respiratory secretions; reduction in urine output resulting in less need for indwelling catheters or bedpan use; and less nausea and vomiting. Dalinis & Henkelman reveal that of particular importance is the lack of any sensations of hunger associated with patients who are near death. Conversely, they report that abdominal pressure and nausea are caused by the provision of food.

SUMMARY

End of life nursing care for the dying alcoholic reflects the same legal implications as with other patients. Informed consent, advance directives, do not resuscitate orders, withholding and withdrawing treatment, and artificial nutrition and hydration can be riddled with legal and ethical questions. It is of utmost importance that nurses be familiar with state laws, statutes, the Code for Nurses, professional guidelines and standards, and organizational policies and procedures affecting delivery of end of life nursing care to the dying alcoholic. It is critical that the nurse use self-reflection to assess his or her ability to honor those treatment decisions made by the patient and reflected in advance directives. If the nurse holds a perspective that opposes the patient's choices, it is imperative that appropriate actions are taken to transfer responsibility for care to another nurse who can support the patient's decisions.

REFERENCES

American Nurses Association. (1980). *Nursing: A social policy statement.* Kansas City, MO: The Author.

American Nurses Association Task Force on the Nurse's Role in End-of-Life Decisions (1994). *Position statement on assisted suicide.* [On-line]. Available: www.nursingworld.org

American Nurses Association. (1985). *Code for nurses with interpretive statements.* Kansas City, MO: The Author.

American Association of Critical Care Nurses. (1999). *Designing an agenda for the nursing profession on end of life care.* [On-line]. Available: www.cityofhope.org.

American Nurses Association Task Force on the Nurse's Role in End-of-Life Decisions. (1992). *Position statement on nursing care and do-not-resuscitate decisions.* [On-line]. Available: www.nursingworld.org.

American Nurses Association. (1998). Report of the House of Delegates. *End of life Decisions.* [On-line]. Available: www.nursingworld.org.

American Psychiatric Association. (1994). Diagnostic and Statistical Manual of Mental Disorders (4th ed.). Washington, D.C.: Author.

Brant, J. M. (1998). The art of palliative care: living with hope and dying with dignity. *Oncology Nursing Forum,* 25(6), 995–1011.

Cassel, C. K. & Foley, K. M. (1999). *Principles for care of patients at end of life: An emerging consensus among the specialties of medicine.* [On-line]. Available: www.milbank.org.

Cassell, E. J. (1991). *The nature of suffering.* New York: Oxford University Press.

Center for Disease Control. (1997). *National Vital Statistics Report,* 47 (19). [On-line]. Available: www.cdc.gov.

Center for Disease Control. (1999). Alcoholic liver disease: Latest guidelines for detecting and managing. *Consultant,* 39(3), 99–104.

Dalinis, P., & Henkelman, W. J. (1996). Withdrawal of treatment: Ethical issues. *Nursing Management,* 27(9), 32–37.

DePalma, D. J. (1996). How race and culture influences advance directive decisions. *Journal of American Geriatric Society,* 44(8), 938–943.

Erlen, J. A. (1996). Issues at the end of life. *Orthopaedic Nursing,* 15(4), 37–41.

Feutz-Harter, S. A. (1997). *Nursing and the law* (6th ed.). Eau Claire, WI: Pesi Healthcare.

Grey, A. (1994). The spiritual component of palliative care. *Palliative Medicine,* 8, 215–221.

Herbst, L. H., Lynn, J., Mermann, A. C., & Rhymes, J. (1995). What do dying patients want and need? *Patient Care,* 29(4), 27–36.

International Council for Nurses (1973). *Code for nurses.* Geneva, Switzerland: Author.

Joint Commission on the Accreditation of Healthcare Organizations (1993). Nursing care standards. *Accreditation manual for hospitals.* Oakbrook Terrace, IL: Author.

Kubler-Ross, E. (1969). *On death and dying.* New York: MacMillan.

Louie, K. (1991). Dysfunctional patterns in families with drug and alcohol problems. In M. A. Naegle (Ed.), *Substance Abuse Education in Nursing,* 1: *Curriculum Modules* New York: National League for Nursing Press.

Marik, P., & Mohedin, B. (1996). Alcohol-related admissions to an inner-city hospital intensive care unit. *Alcohol and Alcoholism*, 31, 393–396.

Mudd, E. R. (1992). Spiritual needs of terminally ill patients. *Bulletin of the American Hospital Association*, 45(3), 1–5.

Palliative Care Task Force of the Last Acts Campaign. (1997). *Precepts of palliative care*. [On-line]. Available: www.lastacts.org.

Parkman, C. A. (1997). The patient self-determination act: Measuring its outcome. *Nursing Management*, 28 (10), 45–49.

Pies, R. W. (1994). *Clinical manual of psychiatric diagnosis and treatment: A biopsychosocial approach*. Washington, DC: American Psychiatric Press.

Puchalski, C. (1999). A spiritual history. *Supportive Voice*, 5 (3), 12–13.

Reighley, W. J. (1988). *Nursing care planning guides for mental health*. Baltimore, MD: Williams and Wilkins.

Rousseau, P. C. (1991). How fluid deprivation affects the terminally ill. *RN*, 1, 73–76.

Shives, L. R. (1998). *Basic concepts of psychiatric-mental health nursing* (4th ed). New York: Lippincott.

Talbott, D. G., & Cooney, M. (1982). *Today's disease: Alcohol and drug dependence*. Springfield, IL: Charles C. Thomas.

Wegscheider, S. (1981). *Another chance: Hope and health for the alcoholic family*. Palo Alto, CA: Science and Behavior Books, Inc.

Unit VII

Management of Specific Terminal Illnesses

Critical Thinking Activities

1. Compare nursing assessments, interventions, and evaluative outcomes of patients dying with cardiopulmonary diseases, cancer, and neurological disorders
2. Compare and contrast the differences between physician-assisted suicide, euthanasia, and self-deliverance suicide

Teaching-Learning Exercises

1. Write a critical path for a patient dying with a cardiopulmonary disease, cancer, or a neurological disorder
2. Develop a community resource support list for patients and families coping with terminal illnesses and pending death
3. Attend a community support group aimed at family members coping with suicide

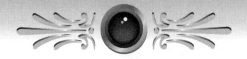

UNIT VIII

ISSUES ACROSS THE LIFESPAN

Learning Objectives

1. Describe essential facts related to growth and development
2. Explain the principles of growth and development
3. Identify Erickson's stages of development
4. Recognize the roles/needs of family caregivers at end of life
5. Identify the physical and emotional roles and relationships and spiritual concerns, needs, and issues of family caregivers
6. Describe nursing measures for end of life care relative to developmental stages of individuals and families
7. Identify common causes of death across the lifespan

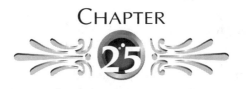

UNSPEAKABLE LOSSES: MISCARRIAGE AND PERINATAL DEATH

Dr. Velma Westbrook

INTRODUCTION

Miscarriage is the loss of a pregnancy prior to 20 weeks gestation or the age of viability. Perinatal death refers to a late-term pregnancy loss typically at 20 weeks or more gestation, a stillbirth, and a newborn death within the first 28 days of life. Miscarriage or perinatal death is never an expected outcome of pregnancy, and few parents are prepared. The unexpected event often leaves families to cope with shattered dreams and aching empty arms. Professional caregivers, including physicians, nurses, and social workers, provide care for families experiencing miscarriage and perinatal loss and are in an ideal position to provide them with direction and support. This chapter will present the incidence of miscarriage, stillbirth, and neonatal death; discuss the response and needs of families experiencing miscarriage and perinatal death; and review the role of professional caregivers.

Miscarriage

The medical terminology used for a miscarriage is *spontaneous abortion*. Most occur early in pregnancy, frequently between the seventh and fourteenth week of gestation. Miscarriage in the first trimester is most often due to chromosomal abnormalities, whereas second trimester miscarriage is more commonly due to an incompetent cervix. In spite of current medical advances and high technology, a direct cause of an individual miscarriage cannot always be determined (Olds, London, and Ladewig 2000).

Incidence. Miscarriage is not a reported occurrence and consequently the prevalence is difficult to assess. Statistics estimate that approximately 10% to 15% of confirmed pregnancies result in miscarriage. When very early unconfirmed pregnancies are considered, estimates increase to possibly 50% to 78% of all pregnancies ending in miscarriage (Coddington 1996).

Symptoms.   Common, reliable symptoms indicating the impending occurrence of a miscarriage or spontaneous abortion include pelvic cramping and backache. Cramping may occasionally be unnoticeable, but more frequently ranges from mild to severe. Usually bleeding is present and may vary from mild spotting to profuse bleeding with the passage of large clots. The actual passage of the products of conception can occur immediately or take several days and can be complete or incomplete. The degree to which these symptoms are present depends on the classification of the miscarriage as threatened, imminent, complete, incomplete, missed, habitual, and septic. Distinguishing between these classifications and the corresponding medical management is beyond the scope of this text. Medical intervention varies depending on the woman's presenting symptoms (Olds, London, and Ladewig 2000).

Stillbirth
Stillbirth is a fetus born dead after 20 weeks gestation or the age of viability. Stillbirths or fetal deaths, also referred to as fetal demise, can be due to unknown causes, compression of the umbilical cord, or complications of pregnancy including pregnancy-induced hypertension, abruptio placenta, placenta previa, diabetes, infection, congenital anomalies, and isoimmune disease (Olds, London, and Ladewig 2000).

Incidence.   Stillbirth or fetal demise occurs in approximately 9 out of 1,000 live births; however, this rate is much higher in certain high-risk groups. Still, nearly one-half of stillbirths occur in women who are not recognized as having a high-risk pregnancy (Catanzarite, Thomas, and Dixson 1994).

Neonatal Death
Neonatal death is the death of a newborn within the first 28 days of life. Causes include prematurity, severe congenital anomalies, and complications of pregnancy.

Incidence.   The National Center of Health Statistics (NCHS) is the federal government's principal vital and health statistics agency that is a part of the Centers for Disease Control and Prevention, U.S. Department of Health and Human Services. The NCHS reports the neonatal death rate as an annual rate per 1,000 live births. For 1996, the reported neonatal death rate by the NCHS was 4.8 neonatal deaths per 1,000 live births (Centers for Disease Control and Prevention, 1998).

RESPONSE TO MISCARRIAGE AND PERINATAL DEATH

A couple's overt behavioral response to a miscarriage and perinatal death may vary. Responses can range from a matter-of-fact, seemingly accepting, life-goes-on response to more commonly one of a life crisis event filled with profound devastation and grief. Influencing factors may include gender differences, whether the pregnancy was planned, if it was the first pregnancy, if complications were present, the relationship of the couple, and various cultural and spiritual beliefs. It is important for health care providers to remember that people react differently to loss, and assumptions cannot be made that a loss at 8 weeks gestation will be easier for the client to deal with than a loss at 40 weeks gestation (Ewton, 1993). Consequently, assessing what the loss means to the client and individualizing interventions based on this assessment is paramount, regardless of at what gestational age the loss occurs.

One might ask, How is a loss due to miscarriage unique compared to a loss later in pregnancy? Although a loss later in pregnancy seems to warrant more sympathy from caregivers than a miscarriage, in many ways, after miscarriage it may be more difficult for the couple to lay their baby to rest as compared with couples who experience a stillbirth or neonatal death. Miscarriages are losses for which society has not formalized with funerals, sympathy cards, mourning, or expression of sympathy. Even in cases of stillbirths or neonatal deaths, burial and funeral arrangements may be meager or undeveloped; in miscarriage, the total absence of these rituals makes the process of grieving complex and lonely. The message parents read from these nongestures is that this was not really an important life event, despite their subjective experiences to the contrary (Malacrida 1999). When a miscarriage occurs, there is no birth or death certificate and no acknowledgement from the outside that a real baby existed, which again implies that the loss was not real or important and adds to the couple's confusion as to why they are feeling so much hurt and pain.

Further, societal beliefs that miscarriage is an event without the potential for significant emotional impact often causes a loss of this type to be misunderstood or minimized by well-meaning caregivers, extended family, and friends. Statements such as, "You're still young, you can try again," "Just thank God for your healthy children at home," "It's God's will," "It's nature's way of dealing with an imperfect fetus," or "It was probably a blessing," do very little to provide support for the couple. These comments negate the parent's prenatal attachment and only further serve to make the couple feel that they have not indeed suffered a real loss. Although well intended, the message is conveyed that the parent's feelings are unimportant or nonexistent and they should not be feeling the emotional pains of disappointment, grief, and anger (Gardner and Merenstein 1986).

Exacerbating the loneliness of a very early miscarriage is that extended family and friends may not be aware that a pregnancy ever existed. The couple may not have had the opportunity to announce the news of pregnancy. Consequently, the couple's support system may not be available to provide emotional support, leaving the couple to face this event alone.

Couples frequently search for reasons to explain why the miscarriage or perinatal death happened and harbor much guilt. It is not uncommon for the expectant couple to wonder if it was something they did or did not do that caused the miscarriage or perinatal death, or perhaps it was something they should have done differently. A great part of the remorse and guilt parents feel stems from uncertainty as to the reasons for the death (Malacrida 1999). These feelings, coupled with depression, anxiety, and sometimes anger are common reactions to miscarriage and perinatal death that can be overwhelming to the couple. Possibly adding to feelings of guilt and blame are the ambivalent feelings the mother normally experiences when she first learns of her pregnancy. These ambivalent feelings are usually worked through in the first trimester. If miscarriage occurs before feelings of ambivalence are resolved, guilt and depression may be compounded. In order for resolution to occur, the couple must acknowledge and understand that the loss of their baby was not their fault and was unrelated to factors within their control. Caregivers should reassure bereaved parents as often as necessary that this was not their fault.

Unlike in a miscarriage, when a perinatal death occurs, there is a tangible baby who can be seen, touched, and held. Caregivers should be aware that providing an opportunity for the couple to see their child can be a first step in assisting parents to begin the hard process of grief work. Researchers report when the beginning of life is so shortly followed by the end, even a short period together gives parents an opportunity to know their child (Gardner & Merenstein 1986). As difficult as it may seem, as soon as feasible, parents should be asked if they would like to see their baby and be given an opportunity to either spend time alone with their baby or have the caregiver present with them. Caregivers often say that they don't know what to say to parents who are saying goodbye to their dead baby. Just being there and saying nothing initially can be supportive. Simply your presence can convey empathy and caring and have a profound impact.

If parents say they are not ready or unable to see the baby because it's too painful, pictures can be taken and kept in a safe place for viewing at a later time. Parents have been known to return as much as one year later to view the pictures in an effort to help bring grief to closure. Malacrida (1999) cited previous research on perinatal loss that has provided insight into gestures by parents that appear to be beneficial to grief resolution. These gestures included keeping mementos or tokens of remembrances of the baby such as footprints, a lock of hair, or a picture; buying clothes and toys for the baby's burial; buying decorations and ornaments to commemorate the baby, such as angel figurines; or having a funeral or memorial service for the baby.

Further, in a study by Radestad, et al. (1996), researchers identified factors that may predict long-term psychological complications among women who have had a stillborn child. Researchers reported it was advisable to induce delivery as soon as possible after the diagnosis of death in utero. Additionally, a calm environment for the woman to spend time with her stillborn child was beneficial, and collecting tokens of remembrances was recommended.

Gender Differences

We also know there are gender differences in response to perinatal loss and grief. The father and the mother may bond differently with the baby and work through their grief in different ways or at different times (Menke and McClead 1990). A factor contributing to these differences may be societal expectations of appropriate behavior (DeFrain, et al. 1990). Traditionally gender roles have allowed for more emotional, expressive crying from women than from men. The expectation that the father remain stoic and strong may affect the timing, amount, and place of his grief. For instance, researchers have reported factors influencing a father's grief response include his attachment and emotional investment in the child (Kimble 1991, Worth 1997), the roles and responsibilities he must carry out after the death, and his relationship with his partner before, during, and after the death (Wallerstedt and Higgins 1996). It is important for caregivers to be aware that in spite of apparent pressure for fathers to be strong, fathers still grieve and need to be allowed to do so (Worth 1997). The incongruent grief response between the couple can be misinterpreted and create conflict in the relationship: The mother may interpret the father's behavior as callous, whereas the father may view the mother as too emotional.

Other reported gender differences regarding response to loss include: (1) men tend to use physical activity and increase involvement in work, avoid talking about the death or obtaining professional support, and some seek pain relief through drinking or smoking and sleep (DeFrain, et al. 1990); and (2) women tend to engage in coping behaviors such as talking about the death and crying, avoiding painful thoughts and feelings by keeping busy and sleeping, reading material on loss and grief, finding meaning in helping others, relying on religious beliefs, and gaining support from groups and professional help (Schwab 1990).

Awareness by professional caregivers of the couple's differences in response to a perinatal loss is important. Each person's experience with death is unique. There is no right or wrong way to grieve, and each person's response to grief should be respected. Research indicates that parents mourn the loss of a pregnancy as deeply as they would mourn the death of an adult loved one. The grief process may take six months to two years (Theut, et al. 1989). Caregivers should use an accepting, nonjudgmental approach that will promote expression of feelings of both the mother and the father. Communication and sharing feelings about the event should also be encouraged between the couple. Open communication will promote understanding and allow the couple to discover their own strength and support each other.

Extended Family

Extended family members are also impacted by a miscarriage or perinatal loss and have a need to engage in expressing their feelings. Not only do the mother and father feel anger, but grandparents frequently feel anger and disappointment about their loss, which may be directed toward the staff, hospital, or friends and family.

It is important for caregivers not to react in a threatened or defensive manner. Rather, remain calm, allow the family to vent their feelings and be heard by understanding nonjudgmental caregivers. To quote Bruder (1997): "Healing from the pain of grief will only come from facing the horse on the dining room table. That means talking—putting words to the anguish of grief. It means touching. It means holding." The loss must be faced. To postpone open communication about feelings toward the loss is to postpone healing.

As caregivers, we must respect the awesome power of emotions and the value of validating them. We must develop a sense of the intensity and depth of pain and loss these parents and families feel. At the same time, we must also be aware of the incredible ability of the human spirit to survive, to heal, and to conquer overwhelming despair (Wolf-Gabor 1997).

Siblings

Siblings are often the forgotten mourners. Age-appropriate activities can be initiated to promote the grief process in siblings. Making toys that can be buried with the baby, collecting mementos, planting a memorial tree, viewing the baby, or looking at pictures of the baby are examples of gestures that can be initiated with siblings. Common grief reactions in children include regression, physical complaints, anger, guilt, fear, and school problems. Children need honest explanations according to their development level and their understanding of the pregnancy loss. Parents and family should avoid statements such as "the baby is sleeping," which can be frightening to children who may fear they too will die if they go to sleep. Age-appropriate books explaining death can be useful for parents (Ewton 1993).

Support Groups

Although many bereaved parents do not want to participate in support groups, hospital-based support groups may be helpful in assisting couples work through the loss of a baby from miscarriage and perinatal death. Sharing with other bereaved parents who have experienced a similar loss may be particularly helpful for couples with little or no social support. A list of support groups should be made available to the couple and follow-up provided by a primary nurse or grief counselor.

Role of the Professional Caregiver and Clergy

Physician

The physician's role is that of informant. It is important to be honest with the couple and sensitive to their needs. The physician should keep the couple informed as soon as information is known or a diagnosis confirmed regarding the status of the fetus or neonate. Be prepared to answer all questions to the best of your ability and avoid using technical, medical terms. It has been stated that direct questions deserve direct answers. Those who ask direct questions are ready for the information (Gardner and Merenstein 1986). Repetition, diagrams, and literature may be helpful for reinforcement of what was said. If the mother is alone, she will want to call her partner or a friend. Arrange for her to make this call. The physician should remember to emphasize that the occurrence of the event was not in the couple's control and not their fault. A follow-up grief conference between the involved medical staff and the parents should be planned four to six weeks after discharge.

Nurse

In addition to providing competent care, the nurse's role is advocating for the parents and assisting them in grief work. Listening and encouraging open communication between the couple and family is paramount. The nurse should reinforce to parents that the event was not their fault. Provide as much time as the couple requires to say goodbye to their baby, and initiate gestures such as collecting mementos and remembrances of the baby. The nurse can also ask if a name was chosen and call the baby by name. These gestures will assist in making the loss real (Ewton 1993). The couple's loss can be acknowledged regardless of gestational age by simply stating "I'm sorry about your loss." If agreeable with the couple, a member of the clergy should be contacted for burial and funeral arrangements and for providing religious and spiritual support. Hospital protocol for bereaved parents should be initiated by the nurse, such as providing booklets on miscarriage or perinatal loss. A list of resources, such as support groups, should be provided upon discharge. Follow-up contacts should be made at one week, four to six weeks, three months, six months, and at the one-year anniversary date of the death. These contacts can be made by home visits or by phone calls and are significant for integrating the death of the infant. Grief conferences should be scheduled for parents to meet with the involved medical staff four to six weeks after the infant's death and after a request from the parents (Wallerstedt and Higgins 1996).

Social Worker

The social worker's role is to provide individual counseling for the couple and siblings as necessary, and to provide follow-up grief counseling after discharge. If indicated, marriage counseling can be provided, scheduled, or referred. It is common practice for the social worker to leave a business card with the family prior to discharge should there be a need for services.

Clergy

The clergy can provide for spiritual counseling, baptize the baby, and assist in arranging for funeral and burial. Religious and spiritual support can help facilitate grief work by providing solace, rituals, and legitimizing the event as significant.

As professional caregivers, physicians, nurses, social workers, and members of the clergy can assist families during a life crisis such as a miscarriage or perinatal death. Through assistance and support, the blow of a tragedy can be softened, even if the tragedy cannot be prevented. Assisting families to heal effectively for their future can be life-changing.

BIBLIOGRAPHY

Bruder, P. (1997). The horse on the dining room table. *Hospital Topics*, 75(4), 8–10.

Catanzarite, V. A., Thomas, S., & Dixson, B. (1994, November). Confronting fetal death. *Contemporary* OB/GYN, 39(11), 29–42.

Centers for Disease Control and Prevention. (1998). National Center for Health Statistics: Vital Statistics of the United States, Vol II, mortality, part H, for data years 1950–96. Washington, D.C.: U.S. Government Printing Office.

Coddington, C. C. (1996). Spontaneous abortion. In K. R. Niswander & A. T. Evans (Eds.), *Manual of obstetrics* (pp. 261–271), Boston: Little, Brown.

DeFrain, J., Martens, L., Stork, J., & Stork, W. (1990). The psychological effects of a stillbirth on surviving family members. *Omega*, 22(2), 81–108.

Ewton, D. (1993). Nurse practitioner. *American Journal of Primary Health Care*, 18(12), 30–36.

Gardner, S., & Merenstein, G. (1986, October). Helping families deal with perinatal loss. *Neonatal Network*, 5(2), 17–32.

Kimble, D. (1991). Neonatal death: A descriptive study of fathers' experiences. *Neonatal Network*, 9(8), 45–50.

Malacrida, C. (1999). Complicating mourning: The social economy of perinatal death. *Qualitative Health Research*, 9(4), 504–519.

Menke, J., & McClead, R. (1990). Perinatal grief and mourning. *Advances in Pediatrics*, 37, 261–283.

Olds, S. B., London, M. L., & Ladewig, P. A. (2000). *Maternal newborn nursing: A family and community-based approach*. New Jersey: Prentice Hall Health.

Radestad, I., Steineck, G., Nordin, C., & Sjogren, B. (1996). Psychological complications after stillbirth—influence of memories and immediate management: Population based study. *British Medical Journal, 312*, 505–508.

Schwab, R. (1990). Paternal and maternal coping with the death of a child. *Death Studies, 14*, 407–422.

Theut, S., Pedersen, F., Zaslow, M., Cain, R., Rabinovich, B., & Morihisha, J. (1989). Perinatal loss and parental bereavement. *American Journal of Psychiatry, 146*, 635–639.

Wallerstedt, C., & Higgins, P. (1996). Facilitating perinatal grieving between the mother and the father. *Journal of Gynecological and Neonatal Nursing: Principles & Practice, 25*(5), 389–393.

Wolf-Gabor, S. (1997, July/September). Perinatal loss: Bridging tragedy with hope. *Nursing Forum, 32*(3), 33–36.

Worth, N. (1997). Becoming a father to a stillborn child. *Clinical Nursing Research, 6*(1), 71–89.

CHILDREN AND
END OF LIFE ISSUES

Gretchen Gaines

We are not inclined to think of death when we think about children. In reality, many children die every year around the world. Children's Hospice International (2000) states that approximately 100,000 children die each year in the United States alone. Children also experience the death of others. Each year, many children lose a parent by death. As other family members die, children continue to be affected by family losses and grieve significant loved ones. According to Corr, Nabe, and Corr (1996), no reliable data are presently available concerning the frequency of these death encounters. Perhaps the impact of these experiences is not perceived as significant enough to warrant gathering this information. Yet it is wise to understand children's responses to grief and to gain insight into the world of dying children.

Children live in family settings. They see that illness and death happen, often to those who are older. At times, the death may be premature, happening in the life of a younger relative. In a family setting, teaching the children about the natural cycle of life and death can be a positive growth experience. The family is also the central potential source of support. Learning about how to support each other and how to cope with crises is another aspect of family life. Silverman (2000, 73) discusses ways in which events in the life of a family shape the children. The experiences cannot be avoided, she says: "We cannot protect children from the pain or disruption of a loss—bereaved children will always experience the fullness of the loss. . . . Children who are seen as participants in the family drama and who are actively involved in it are much more equipped for living."

There are many types of deaths a child may encounter. The death of a grandparent or other older family member is the most likely to occur. The death of a parent happens less frequently but is significant and must be approached sensitively and with skill. The death of a sibling is also significant, needing special attention. Many have noted that the death of a friend during childhood was not recognized as an important loss; nowadays, this loss is receiving more attention, with support being offered. Increasingly, schools and communities have been addressing the losses of individuals or groups of people in the community.

CHILDREN AND GRIEF

Children's grief is a new field of study. Health care providers are developing novel conceptual approaches concerning children's grief, evident in the plethora of new information found in journals, books, and other publications. Adult bereavement concepts cannot be applied to children. The consensus of current knowledge is that children grieve differently than adults. The differences include:

- Children grieve in small increments of time. Typically a child cries for a few moments and then returns to an activity such as playing outdoors or with dolls.
- Children grieve at times in silence.
- Children may grieve privately, at bedtime or other alone times, causing adults around them to think that they are not grieving because they do not see behaviors that indicate grief.
- Children do not have the verbal skills of adults. They may not be able to put their thoughts and feelings into words.
- A child's behavior is a valuable indicator of grief, both feelings and thoughts. Their grief is likely to be expressed as irritability, outbursts of feelings that are difficult to control, and sudden change in mood or expressions, which convey, "I don't feel good about myself." These behaviors may be perceived as childhood behavioral problems, with adults caring for the child saying, "He is such a bad kid lately," or "She never minds me anymore, she is not the same child I knew." Discipline may not be the concern when these changes are seen in grieving children.
- Children have fewer coping skills than adults. They have had fewer opportunities to learn how to cope with the separations and losses of life.

Some similarities in the grief of children and adults are:

- Difficulty concentrating, which may interfere with reading, studies, and daily activities.
- Personal differences, which may be seen in either withdrawal, increased social activity, or increased dependence.

All of the characteristics of grieving children noted above apply to children of all ages.

Defining developmental ages or stages of children varies from author to author. Both before and after a death, grief occurs. Grief, therefore includes anticipatory grief and the bereavement period after the loss. Kubler-Ross (1969) defined the classic understanding of grief as five stages that human beings experience as they are dying: denial, anger, bargaining, depression, and acceptance.

Rando (1984) presents a schema based on the griever's reaction. Rather than stages, she discusses the phases that the griever moves in and out of. These phases are possible responses to a loss—it is important to understand them as some of the many ways people react when confronted by the grieving process:

- **Avoidance phase:** There is a desire to avoid the reality of the loss. This period of shock includes feelings of numbness.
- **Confrontation phase:** Grief is experienced most intensely. The numbness and disbelief begin to wear off and the emotions and other multifaceted reactions begin to seep in. This phase includes the entire range of feelings, from acute feelings with intensity to a surprising lack of intensity, accompanied by new understandings of loss, abandonment, hopelessness, meaninglessness, and a host of other responses.
- **Reestablishment phase:** Grief begins to decline and reentry into emotional and social arenas begin. The loss is not resolved or forgotten, but is woven into the fabric of the griever's being.

Christ (2000) defines the children's stages of development differently. She defines five developmentally derived age groups and the themes identified in each age group concerning how they perceived the illness of a parent and how they grieved. The age groups were 3–5, 6–8, 9–11, 12–14, and 15–17. The children differed in cognitive, emotional, and social-ecological developmental characteristics. Table 26–1 lists a brief conclusion of the age-related reactions of each age group.

A central concept that should be noted is that as years continue and children increase their cognitive, intellectual, and other abilities, they grieve and re-grieve the loss. Moving into and through each developmental stage, the child who has had a loss uses new skills to rework the loss. The feelings of bereavement are never being totally erased or resolved from the fabric of the individual's life. Rather the loss can contribute to the self-concept of the individual. Each time the loss is reworked, there is the opportunity to integrate the death and the construct of the deceased person's memory in new ways.

How do we as professionals assist a grieving child? A grieving child needs safety, security, and support. There are many ways that we can help the child get this assistance. First and foremost, it is our role to help the child's parent give the child the safety, security, and support needed. When that is not possible, professional caregivers assist in providing what is needed.

A Story of a Grieving Child

Nine-year-old Seth was told gently and sensitively by both his parents that his father was diagnosed with lung cancer. He was informed of the plans for chemotherapy, prepared for each hospitalization, visited his father, and

TABLE 26–1   AGE-SPECIFIC REACTIONS TO THE DEATH OF A PARENT

- Three-to-five year olds cannot foresee the loss of a parent and do not instantly comprehend that the parent will not return. After they do understand the finality of the death, they want to see the family restored as soon as possible—for example, a rapid remarriage by the surviving parent.
- Six-to-eight year olds develop incorrect ideas such as believing their thoughts or actions caused the death. This is termed "magical thinking."
- Nine-to-eleven year olds are beginning to comprehend facts and therefore need to know as much as they can about the death to be able to bring more containment to the event.
- Twelve-to-fourteen year olds are beginning to separate from their parents. They are becoming more autonomous and developing a sense of their own individuality. They can become enraged and very frightened when it is evident to them that the parent is dying. Their concentrated self-focus can become exaggerated.
- Fifteen-to-seventeen year olds begin to describe the strong sense of loss that adults feel. The grief experienced by older teenagers was close to the adult experience but lasted a shorter period of time.

Note. G. H. Christ, *Healing Children's Grief.* New York, Oxford University Press, 2000.

learned what equipment was used in the medical treatment. After his father's death, one year after diagnosis, the bereavement counselor visited with his family to see what support was necessary.

Knowing the skilled preparation that the family had received, the interview with his mother and Seth was not revealing, until Seth blurted out, "I want to be told everything! I don't understand why he had to die. At school, the counselor told me, 'He won't die. People don't usually die of cancer.' I think it happened because I didn't stop being noisy. Mother always said, 'If you keep behaving this way, you will be sure to kill your father'." Seth's mother was shocked that her well-informed son was thinking that he caused his father's death. She had seen to it that he was kept informed and included in every step of the illness's progression. In the stress of the caregiving, she did not realize her son's worries were increased by her desire to provide a quieter home for her husband.

Even the well-prepared child can have bereavement needs that are not obvious to those around him. It is imperative that the parents or primary caregivers be aware of cues that the children may exhibit.

What does the grieving child need? The child who is grieving needs information. They have a basic need to know, as fully as possible, what happened at the death. They need to be told how the person died and what the name of the disease is or what caused the death. A child does not need to be told every detail when the description of trauma is difficult.

The grieving child needs to have the closest parental, caring adult available. Physical presence of the adult is a base of security for the child. Touch and physical closeness is vital during times of loss and separation.

Grieving children need to be reassured that they and the family, including the family's lifestyle are safe. Safety can be understood on many levels. Whatever the circumstances, the child needs to be able to depend on the adults.

The grieving child needs to be told who will provide support and how that support will be provided.

Grieving children need to be able to ask questions. Many questions are on their minds. Despite being told what the diagnosis is and despite descriptions of treatments, lifesaving attempts, or other details of the death, children frequently do not understand the words being used or they misunderstand phrases or colloquialisms. Misunderstandings can continue for years if opportunities for asking questions are not available.

Questions that Children Have

Children have underlying psychological concerns that are expressed in these questions:

- Did I cause this (death) to happen?
- Will it (death) happen to me?
- Who will take care of me?
- Will it (death) happen to the person who will take care of me?

Whatever the developmental stage of the child, adults should pay attention to these questions.

ASSESSING NEEDS OF CHILDREN

To assess the need for a referral for a bereaved child, several areas should be addressed to assist the parents or guardians with that decision. Questions to ask include:

- Has the child's normal personality and mood changed?
- Is the child getting support and information from caring adults?
- Are the child's questions being addressed and answered?
- Are there signs of being accident prone or suicidal behavior?

Table 26–2 provides helpful ways to discuss death with a child.

THE ROLE OF THE NURSE

The nurse should guide the parents of a grieving child. Answer all questions from the parents and children openly and honestly. We must let the parents know danger signs that children may present. Just being available or present is

TABLE 26–2 How to Explain Death to a Child.

How Do I Explain Death to My Child?

It is difficult for most adults to discuss death. The subject matter influences our thoughts, particularly when a history of losses has affected us.

Because we want to help children have a positive experience, without preconceptions acquired from our culture or personal histories, it helps to think through some basics when we talk to children about death.

Basic Advice

Give clear information; tell the child the facts about what happened. In simple words explain that "_____" has died. Saying "The illness/disease made his/her body stop working" is a good way to begin.

Questions: Then give the child a chance to ask questions. Silence, without jumping in to fill the silence, is the key here. When the child has no questions, say, "Let me know when you have a question."

Honesty: Sometimes the simplest, most honest response is difficult during an emotional time. Children need honesty to feel secure. It can be hard to tell a child, "I don't know," when you truly don't know the answer to a question, but this response should be seriously considered when you are confused or stumped by the question.

Children need security: When a loss occurs, the pain and fears affect everyone. Even a child who hasn't been told about an illness knows that there are changes because of the effects of the stress on other family members.

The overall goal of contact with children who are experiencing a loss should be to provide a secure environment. An attitude of comfort, warmth, and closeness is a helpful approach for most children. Because a child is dependent on parents (or other adults), they notice cues from the adults around them. These adults should primarily reassure the child in this way:

1. that they will be cared for
2. stating who will care for them
3. giving them an opportunity to say goodbye to the dying person
4. telling them that illness leading to death will not happen to them, but occurred due to age or a special illness or accident

© Gretchen Gaines, M.S.W., LCSW-C 1995

invaluable. The major role of the nurse is to recognize danger signs in the grieving child and refer the child to proper therapists. Referrals should be made if the health care provider has any doubts at all for the safety of the child.

It is important for the nurse to give support, understanding, and continuing love to children in grief. Be willing to listen for as long as they need to talk.

Share happy times with the child. When at a loss for words, appropriate touch is important. Physical displays of love and concern are a great comfort to grieving children (Grollman 1995).

THE DYING CHILD

A child's death is unthinkable for most of us. Children bring to mind the future, and being confronted with the possibility that the child may not have a future is a thought we do not wish to entertain.

Although early research into the young child's understanding of death was done by Nagy (1948), the subject did not gather interest until after the 1970s.

Speech and Brent's study (as cited in Corr, 1995) identified and defined subconcepts which are central elements in children's concept of death:

* **Universality**—the understanding that all living things must die; if it is universal, it must also be inevitable and unpredictable.
* **Irreversibility**—the understanding that once the physical body dies, it cannot be made alive again
* **Nonfunctionality**—the understanding that once a living thing dies, all of the typical life-defining capabilities of the living physical body (walking, eating, seeing) cease
* **Causality**—the abstract concept or understanding that death ultimately results from internal or external causes
* **Noncorporeality**—the notion that some form of personal continuation exists after the death of the physical body

Bluebond-Langner (1978) wrote that children experiencing a life-threatening illness know and comprehend, albeit on some level, that they are dying. She argues that these children have a more mature concept of death than children of the same age who have not experienced a serious illness.

The way children understand the concept of death depends on the developmental level of the child. Children become aware of the fact that they are dying before death is imminent. But the awareness does not just happen. It is developed through a process. Bluebond-Langner (1989) identified the five stages of this process:

* Stage 1: Child learns of the serious illness.
* Stage 2: Child learns of the medications and side effects, understands the seriousness of the illness but believes he or she will get better.
* Stage 3: Child understands the purposes of the numerous treatments and procedures but still believes that he or she will get better.
* Stage 4: Child is able to compile the small pieces of information and put it into a big picture. The disease is experienced as a cycle of remissions and relapses.
* Stage 5: Child realizes that the disease has a terminal prognosis.

Consider the following:

Sean was 6 years old and had been through two years of chemotherapy, bone marrow transplant, radiation, and all side effects of the treatments. He was in remission for 11 months and was found to relapse on a routine checkup. He again began chemotherapy but was very ill from the treatment. His parents discussed prognosis and treatment options with the oncologist and learned that his prognosis was very poor with treatment and death was certain without treatment. Sean was so ill from the treatment that he asked to stop the chemotherapy. He told his parents that he just did not want to be sick anymore. His parents (with a lot of guidance from the health care providers) explained to Sean that if they did stop the treatments, he would be certain to die. Sean opted to stop all treatments.

Sean lived six months feeling very well for the majority of the time. Even though he was six, he was capable of making an informed decision. His parents were thankful that they chose to discuss this with Sean and allow him to be involved in the decision to stop the treatment. Based on the five stages, Sean understood the disease, treatment, illness, and finally the terminal prognosis.

PROVIDING CARE TO THE DYING CHILD

The care provided to the dying child must be family centered. Decisions should be made by all members of the family, such as where the child will die, who will be the primary caregiver, and who will support the family through the experience. Most importantly, the dying child must be included in all decisions. Both the family and the dying child need extensive information to make these decisions.

An important option for the family and child to consider is whether to use hospice or hospital care for the terminal stage of the illness. Hospital care involves the traditional care practices in the acute care setting. Hospice is a concept that provides palliative care to the dying child and can be provided in a facility that employs the hospice concept or in the child's home.

At home children can have their parents at hand; be surrounded by a familiar environment; have the company of brothers and sisters, pets, friends, and relatives; eat what and when they want or are able to; and participate in the normal family activities as much or as little as desired. During the illness, the child often had to be in the hospital, for testing and treatment. Being at home was not possible. However, once treatment has been stopped, as well as in between treatments, health professionals and family members must remember that it is usually far more comforting for the child to be in the familiar surroundings of home and family.

Some parents may also feel better physically and emotionally if they care for their dying child at home—they may feel less helpless and "out of control" than being in a hospital setting.

Regardless of where the child is cared for during the terminal stage of an illness, there are fears experienced by both the family and the child (Wong and Perry 1998) such as:

- fear of what the actual death will be like
- fear of dying alone (child) or not being present (family) when the child dies
- fear of pain

Nurses play an important role in alleviating these fears. Although no one can predict what the actual death will be like, nurses can answer questions that families pose and alleviate misconceptions that they may have.

Pain management for the dying child is the same as for an adult. Pain is prevented as much as possible, therefore pain medications should be given routinely and not on an as-needed basis. It is important to give opioids as required by the child's report of pain. Nonpharmacologic methods of pain management that are effective for the child should also be incorporated into the plan of care (Wong and Perry 1998).

Parents usually express concern about their ability to provide adequate care to the child in the home. With proper support and guidance from the nurse, parents will learn safe and effective methods of providing care for their child. Concern for siblings is also at the forefront. Sibling reactions to the dying child will depend on several factors: the developmental stage of the siblings and their understanding of death, the communication in the family, the communication with other siblings, and the circumstances of the death. Remember, the healthy siblings need to feel the security of parents being with them and to have the parent's support during this troubling time. In assisting the families, the nurse should keep in mind the questions that both parents and siblings will have and address them with honest and caring answers.

WHAT DO THE ADULTS NEED?

Adults who are part of the world of the child who is near the end of life need several important things:

- information about the illness and the treatment plans
- someone to listen to his or her thoughts, feelings, and concerns
- access to others in the family to assist them when they are not available due to treatment schedules and their own need for privacy.

Grandparents and other adults who are part of the child's life will need information and support. Perhaps the amount of information and support they receive will be different than that of the parents. As always, confidentially should be respected, and the parents must be the ultimate decision makers regarding who gets information regarding the illness and treatment decisions.

Volunteers, friends, church and community supporters often want information; the parents should be consulted to see if they need help in giving out information or if they are open to doing so.

FAMILY LIFE

When a child is diagnosed with a terminal illness, the child's life begins to change and at the same time the family changes. Illness enters the life of a family unexpectedly. Changes that occur are out of the family's control. The changes affect the patient, each parent, the siblings, and other family members who may not be living in the same house or community. As a result of all of these changes, the family dynamics also change on every level. The family is accustomed to behaving in a particular way and may or may not be aware of the new dynamics. This lack of control and multilevel change contributes to the family's sense of chaos. The previously mentioned phases of illness help us to follow a family as they move along the course of the illness, from the initial phase, understanding the fact of the diagnosis and its meaning, to beginning to live in the chronic living-dying phase. Change continues during the family's movement along this continuum. Therefore any description of the family and its members must always remain fluid.

Silverman (2000, 119) says "Parents have to make a decision not to assign their children to the role of dying persons when the death is still relatively far off. Living in the present and for the moment is something families learn to value. They develop a routine, compartmentalize to the extent that they can, and begin to find a flexibility that they may not have known they have. The family has to find a way of continuing to live and of including the sick child in the family."

Rando (1984) states that while many of the feelings that the family is experiencing is related to the terminal illness, they may also reflect the family's critical need to take care of itself. Challenging demands often leave parents feeling culpable because there is never enough time or energy to attend to all needs. For example, while at the hospital, they are concerned about the other children at home and while at home, they are concerned about the sick child at the hospital.

Children in the family may begin to resent the time spent caring for the dying child and the lack of attention they receive from their parents. A spouse may resent the time commitment of one parent to the dying child because it interferes with the private, intimate time for the couple. Such resentments are actually quite normal and understandable, but can be a source of tremendous stress and guilt to family members. Therefore these feelings should be acknowledged and discussed so that family members' needs are met within the constraints of the family's resources.

Rando (1984) has defined family coping tasks necessary to maintain the functioning of the family unit. These include:

- addressing denial versus acceptance of the illness
- establishing a relationship with a health care provider
- developing strategies for the task of meeting the needs of the dying child
- grant the dying child permission to experience the feelings generated by the illness, the accompanying losses, and the threat of approaching death

The family must balance support for the patient's increased dependence with the continued need for autonomy. Maintaining a functional equilibrium is a major task for the family, one that must be attended to throughout the illness.

Other parts of life do not stop (siblings' school and sports activities, ongoing community organization and church involvement, work schedules, friendships, and family obligations), although at times these have to be eliminated. Therefore the family cannot be looked at as a static entity. It is and should continue to be a multifaceted center of life for all of the family members. Naturally the focus changes as the dying child approaches death.

Nursing and other professionals need to be sensitive to stresses that the families are experiencing. Re-assessment of the family's needs must be ongoing. The family members' ability to handle the stress of the situation must be considered (Rando 1984).

WORKING WITH THE TEAM

The team consists of the physician, nurses, social worker, nutritionist, art therapist, child life worker, and other staff. From the time of diagnosis and continuing throughout the illness, it is very important that the team members work with the patient and the family. Teams work differently in different centers, but fundamentally the concept of communicating with all staff members who have contact with the patient and family provides a basis for quality care. Communicating about treatment plans and psychosocial information and interventions means that the care will be coordinated and provided efficiently. In most team settings, the physician understands the importance of working alongside a social worker and other staff at the time of diagnosis. Good care begins with gathering all the information possible and giving the family opportunities to meet with several disciplines to assist them in this difficult time. Nurses usually have the opportunity of spending much of their time with the patient. Nurses notice the small details about a child that inform us about his or her personality. Nurses can share these details with other team members, which can contribute to the child's comfort. [At the time of each change in the patient, everyone—family and team—needs to be informed.] Experienced caregivers shared the following story:

A child was dying. Her conditioned changed rapidly and she was transferred to the ICU. The doctor told the child what was happening, why she needed to be taken to ICU and in terms understandable to the child, what was happening to her body. The doctor informed the child and also patiently asked her if she had any questions, as he prepared for the transfer. The new graduate nurse involved with the child's care became very upset. She was angry with the doctor for telling the child what was happening. She thought that this would frighten the child.

In this example, we see a doctor handling a situation with a child very competently. The nurse was not accustomed to informing children of their conditions. Not only do children and their parents need to be informed, but also as the illness proceeds, parents need well-timed information. Being prepared is helpful to everyone, even if they resist knowing of the impending death. This is no time to keep secrets and confuse the patient or the family.

It is the responsibility of the nurse to continue to support the dying child and family. In general, nurses are at the bedside and spend more time with the child and family. When parents react strongly to the nurse, the nurse should not take it personally. Parents behave in many different ways when their child is seriously ill. One may scream, while the other walks away, saying nothing. Parents have the right to act differently and to find their own way to manage the crisis that has suddenly changed their life. These suggestions are offered:

- Be there and listen.
- You don't always need to have an answer for them. Sometimes there is not an answer.
- Allow parents to do what they need to do (within the law, respecting the rights of others, and not being destructive to any persons).
- Support what they do, how they respond.
- Don't be judgmental.

SUMMARY

The death of a child is a life-changing event for the child, parents, siblings, extended family and the health care providers. Nurses are in a unique position to provide invaluable support to the dying child and family. It is important that the nurse maintain a caring relationship with the family and dying child throughout the illness. Being sensitive to the family dynamics and family needs is an important step in providing quality nursing care that the patient and family so desperately require. The potential for self-fulfillment for the nurse is enormous.

REFERENCES

Bluebond-Langner, M. (1989). Worlds of dying children and their well siblings. *Death Studies*, 13(1), 1–16.

Bluebond-Langner, M. (1978). *The private worlds of dying children*. Princeton, NJ: Princeton University Press.

Children's Hospice International. (2000). *Home care for seriously ill children: A manual for parents*. Alexandria, VA: Author.

Christ, G. H. (2000). *Healing children's grief*. New York: Oxford University Press.

Corr, C. A. (1995). Children's Understanding of Death: striving to understand death. In K. J. Doka (ed). *Children Mourning Mourning Children*, pp. 4–7. Washington, D.C.: Hospice Foundation of America.

Corr, C. A., Nabe, C. M., & Corr, D. M. (1996). *Death and dying life and living* (2nd ed.). Pacific Grove, CA: Wadsworth Publishing Co.

Grollman, E. A. (1995). Grieving children: Can we answer their questions. In K. J. Doka, (Ed.), *Children mourning, mourning children* (26). Washington, D.C.: Hospice Foundation of America.

Kubler-Ross, E. (1969). *On death and dying*. New York: MacMillan.

Nagy, M. A. (1948). The child's theories concerning death. *Journal of Genetic Psychology*. 73, 3–27.

Rando, T. (1984). *Dying and death, clinical interventions for caregivers*. Champaign, IL: Research Press Company.

Silverman, P. (2000). *Never too young to know*. New York: Oxford University Press, Inc.

Wong, D. L., & Perry, S. E. (1998). *Maternal child nursing care*. St. Louis, MO: Mosby, Inc.

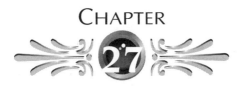

CHAPTER

DEATH AND THE YOUNG ADULT

Randy Bond

Young adults are defined as individuals between the ages of 18 and 40 years. This is a very diverse group undergoing many psychosocial changes as they progress through this stage of development. An understanding of this age group and the changes they encounter are necessary to assess the effect of dying on these individuals, as well as society's response to their death.

PSYCHOSOCIAL ASPECTS OF THE YOUNG ADULT

Young adulthood is characterized by the stage of psychosocial development known as intimacy versus isolation. This stage of development centers on the task of developing an intense lasting relationship with a person, cause, or creative effort. Intimacy requires responsibility, impulse control, the ability to plan, and the ability to trust (Erikson 1963).

Early in this period, the young adult faces pressures to establish a lasting intimate relationship with a significant other and start a career. They often feel a need to find purpose in life. During the early years of this stage, the young adult strives to achieve independence and responsibility (Stevenson 1983). This is a period of great energy in which the individual attempts to find a niche in society. Efforts are centered on establishing financial, personal, and social responsibility. They are faced with choosing a lifestyle, choosing and starting an occupation, selecting a mate, starting a family, and managing a home. Competing demands on the individual's time, creativity, and energy, along with negative feelings about self, can interfere with the ability to achieve these tasks (Stanwyck 1983).

Sexuality is an important part of the young adult's life. Feeling competent in this arena is essential to well being. Perceived inadequacies in this area can result in a loss of self-confidence and an altered concept of self, which can effect all aspects of the young adult's life (Devney and Abbink 2000).

As the young adult progresses through this period, emphasis is placed on maintaining and advancing both personal and professional relationships, as well as meeting the expectations of society. Balancing the demands of family life, the demands of career advancement, and the demands of society can often create conflict at a time when parental responsibility is becoming increasingly difficult. In addition, financial stressors on the young family can cause conflicts.

Toward the end of this period, the young adult begins to reflect on choices made and to face the inevitability of aging. Regret about life choices and the realization that youth is behind them can lead to what is commonly called midlife crisis. The individual may respond to this event by making sudden and drastic alterations in lifestyle or may become very introspective and possibly depressed. In contrast, if the individual believes life up to this point has been productive and had meaning, he or she will be able to move on to the next stage of life without difficulty.

Failure to establish and maintain these personal, professional, and societal relationships during this period of life can result in isolation (Erikson 1963). Isolation can result in alienation and self-absorption, and can prevent the individual from advancing to the next stage of development (Stanwyck 1983).

Society views young adulthood as the productive years. Even though productivity can and does extend well beyond this period, young adults are truly the "worker bees" of society. The young adult is expected to make the transition from childhood—a period in which resources are allocated to nurturing, educating, and protecting—to adulthood—a period in which the individual is expected to contribute to society.

Along with this responsibility, certain norms are established, which society expects individuals in this age group to attain. Failure to conform to these norms can result in society viewing the individual as lazy or irresponsible. For men in this age group, these norms include going to work, getting married, fathering children, and providing for their family. For women, the expectation is getting married, having children, nurturing and rearing the children, and maintaining the home. Despite changes in our society that have altered this reality, these norms, for the most part, remain intact.

HEALTH ISSUES OF THE YOUNG ADULT

Young adulthood is generally seen as a time of health, vigor, and well-being. The diseases of childhood are, for the most part, in the past, and the chronic conditions associated with aging are yet to manifest themselves. Due to this, health is not usually a major concern to the young adult.

Health promotion is centered on exercise, nutrition, and adequate sleep (Davney and Abbink 2000). Social patterns regarding alcohol use, substance abuse, smoking, improper diet, as well as sexual practices can have immediate, as well as long term consequences for the young adult. Men in this age group may have concerns about stress and stress-related disorders, while women in this age group may be concerned about birth control and pregnancy. Both genders may experience sports-related injury and fatigue associated with overactivity and inadequate rest.

MORTALITY OF THE YOUNG ADULT

The concept of death is not always recognized as a part of life for the young adult. This recognition usually begins in the middle-aged adult. The young adult's awareness may begin to increase as the older adults who have a relationship with them begin to develop illness and die (Davney and Abbink 2000). In general, chronic terminal illness is usually seen in the older adult.

In the United States, the leading causes of death for young adults are accidents, violence, acquired immunodeficiency syndrome (AIDS), and suicide (National Center for Health Statistics 1999). These causes of death, with the possible exception of AIDS, reflect the unanticipated nature of death among young adults. In addition, each carries with it the stigma that it could have been prevented or avoided. These types of deaths, in conjunction with the victim's age and society's view of the young adult, are the major factors associated with how we experience the death of the young adult.

Death by Accident

Accidents are a major cause of death among young adults. Men are more likely to die by accident than women, due to risk-taking behavior associated with men of this age (U.S. Bureau of the Census 1999). Accidents by definition are sudden and unplanned events. Survivors are often robbed of their opportunity to say goodbye. This inability to say what they feel to the dying individual often makes closure difficult. They may regret words spoken or unspoken. Death as a result of accident can result in dysfunctional grief.

Often the survivors seek understanding or explanation for the accidental death when none exist. They may want to place blame and often there is no one or nothing to blame. In these cases, God is an easy target. When there is someone to blame, their focus may revolve around punishment of the guilty party. They feel that retribution will ease their loss. In most cases, once retribution is gained, the survivors still feel a sense of unnecessary loss.

Accidents where bodies are destroyed or lost can complicate the grieving process even more. Without a body, acceptance and closure become more difficult. Our society puts great value in memorializing the dead. Grieving at an empty coffin or grave can leave the survivors feeling cheated. This can prolong the grieving process and result in dysfunctional grief (Carpenito 2000).

Death by Violence

Violence is another major cause of death in the young adult. African American men are more likely to die as a result of violence than any other subset of this age group (U.S. Bureau of the Census 1999). As with accidents, the survivors often feel the pain of a senseless and unnecessary death. Again, their feelings may revolve around retribution. If the perpetrator of the violent act is not apprehended, they may feel cheated. They may devote their lives and resources to catching the guilty party. In cases where the guilty is apprehended, they may focus on justice. They may attend the trial, which may drag on for long periods of time, delaying their recovery from grief. The trial may resurrect feelings of grief and loss. If they are dissatisfied with the outcome of justice, they may suffer the pain of loss all over again. They may feel they have let their loved one down. Some may make the cause for justice a crusade, devoting a large amount of their energy to this cause at their expense, as well as the expense of those around them.

Children who lose a parent to violence may suffer unfounded fear. They may be afraid the "bad man" will come to get them. They may have irrational fears of losing the remaining parent to violence. Their fears may be manifested in nightmares, bed-wetting, or irrational behavior such as not wanting to be separated from the remaining parent (Carpenito 2000).

Death As a Result of AIDS

Even though the face of AIDS in the United States has changed since its inception, it is still predominately a disease associated with homosexuality. Society's attitude regarding homosexuality, as well as religious and cultural taboos, have contributed to the stigma associated with AIDS. Certain segments of society will blame the victims for their infection and, as a result, may show them little sympathy. In some cases the victims may be shunned and isolated. Some members of society may respond to the AIDS victim with anger, disgust, or fear (Flaskerud and Ungvarski 1992).

Even though heterosexual women are the fastest growing group of new HIV/AIDS cases, homosexual men still account for the greatest number of persons living and dying with AIDS. This creates unique dilemmas in the grieving process. Support systems usually associated with the dying individual may not be intact. Homosexual men may be estranged from their families. Often they have kept their homosexuality a secret from coworkers and friends. Even in the homosexual community there can exist a stigma between the "positives" and the "negatives." Friends may have already succumbed to the disease, reducing the support system. Concerns over insurance, job, and social standing may prompt the individual to hide the disease from others.

Individuals with AIDS may blame themselves, especially if they have engaged in risky sex without protection. This blame may result in anger towards themselves. They may try to figure out who infected them, in an effort to assign blame, but in many cases may never know the answer. Sometimes their anger may be directed at institutions such as the drug companies, because of the high cost of AIDS medication; the medical system, because they sense a lack of understanding and sympathy; or society at large, for not having accepted them and their lifestyle. Guilt and anger may be intensified if they already have unresolved issues regarding their homosexuality.

Unlike the sudden deaths associated with accidents and violence or the planned death associated with suicide, the AIDS victim usually has many years to contemplate death. This extended death can actually bring on more anxiety. They may have fears regarding loss of income, loss of independence, social isolation, and loss of body image. If they have witnessed the death of others with AIDS, they may be aware that they could face a slow and agonizing death. They may also fear the loss of intimacy with their partner.

Some may be determined to beat the disease, while others may have feelings of hopelessness, which can lead to risky behavior, alcohol or substance abuse, and possibly suicide. They may adopt a "live for the day" attitude, with no regard for the future. Dreams and goals for the future may be abandoned. Some individuals may make their health the centerpoint of their lives, seeking all the knowledge they can about their condition. This can sometimes consume their entire life. AIDS, for them, may become a life mission, prompting activism. Other individuals may show no regard to health at all, figuring there is nothing they can do.

The significant others of the homosexual AIDS patients may find themselves in a precarious situation. Unless special consideration and planning has been undertaken, they will have none of the legal rights afforded a family member (Flaskerud and Ungvarski 1992). This can create problems regarding care decisions, end of life decisions, inheritance, and disposition of the body. Even though time is usually available to make these decisions in advance, avoidance of the issue and denial can sometimes delay preparation.

The grieving process of significant others is not unlike that of spouses; however, they may encounter certain unique problems due to their situation. If the significant others are also HIV positive, they may witness their own death in their partner. If that death is agonizing, it will increase fear and anxiety regarding their death. If they are HIV negative, they may become more fearful of their partner as they witness the devastation of the disease.

There may be resentment between the significant other and the family. Families may blame significant others, who in turn may feel the families are imposing on their territory. The tension created by this conflict can increase anxiety and anger on both sides, and place the dying individual in the middle.

Decisions regarding the end of treatment and hospice care can often fall on the significant other. Sometimes it becomes impossible to care for the individual at home, and decisions regarding institutional care must be made. These types of decisions are often accompanied by second-guessing and guilt, especially if the dying individuals did not make their wishes known.

In addition to the trauma of losing a child, the parents of the homosexual AIDS patient may be forced to deal with unresolved issues. They may be embarrassed that their child is homosexual. They may have regrets that they did not accept their son's lifestyle. The parents may experience guilt over their own feelings regarding homosexuality and AIDS. They may blame themselves that their son is homosexual, feeling they are ultimately responsible for him having AIDS.

Children are sometimes a part of an AIDS patient's life. They may fear the parent with AIDS, especially if they have a limited understanding of the disease. They may suffer the stigma of AIDS, being shunned by friends and classmates.

Death by Suicide

Suicide possesses its own unique stigma in society. Most Western religions, as well as Western culture, have taboos against the taking of one's own life (Dickinson, Leming, and Mermann 1993). The stigma of mental illness is also attached to suicide. It is often seen as a selfish or cowardly act. Some may view it as a weakness of character. Society seeks understanding of suicide by wanting a simple explanation of why. Sometimes the reasons are clear, but often the underlying causes of suicide are complex and not clearly understood. Without a simple and clear reason, society is left confused and closure can be difficult.

Women are more likely to attempt suicide, but men are more likely to complete the act (Dickinson, Leming, and Mermann 1993). The underlying reason for suicide can vary. Some of the life events that precipitate suicide in this age group may be the inability to develop intimate relationships, marital problems, stressors associated with work and career, an unfavorable concept of self, and financial problems.

The individual contemplating suicide experiences the same grieving process as others faced with their own death. They will usually experience depression associated with an overwhelming feeling of hopelessness for the future. In some cases they may make awkward attempts at saying goodbye to loved ones prior to the act, without giving away their intentions. Suicide is usually a planned event, in which the individual picks a time, place, and method of death. Suicide notes are often left, but these can be feeble attempts at explaining or justifying the act, as individuals are often not completely aware of all the dynamics associated with their decision to end life.

The spouse of a suicide victim is often faced with a need to publicly grieve, which conflicts with embarrassment over the suicide of their loved one. They may feel a sense of responsibility and guilt resulting in close examination of all their actions prior to the suicide. They may feel that they could have and should have done something to prevent the suicide. Often they will have anger directed toward the suicide victim. In trying to understand their loss, they will seek to place blame, sometimes on the victim, sometimes on themselves, and sometimes on outside factors or persons. Due to their embarrassment, as well as the uncomfortable feelings of others, personal support systems may not be readily available.

Children of suicide victims are very vulnerable to blame and guilt. They often believe they are the reason for the suicide. Along with this, they may feel a sense of abandonment. These feelings are often expressed as regression or behavioral changes. Older children may want to blame the surviving spouse, driving a wedge between them at a time when they need each other the most. Children may also be the victims of embarrassment. They may suffer ridicule and isolation from their peer group. Sometimes the adolescent male may see the suicide of a father as a heroic act (Dickinson, Leming, and Mermann 1993). They may identify with some of the same feelings of hopelessness and despair. These individuals are at high risk of following in their parent's footsteps. They may first express their desire to die through reckless, risk-taking behavior, coupled with alcohol or substance abuse.

THE GRIEVING PROCESS

Grief is a transitory response to loss. The process of grief includes denial, anger, bargaining, depression, and acceptance (Kubler-Ross 1969). These may occur in varying degrees, and the sequence may vary as well. Many factors can effect the grieving process, such as culture, age, race, gender, type of death, and religion.

Dysfunctional grief is grief that is unusual in intensity or duration, considering the individual's culture and religion. It can be pathological, causing physical or psychological illness, or a disruption in the individual's ability to return to normal functioning after an appropriate time (Carpenito 2000).

Grief and the Young Adult

Many factors regarding the grieving process in relation to young adults can vary, such as race, culture, religion, and gender. In order to have a general discussion of grief and the young adult, it is necessary to focus on generalities such as age group, psychosocial development, their place in society, and the type of death. As is the case with most human endeavors, death impacts not only the dying, but a cast of individuals as well.

DYING YOUNG

Death is not the same at any age. Society views the death of the young quite differently than it does the death of the elderly. Young adults are viewed by society as being at their prime, in their most productive years. When a young adult dies, it is often seen as the loss of an unexplored potential. This view can often heighten the sense of loss, making acceptance harder. The death of young adults are often met with a sense of disbelief.

The young do not expect to die. As a result, they have neither contemplated their death, nor have they prepared for it. If death is sudden, which is often the case with the young adult, they are robbed of the opportunity to prepare for death. This can often leave unresolved issues and problems for the survivors. Sudden and unexpected death can be a cause of dysfunctional grief (Carpenito 2000).

Denial is often the first reaction a young adult will have toward their own dying. They may feel that someone made a mistake. Often they feel that this can not be happening to them. They may rationalize that they are young and strong enough to overcome anything. If they have been otherwise healthy up to this point, this feeling of invincibility may be increased.

Once the fact that they are going to die is accepted, they may experience a heightened sense of anger. They may feel cheated of a future they will never have. Regrets concerning paths taken or not taken may increase this anger. They may question why they planned for the future, instead of living for the day; or they may wish they had planned better, assuring the financial future of their children or spouse, and be angry at themselves for not having made arrangements.

If their condition is debilitating, they may grieve the loss of sexual intimacy with their partner. If their condition results in body changes, they may grieve the change from strong and vital to weak and frail. The loss of independence may increase this feeling. They may bargain with God for time. Often this will be centered on wanting to see children grown and independent. In contrast, if they do not have children, they may regret that they will not have the opportunity to leave behind a legacy. They may experience a loss of control over their life and destiny, leading to a feeling of helplessness and depression. They may want to place blame; God is often the object of this blame.

The spouse or significant other of the young adult will have issues as well. They will fear the loss of intimacy. It may seem that they are losing the only individual with whom they will ever be able to share a relationship. Their anger may be displaced toward the dying individual. They may feel a sense of abandonment and isolation. Fears regarding their future and the future of their family will compound their sense of loss. The realization that they will be a single parent, coupled with financial worries, will cause them to view the future very dimly. They will question what will happen to them and then may feel guilty for being concerned about their needs while their spouse is dying. They may also feel that there should have been something they could have done to prevent their loved one from dying. They may ask, "What if I had only done. . . ." which will increase their feelings of guilt. They may see themselves as the martyr, a job that requires acceptance of their lot in life without complaint or regard for themselves. Responsibility for children may cause them to hide their own grief for fear they may upset the children. Time becomes precious to them, prompting them to resent anyone who "steals" time with their spouse from them. Often they feel the need to assume all responsibility for the dying, robbing what independence their dying spouse has left. They may assume the role of parent rather than spouse.

Parents expect to be survived by their children. When a young adult dies, their parents are often still alive, which can result in guilt on the part of the parents. The death of a child of any age can result in dysfunctional grief for the parents. The parents often question why their child died and not them. Additional grief can be experienced if the young adult has not yet had children. The parents see this as an end to a legacy and may feel robbed of the potential to be grandparents.

Young adults are often parents of young children. The loss of a parent may be the child's first experience of loss. Immature attitudes regarding death may result in misplaced anger towards the deceased parent. The child may feel abandoned. Regression of development, such as bed-wetting, is not uncommon when this happens. Older children may act out and have sudden and drastic behavior changes (Carpenito 2000).

In contrast, children may deify the lost parent. They may feel an obligation to live for the deceased parent, trying to fulfill that parent's wishes and dreams, instead of pursuing their own. They may also feel a sense of responsibility for the parent's death. They may feel that if they had been better, this would not have happened. Children may focus on times when, in anger, they wished their parents dead and now feel responsible for the death. They may fear for the life of the remaining parent. An overexaggeration of fear for the remaining parent's well-being may occur, in which they do not want to let them out of their sight. In addition, they may feel an obligation to the remaining family members, taking on adult responsibilities and maturing faster than otherwise expected. Young children who lose a parent can experience dysfunctional grieving (Carpenito 2000).

Siblings and peers of the young adult will most likely be in the same age group. The death of the young adult will prompt them to question their own mortality. They may feel lucky that it's not them and yet feel guilt for the same reason. These individuals may feel an obligation to assume responsibility for the spouse and children of the dying. Often they feel a sense of injustice that someone just like them could be taken. They may question their own values and take inventory of their life accomplishments. This may result in a shift in their priorities.

ASSISTING WITH GRIEF OF THE YOUNG ADULT

When dealing with the grieving individual, it is important to remember that no two persons experience grief the same. Our expectations of grief are based on our experiences and may not be shared by the individual with whom we are dealing. In addition, factors such as race, gender, religion, culture, and age can greatly alter an individual's response to loss. The type of loss can also be a factor in how grief is expressed.

In our society, we often feel a need to express our sympathy through verbal expressions of sadness. Often the best thing we can do is simply listen, allowing the individuals the opportunity to express their feelings and work through the phase of grief they are experiencing.

Certain strategies may assist the grieving individual. Easing the grieving person back to a normal routine may help to alleviate or lessen grief. Physical exercise can relieve anxiety and tension associated with grief and help the person sleep. Family and friends can provide opportunities to voice feelings as well as helping with mundane tasks, allowing the individual time to grieve. More structured support systems, such as community support groups, can provide unique opportunities for the grieving individual to share feelings with other individuals who have experienced similar losses. Professional counseling can provide an opportunity to express in private feelings that the individual may not wish to express in public. Hospice can be of assistance, especially in situations of prolonged death. Services can be provided that allow the patient to die at home, or, when necessary, inpatient hospice services can be utilized. With the exception of AIDS victims, young adults make excellent organ donors. Some people may be opposed to organ donation, but for those who are willing, donating organs may give them a sense of helping others, as well as the feeling that part of them may survive their death. Medications such as psychotropic drugs should be avoided, as they may only delay the feelings of grief (Carpenito 2000).

SUMMARY

Even though generalities can be drawn between young adults and the cast of individuals surrounding them, it is important to note that they are unique individuals. Each one experiences grief and death in a different way. The best strategy in dealing with this issue is to learn as much about the individual as possible before drawing any conclusions and allow them to express their feelings. Characteristic problems associated with this age group will be related to the often sudden and unexpected nature of their deaths, as well as the lack of preparedness for death.

REFERENCES

Berkow, R., and Fletcher, A. (1992). *The Merck manual of diagnosis and therapy*. Rahway, NJ: Merck.

Carpenito, L. (2000). *Nursing diagnosis: Application to clinical practice* (8th ed.). Philadelphia, PA: J. B. Lippincott Co.

Devney, A. M., & Abbink, C. R. (2000). Adult development. In S. M. Lewis, M. M. Heitkemper, & S. R. Dirksen, (Eds.), *Medical surgical nursing* (5th ed., pp. 35–36). St. Louis, MO: Mosby, Inc.

Dickinson, G., Leming, M., & Mermann, A. (1993). *Dying, death, and bereavement* (Annual ed). Guilford, CN.: The Dushkin Publishing Co.

Erikson, E. H. (1963). *Childhood and society* (2nd ed). New York: W. W. Norton Co. Inc.

Flaskerud, J., & Ungvarski, P. (1992). HIV/AIDS: A *guide to nursing care* (2nd ed). Philadelphia, PA: W. B. Saunders Co.

Kubler-Ross, E. (1969). *On death and dying*. New York: Macmillan Publishing Co.

National Center of Health Statistics. (1999). *Mortality statistics in the United States*. Report No. 155. Washington, DC: U.S. Public Health Service.

Stanwyck, D. (1983). Self esteem through the Life-Span. *Family Community Health*, 6 (2), 11–28.

Stevenson, J. (1983). Adulthood: A promising direction for future research. In H. Wherley, J. Fitzpatrick, and R. Taunton (Ed.), *Annual Review of Nursing Research* (Vol. 1, 52–64) New York: Springer Publishing Co. Inc.

Uphold, C., and Graham, M. (1994). *Clinical guidelines in family practice* pp. 52–64 (2nd ed). Gainsville, FL: Barmarrae Books.

U.S. Bureau of the Census. (1999). *Statistical abstracts of the United States* (Annual ed). Washington, DC: U.S. Government Printing Office.

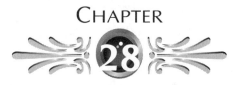

THE END OF LIFE FOR
THE OLDER ADULT

Dr. Thomas Smith

INTRODUCTION

Aging, or senescence, is the process of growing old. This process is individualized, inevitable, and irreversible. As people age, they experience a succes-
sion of losses: physical losses such as male hair loss, psychological losses such
as age-associated memory impairment (AAMI), and social losses such as those
brought on by retirement from the workforce. Typically, the older the person,
the greater the number of losses experienced in life (Snyder and Miene 1994).
The ultimate loss is the loss of life. Although the end of life can occur at any
age, it more commonly occurs in and is associated with "old age"; in short,
older adults are "closer" to death (Marshall 1980).

While death at an earlier age tends to be unexpected and traumatic, death
in old age is more expected and generally considered to be somewhat less
traumatic. Older adults have more time and inclination to anticipate their
deaths than younger persons who "suddenly" died. Therefore for older adults,
end of life is a process with the actual death being an anticipated terminal
event (Doka 1989). Barring outright denial or cognitive impairment, older
adults know that life is drawing to a close. This realization allows them to better make end of life decisions, maximize their control over life and dying, and
prepare themselves and their significant others for death, the inevitable and
impending loss (Krisman-Scott 2000).

The discussion of end of life for older adults is a most relevant topic, especially in this textbook, which addresses end of life care across the lifespan.
This chapter will first briefly overview the life of the older adult, with a focus
on "successful" aging. Next, end of life for the older adult will be analyzed in
detail, along with both general and specific considerations for health care
providers engaged in end of life care. Throughout, emphasis will be placed on
implications, interventions, and appropriate education guidelines impacting
end of life care for older adults and their significant others.

THE LIFE OF THE OLDER ADULT

Older adults, having lived six to seven decades, tend to be more individually distinct than younger adults, as they have had longer to develop unique lives (Neugarten 1990). Hence, one enters and progresses through "old age" with a unique and ongoing accumulation of experiences, changes, information, and losses. To the extent that an older adult can sift through all of these and determine that his or her life has been and is "good," we say that that person has aged "successfully." By way of contrast, if an older adult determines that life has been and is less than good, this person has aged less successfully. Regardless, this sorting through and determination is a very individualized, value-laden process (Brock 1997).

Likewise, when Erickson (1982) labeled the developmental task of the last stage of life to be ego integrity versus ego despair, successful aging was the implied "task." Those older adults who reviewed their respective lives and found that, for the most part, they had achieved their goals, recognized success or "ego integrity." On the other hand, those older adults who fell short on life goal achievement fell short of success and, since they perceived that it was no longer possible to achieve these goals (e.g., time was no longer on their side), they experienced "ego despair." Obviously, ego integrity and ego despair are the endpoints of a line continuum, and the number of points on that line in between these two extremes is at least equal to the number of older adults who have ever lived, are living, and will ever live (Lawton, Moss, and Glicksman 1990).

Hence, what constitutes "successful aging" varies among older adults. Central to the end of life care of older adults is the respective perceptions of the relative "success" of their individual lives. "After one has lived a life of meaning, death may lose much of its terror" (Butler 1975). Before we can provide any care to older adults at the end of life, we must assess how they view their lives as experienced before they reached this point in time (Kalina 1993).

THE END OF LIFE OF THE OLDER ADULT

As people age, they tend to "lose things." Older adults typically have less resources, particularly money, less available family, less functioning, and less health than when they were younger. Multiple illnesses and an increased chance for health care institutionalization are associated with less self-care, less safety, impaired nutritional status, polypharmacy at a time of faltering pharmacokinetics, and a host of other decrements (Sokolovsky 1990). Loneliness, depression, and references to death are endemic in the older adult population (Roberto and Stanis 1994). Oftentimes, older adults prefer death to a life of actual or perceived inactivity, uselessness, deterioration, discomfort, or "becoming a burden" (Marshall 1980). In addition, society as a whole, although providing support programs for the elderly such as Social Security and Medicare, appears to want to usher them out; their "place" in society is unclear and the dictum to "age gracefully" is a mantra (DeSpedler and Strickland 1999).

The older adult's end of life is just like the life that has preceded: It is very individualized based upon varying life experiences, past and present needs, values, and perceptions (Sapolsky and Finch 1991). Age alone is a poor predictor of how an older adult has aged (Hope 1994). Therefore, what will constitute end of life care will vary from one older adult to another and will be determined after analysis of that adult's life.

GENERAL CONSIDERATIONS: LIFE REVIEW

There are many phases, tasks, or aspects of the end of life care of older adults. Since their prior lives will mold their current care, it is important to first review their lives with them and help them put the past in perspective (Weenolsen 1996). Formal or informal life review or reminiscing will help older adults to determine their relative position on the "ego integrity-ego despair," or successful aging, continuum, while identifying both accomplishments and failures, coping mechanisms, and support systems (Kaufman 1995).

This life review can be conducted by older adults either alone or in groups, with or without a professional facilitator. Some like to be alone to "think their thoughts," while others like to discuss and interchange within a peer group. Some prefer one-on-one interaction with a health care provider, while others prefer to be in a group led by a health care provider. Which of these four possibilities is best is determined by trying each one and assessing which one elicits the most life review and changes over time. Also, at any point in time, any combination of the four possibilities may be the best (Brown and Ellis 1975).

Regardless of how the older adult conducts the life review, it is important for the health care provider to encourage and support this process (Chi and Lubben 1996). Be available to older adults via brief but frequent visits or communications, display a nonjudgmental attitude, and offer the use of therapeutic touch. These are all keys to facilitating the life review.

Focus on Present

The life review is an ongoing process, which will conclude only upon the death of the older adult. Although this life review is very important, the older adult will become preoccupied with the past (Heinlein, Brumett, and Tibbals 1997). This focus on the past allows the older adult to escape the present, which is focused on end of life. Therefore, while facilitating the life review, it is important for the health care provider to engage the older adult in the present, to maintain balance. (Stillion 1985).

Older adults who are overly focused on the past tend to display less motivation in and more detachment from the present. Various individual or group activities, whether formal activity or exercise sessions, get older adults active and involved in the present, while increasing both self-esteem and overall health. Recreational activities, outings, discussions, and spending time with family and friends also help. Throughout, a focus on topics or activities of interest to the older adult is central to keeping them in the present (Scrutton 1995).

Preparation for Death

Finally, while assisting the older adult to balance the present with the past, the older adult must be formally supported to prepare for death. Invariably, involvement of the older adult's significant others in death preparation is key to achieving this goal (Kastenbaum 1979). The older adult, significant others, health care providers, and others are all members of an end of life care team. Concealment or nondisclosure of any information among team members impairs care (Krisman-Scott 2000). Full, fluid, open, and ongoing communication is essential to effective end of life care.

As with all other aspects of end of life care, preparation for death will be a highly individualized matter varying with older adults' needs, values, and perceptions (Osterweis, Solomon, and Green 1984). They should be encouraged to spend private time with family, friends, significant others, and themselves. The health care provider should be available to and anticipate the concerns of both the older adult and significant others. Formal assistance with planning the place of death (home or institution, to the extent possible), funeral and burial arrangements, and estate matters prepare the older adult to end life. Older adults should be encouraged and assisted to get their affairs in order (Weenolsen 1996).

The deaths of the older adult's friends or fellow residents should be formally explored via discussion, a memorial service, or the like. Any death, but particularly the death of those of similar age or situation, reminds us of our own mortality (DeSpedler and Strickland 1999). Spiritual guidance or counseling should be available. Throughout, health care personnel should be supportive, honest, and attentive listeners and care providers. It is most important to remain calm and objective, verbally reassure the dying elders and their significant others, and not rush their natural, necessary grief reactions accompanying dying and death (Leash 1994).

As older adults and their significant others prepare for death, emotions are many and tend to run high. Guilt, denial, resentment, and anger are typical, and should be understood by the health care provider and others for what they are: natural humanistic ways to cope with the anticipated end of life (Brice 1982).

Immediate Post-Mortem Interventions

Upon the actual death, the significant others should be encouraged to view, even touch, the dead body. Full, open grieving should be promoted [and facilitated with a viable support system or coping mechanism] (Leash 1994). Health personnel should assist the significant others to implement the funeral arrangements previously discussed and agreed upon prior to the death.

SPECIFIC CONSIDERATIONS: HOSPICE

Hospice is not a place, it is a concept which represents all of the care provided to dying persons and their significant others (Buckingham 1996). Hospice care is essentially synonymous with end of life care; it occurs wherever the dying person is located and is conducted in a manner determined by the dying person and the significant others. Open communication, emotional outlets, and following the dying person's lead are all hallmarks of hospice care (Beresford 1993). Provision and maximization of holistic comfort coupled with preparation for death are the twin goals of hospice (Infield 1995).

Comfort

Mental and social comfort, as previously discussed, come from emotional support, private times with significant others, etc. Physical comfort is achieved by either controlling pain or managing discomforts such as nausea and vomiting, excessive intestinal flatulence, and pruritis. While mental and social discomforts are inevitable with aging and end of life, physical pain and discomfort are not. Hence, assessment for pain or other physical discomforts is necessary (Pruncho 1995).

Physical pain is oftentimes difficult to assess and treat in older adults. Many times their pain presents with vague or varying symptomatology, or is delayed or atypical in presentation. Frequently older adults are unable or unwilling to report their pain or, when they do, have difficulty accurately communicating it (Hope 1994).

Complete, thorough assessment of the older adult in general and specifically of any suspected or reported pain is the first step. This assessment should include the pain's impact on functioning, pain behaviors, and the relative success of pain control measures.

Pain management can be pharmacologic, nonpharmacologic, or a combination of both. Regardless, due to the impairment of all aspects of pharmacokinetics accompanying aging, nonpharmacologic measures—such as relaxation techniques, guided imagery, bio-feedback, and hypnosis—should be attempted before pharmacologic measures—nonsteroidal anti-inflammatory agents, nonopiate and opiate analgesics, psychotherapeutic agents (e.g., valium, antidepressants, haldol, etc.), and other adjunctive medications. However, since maximization of comfort is the goal, prolonged dawdling with nonpharmacologic measures producing only minimal, if any, pain relief is not desired; rather, efficient and judicious use of pharmacologic agents is encouraged to minimize, if not eliminate, pain in the dying older adult (Snyder and Miene 1994).

Besides pain, other physical discomforts are dealt with by determining and eliminating or controlling their respective causes. For example, if eating sausage or other pork products is creating excessive flatulence, simply limiting them in or removing them from the diet will promote comfort. Other discomforts such as constipation, pruritus, and other skin discomforts may be similarly controlled.

Two related physical discomforts in dying older adults require special consideration: fatigue and dyspnea. Fatigue is an overwhelming sense of exhaustion, which markedly limits all activity and cannot be eliminated by rest. Dyspnea is a subjective awareness of breathing, accompanied by a feeling of uncomfortable breathing or breathlessness. Typically, dyspneic older adults are fatigued, and vice-versa, and their occurrence promotes a vicious downward spiral over time. Although rest, relaxation, and other oxygen-and energy-conserving measures help, supplying oxygen and energy is even more beneficial with older adults. Oxygenation can be maximized by breathing techniques, using fans, getting more fresh air, or using oxygen delivery mechanisms (e.g., oxygen tanks with nasal cannulas). Energy can be maximized by small, frequent, nutritious snacks (granola bars, mixed nuts, fresh fruit, etc.) or fluids (fruit juices, milk, etc.). Rarely, are fatigue or dyspnea eliminated as sources of physical discomfort; hence, the goal is to mitigate their impact on the end of life of the older adult (DeSpedler and Strickland 1999).

QUALITY VERSUS QUANTITY OF LIFE

At any age, it is not possible to "have it all" or to "have it both ways," and this becomes especially true as one ages. Mortality has been decreased, thanks to technology; consequently, human longevity, the quantity of life, has been increased. However, to date, technology has not proportionally decreased morbidity, resulting in increasing debilitation and dysfunction with a decreased quality of life in old age. Therefore, one of the major questions in the end of life of an older adult is at what point does the consideration of the quality of life exceed that of the quantity of life. This discussion of increased morbidity and decreased quality of life is central to that of the current social debate of assisted suicide and euthanasia (Morgan 1996).

Obviously, this is a very important and individual matter encompassing a host of factors, and is beyond the scope of this chapter. When older adults no longer perceive sufficient quality of life to justify the quantity of life, morbidity is a more salient consideration than is mortality; in fact, death or mortality can be viewed as a "solution," even a "blessing." The role of the health care provider in this situation is to promote and support the informed decision of the older adult within established ethical, legal, and professional guidelines or standards.

DIRECTIVES

Central to this informed decision is an understanding by the dying elder and the significant others of the concepts of advance (before end of life) directives (i.e., living wills) and actual end of life directives (i.e., do not resuscitate orders). All adults, regardless of their respective ages or proximity to death, need to be oriented to and complete one or more written advance directives before the inevitable end of life (Jecker and Schneiderman 1994). Living wills, health powers of attorney, and durable powers of attorney are forms of these advance directives. Adults need to know that these advance directives exist, what they are, and how important they can prove to be at the end of life. Invariably, adults want either "everything" or "nothing" done at the end of life, without knowing either what "everything" entails or what necessary comforts and supports "nothing" excludes. Clearly, health care providers need to fully inform adults of both "ordinary" means of continuing the quantity of life (e.g., nutrition, hydration, comfort measures) as well as "extraordinary" means (e.g., intubation, cardio-pulmonary resuscitation) The informed wishes of the adult should be documented in writing according to the laws of the state in which the adult legally resides, and copies shared with all significant others, health care professionals, and legal representatives (Beresford 1993).

As previously mentioned, actual end of life directives encompass phrases like "do not resuscitate," "do not intubate," and "chemical resuscitation only."

As with the advance directives, support of actual directives by dying elders or their significant others is key. Hopefully, the existence of a valid advance directive will preclude the need to make any of these end of life decisions.

CAREGIVERS AND CAREGIVING

Most older adults remain relatively healthy, active, and independent up to very close to the time of death. For this majority of older adults, family members and significant others merely provide supportive care at or about the end of life (DeSpedler and Strickland 1999). For a minority of older adults, greater amounts of care, physical and otherwise, are required, with these amounts increasing at or about the end of life. Traditionally, family homes have been the principal sites and family members the principal providers of care for aging relatives. However, some older adults require professional care services, if not in the home then in an institutional setting—invariably a nursing home or similar long-term care facility. The placement of an older adult in such a facility is typically a difficult experience for both the elder and family members (Pruncho 1995).

Caregivers, familial and professional, need to keep in mind at least two things in providing end of life care:

1. Growing old is not a disease. Therefore, the care for the symptomatology of and the disease itself is distinct from end of life care.
2. Care of the caregiver is paramount; if we lose the caregiver, we also lose the older adult recipient of care.

Stress, burnout, burden, disease, and infirmity are commonplace among caregivers, who are invariably family members. It is important to maintain and support them for their own benefit as well as for that of the elders they serve (DiGiulio 1989).

SUMMARY

Aging is conceptualized as a series of losses, with the ultimate loss being the loss of life. Older adults are "closer" to death, but have more time and inclination to anticipate their deaths than younger persons. Hence, with older adults, the end of life tends to be an anticipated event for both themselves and their significant others. How successful one has aged impacts how the end of life itself, as well as its inherent care, will transpire. General considerations for care include facilitating life review, preparing both the elder and significant others for the impending death, and providing care at and immediately after the actual time of death. Hospice, comfort measures, directives, and concerns for caregivers are among the specific considerations for care. A team approach involving the older adult, significant others, and health care providers—characterized by open, honest, and ongoing communication—is critical. Holistic support, coupled with a positive focus, are the minimum criteria for a quality end of life experience.

REFERENCES

Beresford, L. (1993). *The hospice handbook: A complete guide.* Boston: Little, Brown.

Brice, C. (1982). Mourning throughout the life cycle. *American Journal of Psychoanalysis,* 42(4), 320–321.

Brock, I. (1997). *Dying well: The prospect of growth at the end of life.* New York: Riverhead.

Brown, L., & Ellis, E. (1975). *Quality of life: The later years.* Acton, MA: Publishing Sciences Group.

Buckingham, R. (1996). *The handbook of hospice care.* Amherst: Prometheus.

Butler, R. (1975). *Why survive? Being old in America.* New York: Harper and Row.

Chi, I., & Lubben, J. (1996, July). Patterns of aging: A special report. *Science,* 273: 41–79.

DiGiulio, R. (1989). *Beyond widowhood: From bereavement to emergence and hope.* New York: Free Press.

DeSpedler, L., & Strickland, A. (1999). *The last dance: Encountering death and dying.* Mountain View, CA: Mayfield.

Doka, K. (1989). The awareness of mortality in midlife: Implications for later life. *Gerontology Review*, 2(1), 19–28.

Erikson, E. (1982). *The life cycle completed: A review*. New York: Norton.

Heinlein, S., Brumett, G., & Tibbals, J. (Eds.). (1997). *When a lifemate dies: Stories of love, loss, and healing*. Minneapolis: Fairview Press.

Hope, R. (1994). *Oxford handbook of clinical medicine*. Oxford: Oxford University Press.

Infield, D. (1995). *Hospice care and cultural diversity*. Binghamton: Haworth.

Jecker, N., & Schneiderman, L. (1994). Is dying young worse than dying old? *The Gerontologist*, 34(1), 66–72.

Kalina, K. (1993). *Midwife for souls*. Boston: Puline.

Kastenbaum, R. (1979). Exit and existence: Society's unwritten script for old age and death. In D. Tassel (Ed.), *Aging, Death, and the Completion of Being* (pp. 69–94). Philadelphia, PA: University of Pennsylvania Press.

Kaufman, S. (1995). *The ageless self: Sources of meaning in later life*. Madison: University of Wisconsin Press.

Krisman-Scott, M. (2000, First quarter). An historical analysis of disclosure of terminal status. *Journal of Nursing Scholarship*, Vol. 32, 47–52.

Lawton, M., Moss, M., & Glicksman, A. (1990). The quality of the last year of life of older persons. *Milbank Quarterly*, 68, 1–28.

Leash, R. (1994). *Death notification: A practical guide to the process*. Hinesburg, VT: Upper Access.

Marshall, V. (1980). *Last chapters: A sociology of aging and dying*. Monterey, CA: Brooks/Cole.

Morgan, J. (1996). *Ethical issues in the care of the dying and bereaved aged*. Amityville, NY: Baywood.

Neugarten, B. (1990, November). Growing as long as we live. *Second Opinion*, 15, 42–51.

Osterweis, M., Solomon, F., & Green, M. (Eds.). (1984). *Bereavement: Reactions, consequeces, and care*. Washington, DC: National Academy Press.

Pruchno, R. (Ed.). (1995). Death of an institutionalized parent: Predictors of bereavement. *Omega: Journal of Death and Dying*, 31(2), 99–119.

Roberto, K., & Stanis, P. (1994). Reactions of older women to the death of their close friends. *Omega: Journal of Death and Dying*, 29(1), 17–27.

Sapolsky, R., & Finch, C. (1991, March/April). On growing old. *The Sciences*, 31, 30–38.

Scrutton, S. (1995). *Bereavement and grief: Supporting older people through loss*. London: Edward Arnold.

Sokolovsky, J. (1990). *The cultural context of aging: Worldwide perspectives*. New York: Bergin & Garvey.

Snyder, M., & Miene, P. (1994). Stereotyping the elderly: A functional approach. *British Journal of Social Psychology*, 33, 63–82.

Stillion, J. (1985). *Death and the sexes: An examination of differential longevity, attitudes, behaviors, and coping skills*. Washington, DC: Hemisphere.

Weenolsen, P. (1996) The art of dying: How to leave this world with dignity and grace, at peace with yourself and your loved ones. New York: St. Martin's.

UNIT VIII

ISSUES ACROSS THE LIFESPAN

Critical Thinking Activities

1. Compare end of life issues across the lifespan
2. List 10 intrinsic and extrinsic factors that determine the impact of death and dying on the family or caregivers
3. Apply Maslow's hierarchy of human needs relative to perinatal death, children's death, and the young and older adult death

Teaching-Learning Exercises

1. Develop a family assessment guide for end of life care including family structure, family roles and functions, health status of family in general, communication patterns, family values, and coping resources
2. Apply a growth and development theory to an actual patient situation

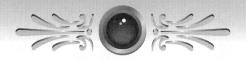

UNIT IX

THE END OF LIFE

Learning Objectives

1. Discuss physical changes at the time of imminent death (the last 48 hours)
2. Describe signs and symptoms of impending death
3. Discuss the role of the nurse at the time of death
4. List nursing interventions immediately following death
5. Discuss historical events relative to current end of life care concepts and practices

CHAPTER

THE PATHOPHYSIOLOGY OF DEATH AND THE DYING PROCESS

Dr. Gary Arnold

In today's world, there are very few people past the age of three years who do not have some understanding of the concept of death. Every member of society has experienced death on some level. It may take the form of the death of a loved one, a relative, a neighbor, or a pet, or it may only be experienced passively as a bystander at the death of strangers. Indeed, in today's society, people have difficulty avoiding issues surrounding death. The media seem to have a fascination with suffering and death, presumably because of the sensationalism it holds for a death-oriented public. Religious leaders are continually reminding the faithful of the concept of life after death and the importance of the personal preparation for this inevitable event. Artists and poets through the ages have attempted to romanticize and glorify death, either overtly or subtly, through craftily created symbolism. Philosophers, and indeed all individuals in their own way, have striven to unlock the mysteries surrounding death and to seek a deeper meaning for that which all must eventually face.

Throughout recorded history, there has been a continual evolution in society's attitudes about death. Before the era of modern medicine, death was a frequent occurrence within every household. The majority of deaths resulted from infectious diseases and occurred in what today would be considered children and young adults. Many of these infectious diseases reached epidemic proportions, killing thousands of people at one time. The decentralization of health care common in those times meant that the majority of people dying did so at home and in the company of their friends and family. Survivors of these epidemics and of the other causes of death had ample opportunities to personally care for these individuals and to witness death firsthand. Under these circumstances, the dying process was very visible and was experienced on an intimate and personal level. Death came to be viewed and accepted as a natural part of life. It was understood both as a spiritual event and, very clearly, as a physical phenomenon with a definite and often predictable pattern. Those family and friends who attended the dying individual got to witness death from the front row, and the anatomical and functional aspects of death were very apparent to them.

With the dawn of modern scientific medicine, not only did the mechanisms of illness and death change but the practice of medicine became relocated to a more centralized, hospital-oriented system of health care delivery. People began to survive to "old age," but by doing so they developed new and markedly different diseases and health-related problems. People became ill from these conditions and were transported to hospitals where many of them died. This change in the methodology of health care delivery had two significant consequences that impacted the attitudes about death. First, it allowed opportunity for trained medical personnel to witness and study death in ways never before possible. A direct result of this study was a change in the attitude of medical personnel about death and a better understanding of the physical aspects of death. They began to look at death and the dying process as a pathophysiological event, and in doing so learned better and more efficient ways to preserve life. The second consequence of this change in health care was that it separated the dying individual from family and friends. Death and dying became a solitary hospital event occurring in the presence of health professionals, with the family observing short segments of the dying process only at visiting hours. Death became more associated with old age and the diseases that afflict the elderly.

Not being able to witness death as intimately as before, attitudes of the nonmedical public about death began to change. Death and dying became much more mysterious and threatening. It no longer was considered a natural life event, but rather something to be feared and avoided. This mystery and fear of death led to suspicion and denial about its appropriateness as a natural phenomenon, an attitude that, for some, still exists today. A consequence of this attitude about the dying process has also led to an aversion to the aging process. Even a casual review of the entertainment and advertising industries will reveal numerous examples of the youth-oriented practices that define modern society.

Today, death is understood and confronted on two levels. In a traditional sense, it is experienced as a spiritual or religious event, embellished both with theological and secular trappings. Religious services are provided for the dead and dying, even for those individuals who were not particularly religious before the final event. The secular aspects of the final event are manifested by a variety of mourning rites and funeral customs utilized primarily by the bereaved to help them cope with the loss of a loved one. In the scientific sense, death and dying are today viewed as a physical and physiological event. By viewing death in this way, it has become accepted as a normal part of life.

Beginning in 1974 with the genesis of the hospice movement, care of the terminally ill has, once again, been returned to the home setting and to the capable hands of family, friends, and hospice professionals. As a result, the attitudes of nonmedical personnel and society at large have again evolved. The general public has come to appreciate that death is a physical as well as a spiritual process (Kalina 1993). The combined efforts of both health professionals and the public in studying death as a living event has promoted a general understanding of the pathophysiological processes that characterize this terminal stage of life. Ironically, by studying death from a pathophysiological perspective, what has been learned has helped to achieve the ultimate goal of the general public: the avoidance or, at least, the postponement of death. By studying death in this way, enormous strides have been made toward a better understanding of life. It has led to the development of modern techniques that have enabled health care professionals not only to save lives but also to actually prevent illnesses and diseases that in the past have inevitably led to death. In fact, these same techniques and the results of their application have caused modern society not only to look at death in new ways but have required a reevaluation of the very definition of death.

DEFINITIONS OF DEATH

In its most simplistic sense, death can be defined as the absence of life. While this definition is technically accurate, it is limited in scope and views death as a simple, one-dimensional state that exists only after life is ended. It fails to recognize death as a process that begins even before there is an absence of life. This dying process of physical death begins during life and can be viewed as a dynamic and functional living process, albeit one that ends, that defines the limits of life. Until the 1960s, there was general agreement on the definition of death. Death was succinctly and accurately defined as the cessation of circulation and respiration (Perper 1993). Determinants of the cessation of these functions were made by simple observation of patient movements (i.e., physical efforts to breathe) and by basic measurements with whatever medical instrumentation was available at the time. Originally, stethoscopes and electrocardiograph machines were used to detect the presence of a heartbeat and the electrical activity of the heart muscle. Blood pressure cuffs were used to detect evidence of pressurized blood flow to peripheral parts of the body.

Not only was this concept of death accepted by the general public, but the medical and the legal professions easily recognized that circulatory and respiratory functions were the essential defining characteristics of life, the absence of which consequently defined death. The 1968 edition of *Black's Law Dictionary* defined death as "the cessation of life; the ceasing to exist, defined by physicians as the total stoppage of the circulation of the blood and cessation of the vital functions consequent thereon such as respiration, pulsation, etc." (Black 1968, 488).

During the 1960s, however, two major breakthroughs in medicine occurred that dramatically and permanently altered the landscape of medicine and its definition of death. These two advances were the development of cardiopulmonary resuscitation techniques (CPR) and the development of instrumentation that enabled circulatory and respiratory functions to be "artificially" continued even if removal of the instruments would result in the cessation of the essential life processes. Successful recovery of patients with CPR following cardiopulmonary arrest required a reassessment of what constituted death. No longer was simple cessation of circulatory and respiratory functions adequate to define all cases of death. Since successful CPR enabled some patients to continue to live after what appeared to be the temporary cessation of circulation and respiration, the term "irreversible" was added to the definition of death to exclude those patients who were successfully resuscitated. Now death had to be defined as the irreversible cessation of circulation and respiration (Perper 1993).

The instrumentation that allowed circulatory and respiratory functions to be artificially maintained included ventilators and cardiopulmonary bypass machines. As these machines became more and more efficient, it was soon discovered that the vital life functions of respiration and circulation could be indefinitely sustained artificially. The question then had to be asked, if patients could have circulatory and respiratory functions maintained by machines for indefinite periods, could they be considered clinically dead if, by turning the machines off, these vital functions would cease? This concept assumed increasing importance as the practice of organ transplantation became a reality.

The earliest source of human organs for transplantation into living patients was from human cadaver donors. The organs were harvested soon after the donor was pronounced dead. As experience was gained, it became apparent that the sooner the organs were harvested from the donor, the greater was the likelihood of successful functioning of that organ in the recipient. This required that the timing of the pronouncement of death be very precise so as to signal the optimum time for removing the organs. This practice necessitated yet another refinement to the definition of death. The phrase "irreversible cessation of circulation and respiration" could no longer be used to define the death of potential organ donors. A new concept of death had to be developed to cover those patients who "ceased to exist" but did so with sustainable circulation and respiration.

Although it was important to use organs from patients with functioning circulation and respiration, it was not essential that the potential organ donor have a functioning central nervous system. From a medico-legal standpoint, it became important to declare a person clinically dead by using a different set of criteria. This initiated the idea of brain death, which recognized that a person could be functionally dead and still have intact circulatory and respiratory functioning (Powner, DeJoya, and Darby 2000; Power & Van Heerden 1995). In 1968, an ad hoc committee of the Harvard Medical School was the first to define brain death using the following criteria (Beecher, et al. 1968):

- Unreceptivity and unresponsivity including a lack of response to the most intense, painful stimuli.
- No movement or spontaneous respiration, defined as no effort to breathe for three minutes off the respirator with the patient's carbon dioxide normal and room air being breathed for 10 minutes prior to the trial.

* No reflexes; fixed, nonreactive pupils and a lack of cranial nerve reflexes (corneal, pharyngeal, ocular movements in response to head turning and irrigation of the ears with ice water, etc.).
* Isoelectric electroencephalogram.

In other words, brain death is defined by both physical observations and by measurements with scientific medical instrumentation. The physical observations include a lack of a purposeful protective withdrawal from a source of obvious intense pain (such as a pin prick), a lack of physical effort of chest muscles to breathe, and a lack of the body to respond in a normal way with the involuntary reflexes that are controlled from the most primitive part of the brain (the brain stem). The pupils should constrict when a bright light is shined into the eyes. The eyes should close (blink) in a protective manner when an object is touched to the cornea. Small muscles in the eyes should move the eyeballs in response to a sudden change in head position or a sudden change in the temperature inside the ear. If these actions are absent and there is no other explanation for their absence such as the presence of central nervous system depressant drugs or extremely cold body temperature (hypothermia), the brain stem is considered to be dead. If this, the most primitive part of the brain is dead, then it is assumed that the higher cognitive cortical area of the brain is also dead.

The scientific instrumentation used to measure brain activity is the electroencephalogram or EEG. Because a living brain generates a type of electrical current, EEGs are used to measure this current as evidence of viable, functioning brain cells. An isoelectric EEG refers to the absence of a normal electrical current and is scientifically accepted as evidence of brain death if there are no other explanations for its absence.

In 1977, the National Institute of Neurological Disease and Stroke reemphasized these points by defining brain death as (1) coma and cerebral unresponsiveness, (2) apnea (absence of breathing), (3) dilated pupils, (4) absent cephalic (brain stem) reflexes, and (5) electrocerebral silence (isoelectric EEG). It further required that these manifestations be present for 30 minutes at least six hours after the onset of coma. Although the wording may vary, the basic clinical elements defining brain death are the same in other countries around the world (Power and Van Heerden 1995).

It will be noted that this definition of brain death does not include the absence of the circulation. It also stipulates that artificial means of maintaining respiratory function must be excluded. It is this apparent dichotomy within the definition of death that had to be resolved in order to provide a medicolegal basis for both the pronouncement of death and the feasibility of organ transplantation. This dichotomy began to be reconciled in 1980 by an attempt to codify a legal definition of death. In that year, the American Bar Association in a joint statement with the National Conference of Commissioners of Uniform State Laws agreed that a model definition of death should declare that "an individual who has sustained either (1) irreversible cessation of circulatory and respiratory functions or (2) irreversible cessation of all functions of the entire brain stem, including the brain stem, is dead. A determination of death shall be made in accordance with accepted medical standards" (Perper 1993, 15). This concept of death has been universally accepted and is exemplified in revised Louisiana statutes (1976), which defines death as follows:

> A person will be considered dead if in the announced opinion of a physician, duly licensed in the state of Louisiana based on ordinary standards of approved medical practice, the person has experienced an irreversible cessation of spontaneous respiratory and circulatory functions. In the event that artificial means of support preclude a determination that these functions have ceased, a person will be considered dead if in the announced opinion of a physician, duly licensed in the state of Louisiana based upon ordinary standards of approved medical practice, the person has experienced an irreversible cessation of brain function. Death will have occurred at the time when the relevant functions ceased. In any case when organs are to be used in a transplant, then an additional physician, duly licensed in the state of Louisiana not a member of the transplant team, must make the pronouncement of death. (Definition of Death, 1976, p. 37)

This definition of death embodies both concepts of death: the cessation of circulatory and respiratory function on the one hand and the cessation of brain function on the other. It also provides for their mutual exclusion.

THE CONTRIBUTIONS OF FORENSIC SCIENCE

Much of what has been learned about the pathophysiological events surrounding death has resulted from the scientific investigations of forensic scientists (DiMaio and DiMaio 1993, Perper 1993). The term *forensic* means pertaining to or applied to legal proceedings. Forensic scientists are those medical and legal specialists who study death from all angles and include highly skilled persons such as pathologists, biochemists, physical chemists, criminologists, and psychologists. These scientists have enlarged the body of knowledge about death and the dying process by examining death in three ways: (1) the causes of death, (2) the mechanisms of death, and (3) the manner of death.

Cause of Death.   The cause of death is defined as any injury or disease that produces physiological derangement in the body that results in an individual dying. These may be such things as cancer, heart attack, pneumonia, stroke, or gunshot wound. It is usually one of these conditions that is medically and legally recognized as the event that directly results in the cessation of circulation, respiration, or brain function. It is the term that is entered on the death certificate as the cause of death.

Mechanism of Death.   The mechanism of death is the physiological derangement or derangements produced by the cause of death. For example, a heart attack damages the muscles of the heart to such an extent that the heart no longer has the power to pump blood around the body to the vital organs such as the brain, lungs, and kidneys. With the cessation of the circulation of oxygenated blood to these organs, their functions cease and, in the case of the brain, brain function ceases. The mechanism of death in this case is deficient supply of oxygenated blood to vital organs.

In a similar way, pneumonia or lung injury from trauma may prevent adequate oxygen delivery from the air into the blood. If oxygen cannot enter the blood by way of the lungs, there can be no oxygenated blood supplied to vital organs. In this case, the mechanism of death is the same even though the cause of death is different. One mechanism of death can result from many different causes of death. Likewise, a single cause of death can be responsible for several mechanisms of death.

Manner of Death.   The manner in which a person dies is an explanation of the nonphysiological circumstances by which the death comes about. The manner of death may be stated as natural causes, homicide, suicide, accidental, or undetermined. The terms *homicide, suicide,* and *accidental* (often referred to as violent deaths) usually refer to manners of death which are sudden and clearly result from external physical forces which, in turn, are caused by traumatic injuries to any number of vital organs. Manners of death classified as natural causes or undetermined typically result from disease processes which may or may not be diagnosed and which may occur suddenly or take place over a long and protracted period of time.

Those manners of death that are the result of chronic or terminal illness can represent a wide array of causes and mechanisms. There are so many different disease entities that can progress to a fatal outcome that it is almost impossible to make any generalizations about their mechanisms. Sudden deaths resulting from natural causes or undertermined can, however, be classified into relatively few patterns of cause and mechanism. By definition, *sudden death* is that terminal event which is unexpected and, if it is accompanied by symptoms, typically occurs within 1 to 24 hours of the onset of the symptoms. Sudden death can be further classified as instantaneous, sudden but not instantaneous, and "individual found dead."

No matter which of these categories applies, the causes of sudden death are typically limited in number (DiMaio and DiMaio 1993). More than 80% are the result of sudden disturbance in the electrical activity of the heart (dysrhythmia), which, in turn, is the direct result of diagnosed or undiagnosed disease in the coronary arteries supplying blood to the heart muscle. This sudden electrical disturbance can take the form of excessively rapid firing of the nerves in the heart (ventricular tachydysrhythmia or ventricular fibrillation), excessively slow firing of those nerves (bradydysrhythmia), or even complete cessation of electrical activity (asystole). The end result of any of these events is insufficient pumping of blood by the heart and usually sudden cessation of effective oxygenated circulation to all other organs.

Sudden death can also result from diseases in organs other than the heart. It has been caused by brain diseases such as epilepsy, brain hemorrhage, brain infections (meningitis), and brain tumors. Sudden death can result from respiratory diseases like asphyxia (suffocation), hemorrhage, lung collapse, and lung infections. Overwhelming infection (sepsis) from any source in the body can be the explanation of sudden death. Whatever the explanation, sudden death occurs too rapidly for it to be studied in depth as a pathophysiological process. Although those who witness sudden death easily recognize it as a form of the dying process, comprehension of it in this way only occurs after the fact and, in many instances, is never completely understood.

THE PATHOPHYSIOLOGY OF DEATH

It is in those cases of death from chronic, terminal illnesses (including death from "old age") where a more complete understanding of the pathophysiology of the dying process can be appreciated. As death and the dying process are investigated as the final life event, there is an acceptance and a realization that death, despite its terminal nature, has physical aspects that are predictable and easily recognized. In many ways, they are welcomed not only by the dying individual but also by the caregivers, family, and friends who attend that person in the final months, weeks, days, or hours of life (Kalina 1993).

In studying the physical and the pathophysiological aspects of the dying process, attention must be paid not to death as a single final life event but rather as a series of events that can take many forms and that can develop over a wide range of time intervals (Kemp 1999). In viewing death as a process, it can be studied on two levels: on a microscopic level, death of individual cells or groups of cells is referred to as cellular death; on a larger scale, death of the entire person is called somatic death (Cotran, Kumar, and Collins 1999; McCance 1998; Banasik 2000).

Cellular Death

If there was ever any doubt that death is a life event, that thought was dispelled by work begun in 1972 by John Kerr, Andrew Wyllie, and Alastair Currie on tumor cells. Their work and then subsequent work of others led to the concept of apoptosis or programmed cell death (Tran and Miller 1999). Many, if not all, cells have within their genetic codes instructions for activating the chemical and structural processes that eventually result in their own deaths, even though the cells are perfectly healthy. In a sense, apoptosis is a phenomenon in which cells are genetically programmed for cellular suicide. As confirmatory evidence that apoptotic cell death is an essential life event, it has been documented in a variety of normal physiological processes (Cotran, Kumar, and Collins 1999). Apoptosis is a required function in such processes as embryonic and fetal development, maintenance of a stable population of cells in normal healthy tissues and organs, protective functions such as inflammatory and immune functions, and the aging process. Each of these processes is possible only because of the normal death of healthy cells to either "make room" for more essential cells or to be replaced by healthier, more active cells.

Apoptosis is manifested by both structural and functional changes in cells that are initiated by a series of chemical (enzyme) changes inside the cell (Tran and Miller 1999; Cotran, Kumar, and Collins 1999; McConkey and Bold 2000). These enzymes drive a chain of events that damage cellular proteins in a slow and organized manner by disrupting the proteins that comprise the internal structures of the cell. The solid (i.e., nonwatery) parts of the cell condense into nonfunctional clumps. No longer able to carry out normal cellular functions, the cells shrink, presumably by the loss of water, and are eventually attacked and dissolved by the process of phagocytosis. Apoptosis typically occurs in isolated individual cells without affecting any of the surrounding cells. It occurs in many cells in the absence of any disease and actually occurs in everyone on a periodic, even daily, basis. It is responsible for such normal physiologic events as loss of the uterine lining (endometrium) with each menstrual period, the development of fingers and toes in a developing fetus, the continual loss of older skin cells and their replacement with healthier cells, and the loss of many older damaged cells that might eventually form cancers.

A second form of cellular death is that which typically occurs as the result of noxious influences (sometimes called environmental stressors) that injure the cell. These injurious events are generally unpredictable and are often an integral part of some disease process. If the noxious influence is severe enough and sufficiently prolonged, the cell or cells will no longer be able to carry out their normal metabolic functions and will begin the process of cellular death called necrosis. Whereas apoptosis is an expected and planned event that occurs slowly even in normal healthy cells, necrotic cell death results from cell injury caused by external stressors and typically occurs rapidly in groups of cells and in a disorganized manner.

There are several types of stressors that can injure cells. These include hypoxia (lack of oxygen), physical factors or chemical substances, biologic agents (bacteria, viruses, etc.), damage to the cell's chromosomes, nutritional injury from poor dietary intake, and even immunologic and inflammatory mechanisms that ordinarily protect a cell from injury. These stressors, if they result in the death of the patient, correlate well with the statements forensic scientists use for the cause of death. For example, forensic scientists may state that the cause of death was asphyxiation secondary to drowning. This correlates well with cell injury resulting from the stressor of hypoxia.

In contrast, necrotic cell death, often referred to as irreversible cell injury, is the end result of the types of events classified by forensic scientists as the mechanisms of death. No matter which of the stressors initiate the sequence of events that result in cellular necrosis, the end result could be the death of the patient. Clinical death, therefore, is often the result of a culmination of necrotic processes that begin at a cellular level and extend through tissues, organs, and organ systems to prevent the continued functioning of the circulatory and respiratory systems and the brain.

Those pathophysiologic processes that characterize necrotic cell death typically progress rapidly within an individual cell and extend to involve adjacent cells. The environmental stressors that activate the necrotic dying process attack vulnerable cells at three separate but not functionally independent points. First, the plasma membrane of the cell becomes injured, leading to leakage of electrolytes (sodium and potassium) and water through the membrane. Second, the energy-producing parts of the cell (mitochondria) are damaged, which robs the cell of the chemical energy it requires for its vital functions. Third, protein-synthesizing parts of the cell (endoplasmic reticulum) are damaged, resulting in the inability of the cell to produce the proteins it needs to repair the damaged areas of the cell and prevent its own death. These injuries, all occurring simultaneously, lead to increasing acid content of the cell, cellular swelling, and the release of digestive enzymes within the cell. The cell begins to digest its own structures (autodigestion) and eventually the cellular swelling results in lysis or splitting-apart of the cell as the terminal event. As each of these events occur, the progress of the dying process at the other sites is promoted. Cell necrosis, therefore, can be thought of as a cascading of interrelated destructive processes occurring on a subcellular level but which clinically are recognized as the acute, chronic, or terminal illnesses that are well known to medicine.

Somatic Death

Although apoptosis and necrosis are real events that characterize both healthy and disease states, they are individual cellular events that do not necessarily result in death of the person. Apoptosis is an essential part of normal growth and development and occurs throughout the lifespan of an individual without causing the death of that individual. Necrosis can be limited to small groups of cells or even an entire organ and yet, with proper medical care, will not result in the death of the person. These processes are often categorized as localized death. Those dying processes that affect all of the tissues, organs, and organ systems of a person simultaneously are collectively referred to as *somatic death*.

Somatic death is the series of events in which all life processes in a person end and correlates most closely with the original definition of death—the cessation of circulation and respiration. Somatic death should not be confused with clinical death. The term *clinical death* can be used to refer to somatic death in which all life processes are ended but it is also used to refer to patients who are brain dead and in whom circulatory and respiratory functions are artificially maintained. The return of care of the dying patient to the home setting has led to a greater understanding of the pathophysiologic events that characterize somatic death. The ability to witness the somatic dying process within the context of hospice care has helped to remove the mystery surrounding the way in which life processes end.

The physical aspects of the somatic dying process are definite but may manifest themselves in a variety of ways. Because somatic death is death of all life processes, physical signs, although originating in one organ or organ system, will eventually be manifested as derangement in other body systems. Depending on the speed of the dying process, these physical signs may appear gradually over the course of weeks or months and seem to be isolated events. In other cases, the dying process may progress very rapidly over the course of a few days. When death occurs quickly, the full expression of the pathophysiologic changes may be less obvious or not manifested at all. Furthermore, in those cases where death is prolonged, the physical signs may change as the dying process progresses from the general deterioration associated with a chronic illness, through the state of impending death (survival of less than four weeks), and finally to imminent death (survival of less than one week).

The pathophysiological aspects of somatic death will vary considerably depending on the cause of death, but there are some generalizations that can be made about the multisystem organ failures that will present in most cases of death (Kalina 1993, Kemp 1999). Each of the physical deteriorations noted within a body system can be the initiating cause of changes noted in distant sites, or they can be the result of changes that originated in other organ systems.

Cardiovascular System Changes. Within the time periods defined as *impending* and *imminent death*, the changes in cardiovascular functions can be quite dramatic. Most of these are the direct result of a gradual reduction in the pumping efficiency of the heart, called decreased cardiac output. The heart muscle becomes too weak to pump even well-oxygenated blood to all other organs of the body. The pulse becomes weaker and the skin temperature becomes cool to the touch, especially over the knees, elbows, and nose. As the heart muscle grows weaker, blood pressure falls, the pulse rate becomes faster and irregular (dysrhythmia) and, as blood supply (perfusion) to the skin decreases further, the skin becomes pale and occasionally yellowish. Cyanosis (bluish discoloration) may develop in the feet, hands, and lips and, as death becomes imminent, the skin assumes a waxy appearance and reddish-purple splotches may develop on the knees, lower legs, and arms. Occasionally edema (fluid accumulation) may be noted in the skin tissues of the lower legs as a result of increased permeability of capillaries to water that leaks out of dilated blood vessels (vasodilatation).

Respiratory System Changes.   The physical signs associated with the respiratory system relate primarily to the effectiveness of breathing. The pathophysiologic events most responsible for impaired breathing are decreased cardiac output and generalized weakness of the chest (breathing) muscles. As the cardiac pumping efficiency begins to fail, more and more of the blood becomes "backed up" in the lungs. Not only does this slow the flow of blood through the lungs, but also the pressure of the blood in the pulmonary capillaries increases. This results in increased permeability of the capillaries and leakage of water into the air spaces of the lungs (pulmonary edema). There is then an increase in the amount of pulmonary secretions formed in the air spaces of the lungs that become increasingly difficult to clear with coughing. As the dying process advances, the generalized weakness of the chest muscles needed for the cough effort become weaker, making the secretions even more difficult to clear. They accumulate to the point where they interfere with the airflow into the lung and the proper oxygenation of the blood. Eventually, these impaired mechanics of breathing lead to inadequate oxygenation of the blood and the patient develops labored breathing (dyspnea). Because of the generalized muscle weakness, however, the patient lacks the energy and muscle strength required to breathe. Poor oxygenation of the blood also affects cardiovascular functioning in that the weakened heart muscle does not receive the oxygen it needs to pump effectively.

Neurological System Changes.   Neurological (brain and nerve) manifestations are functionally and temporally related to deterioration of the cardiovascular and respiratory systems. As oxygenated blood supply to the brain becomes compromised, the brain (and to some extent the peripheral nerves) develop a series of cognitive (thinking processes), voluntary, and autonomic (automatic) functional disturbances. The initial neurological manifestations typically present themselves as altered cognitive function in which ordered, logical patterns of thinking becomes abnormal. Social withdrawal is common. The ability to communicate, verbally or otherwise, may diminish and periods of lucidity may alternate with periods of confusion and even hallucinations and delusions.

As death becomes impending and then imminent, the more basic functions of the brain deteriorate. There may be a loss of nerve function to various peripheral parts of the body (altered sensation to pain, touch, and temperature) as well as reduction in sensitivity of some of the basic senses (taste, smell, and sight). The loss of visual acuity may also be related to a decrease in blood flow to the retina.

As brain function continues to deteriorate, in part, from a lack of adequate oxygenated blood flow, there is an increasing tendency for drowsiness and periods of unresponsiveness. Multifocal myoclonus (small convulsions) may be noted in different isolated muscle groups. Infrequent blinking of the eyelids leads to a glazed, blank stare. Occasionally, especially as death becomes imminent, there may be a period of terminal restlessness, moaning, agitation, and possible delirium. Eventually, often associated with the development of a coma, there is a loss of basic brain stem control functions and brain stem reflexes. The loss of brain stem control of the cardiovascular system leads to further compromise of heart and blood vessels functions. Without proper brain stem control of respiratory functions, breathing patterns become altered, with irregular rates of breathing and even periods of apnea (absence of breathing). The loss of basic life-sustaining brain stem reflexes such as the cough reflex, the gag reflex, and the corneal (blinking) reflex prevent the person from responding to the need to protect the lungs and the eyes from injury. The loss of the cough and the gag reflex, together with weakness of the pharyngeal (throat) muscles, allows secretions to accumulate in the throat, creating a noisy gurgling sound with breathing called the "death rattle."

A final physical sign of deteriorating neurological function is loss of control over the processes of fecal and urinary elimination. This may present in some individuals as diarrhea and inappropriate urination (urinary incontinence). More often, however, it results in constipation and urinary retention.

Gastrointestinal System Signs. As a vital component of life processes, the gastrointestinal system also undergoes obvious changes that are commonly witnessed in the somatic dying process. At first, the only change may be the loss of appetite (anorexia) which may also be a manifestation of neurological deterioration. The anorexia may initially be limited to an intolerance of solid food only but eventually extends to a loss of desire even for liquids and water. Inadequate intake of the proteins and calories derived from solid foods leads to weight loss and decreased protein synthesis at the cellular level and nutritional injury to all cells, especially apparent in muscle cells. Without an adequate supply of dietary or cell-synthesized proteins, muscles lose the ability to contract. This affects not only the heart, respiratory, and skeletal muscles, but also the muscles of the gastrointestinal tract itself. There is, consequently, a loss of ability to swallow solids and liquids and to move food through the intestinal tract. The inability to swallow complicates the anorexia, and the lack of sufficient intestinal muscular movements (peristalsis) leads to constipation.

As gastrointestinal function continues to deteriorate, the inability to swallow liquids is further complicated by a lack of the sensation of thirst (also a manifestation of neurological dysfunction). Insufficient intake of water results in dehydration, deterioration of the blood volume, decrease in blood pressure, and impaired perfusion of all organs with blood. Dehydration also leads to gradual decrease in urinary output and kidney function. This eventually results in the loss of the kidney's ability to eliminate nitrogen waste products from the blood. These waste products are toxic to brain cells and will accumulate and cause further damage to an already deteriorating neurological system.

Musculoskeletal System Changes. As already noted, there is a general loss of muscle strength in many areas of the body. Loss of skeletal muscle strength is perhaps the earliest of the physical signs of somatic death. Muscle weakness begins in the legs and results, in turn, in an inability to walk, then to simply stand, and finally to move in bed. The generalized muscle weakness extends to the arms, the chest muscles and even to the muscles producing the volume of the voice. As the muscles weaken further and protein synthesis becomes reduced, weight loss from muscles is a major problem. Muscle bulk (size) becomes markedly decreased, further reducing their strength and their ability to even move the extremities and the joints. The joints stiffen, and even passive movement by attendants becomes painful, leading to a continued reduction in general body movement.

Other Physical Signs.   As somatic death becomes imminent, the physical signs of approaching death are unmistakable. Dehydration results in a loss of skin turgor (resiliency) and a sharpening of facial features (face, nose, and chin) as water is lost from these sites. Earlobes and ears lose fullness and lie flat against the head. Neurological control of body temperature is lost, with possible high fever (especially if infection is present) or, more likely, very cold body temperature consistent with the temperature of the air in the room. The neck may hyperextend. The eyes become sunken as dehydration and weight loss continues, and the eyelids often remain in a half-open position. Eventually, apnea and cardiac arrest signify the final life event. At this point, the physical signs satisfy any definition of death.

SUMMARY

As society has assumed greater interest and participation in the final events in the lives of their friends and family, a greater appreciation and understanding of death and the dying process has been gained. This has led to an improvement not only in the care of the dying, but also in the prolongation of life. While there remains for some much uncertainty regarding the spiritual aspects of death, the veil of mystery surrounding the physical aspects of death is gradually being lifted. The more society accepts death as a physical life process, the more it will come to realize and address the physical and emotional needs and the desires of the dying. Members of society who strive to reach this level of understanding for others will, eventually, come to a better understanding of their own final life event.

REFERENCES

Banasik, J. L. (2000). Cell injury, aging, and death. In L. C. Copstead & J. L. Banasik (Eds.). *Pathophysiology: Biological and behavioral perspectives* (2nd ed., pp. 79–90). Philadelphia, PA: W. B. Saunders, Co.

Beecher, H. K., Adams, R. D., Barger, A. C., et al. (1968). A definition of irreversible coma. JAMA, 205(6), 85–88.

Black, H. C. (1968). *Black's law dictionary* (4th ed.). St. Paul, MN.: West Publishing Co.

Cotran, R. S., Kumar, V., & Collins, T. (1999). *Robbins—Pathologic basis of disease* (6th ed.). Philadelphia, PA: W. B. Saunders Co.

Definition of Death, 9 LA Stat. Ann. §§ 233, 1 (1976).

DiMaio, D., & DiMaio, V. (1993). *Forensic pathology.* Boca Raton, FL: CRC Press, Inc.

Kalina, K. (1993). *Midwife for souls.* Boston: Pauline Books and Media.

Kemp, C. (1999). *Terminal illness: A guide to nursing care* (2nd ed.) Philadelphia, PA: Lippincott Williams & Wilkins.

McCance, K. L. (1998). Altered cellular and tissue biology. In K. L. McCance, & S. E. Heuther (Eds), *Pathophysiology: The biologic basis of disease in adults and children* (3rd ed., pp. 44–79). St. Louis: Mosby Year Book, Inc.

Perper, J. (1993). Time and changes after death. In W. Spitz, (Ed.), *Spitz and Fisher's Mediocolegal investigation of death* (3rd ed., pp. 14–16). Springfield, IL: Charles C Thomas Publishers.

Power, B., & VanHeerden, P. (1995). The physiological changes associated with brain death: Current concepts and implications for treatment of the brain dead organ donor. *Anaesth Intens Care, 23*, 26–36.

Powner, D., DeJoya, G., & Darby, J. (2000). Brain death: Definition, determination and physiologic effects on donor organs. In W. Shoemaker, S. Ayers, A. Grenvik, & P. Holbrook, (Eds.), *Textbook of critical care* (4th ed., pp. 1894–1898). Philadelphia, PA: W. B. Saunders Co.

Tran, P., & Miller, R. (1999). Apoptosis: Death and transfiguration. *Science and Medicine, 6*(3), 18.

Unit IX

Pathophysiology of Death and Dying Process

Critical Thinking Activities

1. List measures to include family and loved ones in the care of the dying person at the time of death
2. Discuss issues and concerns that impact the nurse in caring for the dying
3. Identify barriers to effective care at the time of death

Teaching-Learning Exercises

1. Write a description of the dying process based on past experiences
2. Develop personal strategies to assist caregivers in providing care at the time of death

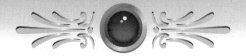

UNIT X

Caring for the Caregiver

Learning Objectives

1. Discuss the role of the nurse providing end of life care in the acute critical care settings
2. Discuss rights and obligations of patients and medical personnel in the acute care areas relative to death and dying
3. Define stress, burnout, and compassion fatigue

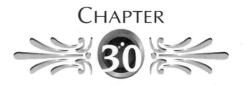

EXTENDING THE CIRCLE OF CARE WHEN DEATH IS IMMINENT

Dr. Sarah Brabant

I never look at the masses as my responsibility. I look at the individual. I can love only one person at a time. I can feed only one person at a time. Just one, one, one.

Mother Teresa

INTRODUCTION

The degree to which the inclusion of family and friends is an important component in nursing care, especially when death is imminent, is dependent in large part on the site of both nursing care and death. In the early part of the 20th century, death in a hospital was limited to those without financial or social resources. Sick individuals with sufficient resources recovered or died at home among family and friends (Corr, Nabe, and Corr 1997). The need to include family and friends in the patient's circle of care is reflected in the suggested code of ethics, presented to the American Nurses Association in 1926 (ANA 1926, 600):

> Therefore the nurse must broaden her thoughtful consideration of the patient so that it will include his whole family and his friends, for only in surroundings harmonious and peaceful for the patient can the nurse give her utmost of skill, devotion and knowledge, which shall include the safeguarding of the health of those about the patient and the protection of property.

By 1990, close to 80% of all deaths in the United States took place in an institutional setting (Corr, Nabe, and Corr 1997). Advances in technology and drug therapy and the concomitant division of labor into ever narrowing specialties minimized both the time with and opportunity for interaction between the professional health care provider and the patient's family and friends. Indeed, it was not uncommon for nurses to regard their expertise with machinery as part of and even the ultimate expression of nursing care (Barr and Bush 1998). The care of family and friends was delegated to others—e.g., social services or pastoral care. The most recent code of ethics includes family in the circle of care only when death is imminent (ANA 1985, 4):

> The measures nurses take to care for the dying client and the client's family emphasize human contact. They enable the client to live with as much physical, emotional, and spiritual comfort as possible, and they maximize the values the client has treasured in life.

The hospital's primary mission, however, is to treat, cure, and send home. In such a setting, death is a failure. Aries (1981, 586) notes:

> When death arrives, it is regarded as an accident, a sign of helplessness or clumsiness that must be put out of mind. It must not interrupt the hospital routine, which is more delicate than that of any other professional milieu. It must therefore be discrete.

In contrast to "the cure-centered, often impersonal approach of the general hospital" (Kalish 1985, 293), hospice care, first initiated in the United States in 1974, focuses on palliative measures when there is consensus death will occur in the near future (e.g., six months) and reversal of the dying process is improbable. Inclusion of the family as an integral part of the care unit is a basic objective (Zimmerman 1981, 5–6). For a variety of reasons, ranging from availability to personal preference, hospice care is limited to less than 20% of the population (Corr, Nabe, and Corr 1997). Thus, with the exception of the relatively small number of Americans who die instantly as the result of trauma or system failure (less than 10%), most Americans can expect to die in an institutional setting.

Although the notion of hospice care for all dying patients has been questioned (Logue 1994), the cultural emphasis on "the good death" as reflected in movies and television has resulted in considerable pressure on hospitals in general and nurses in particular to provide hospice-like care when death is near. The critical care setting itself, however, makes this idealized death problematic. Chapple (1999, 25) writes:

> In reality, death in the intensive care unit (ICU) is neither simple nor natural. [Nurses] would like this to happen "naturally," but our interferences in Nature's course up to the point of making the decision to withdraw life support have eliminated the possibility.

Chapple compares the often abrupt shift from aggressive care to palliative care to trying to "play baseball on the gridiron while the football game is in full swing." In such a situation, "a top priority is to avoid being trampled" (p. 28). This notion of game shift warrants attention. Social psychologist Erving Goffman offers a dramaturgical metaphor in his analysis of human interaction. Grounded in a recognized theoretical model, i.e., symbolic interaction, Goffman's use of the theatrical performance as analogy provides additional insight. Goffman (1959, Preface) writes:

> I shall consider the way in which the individual in ordinary work situations presents himself and his activity to others, the ways in which he guides and controls the impressions they form of him, and the kinds of things he may or may not do while sustaining his performance before them.

Using this approach, we will examine differences between institutional end of life care (particularly in critical care settings) and hospice end of life care, with respect to the drama, the stage, the script, the supporting cast, and the lead actors.

HOSPICE AND HOSPITALS AS THEATERS

The Drama

The phrases "letting nature take its course" and "aggressive intervention" characterize a fundamental difference between the hospice philosophy and other types of health care, particularly health care in critical care settings. The first is process oriented; the latter is event oriented. As such, the enacted dramas are quite different. The first calls for a "wait and watch" performance. There is no specific goal other than pain control. Timing is unimportant. The process of dying is allowed to proceed at its own pace. In contrast, the critical care unit focuses on the immediate event in order to maintain, stabilize or improve the patient's condition as quickly as possible. Although both performances demand skill, the first requires an ability to watch without doing; in contrast, the second requires an ability to assess and respond quickly.

The Stage

Hospice care takes place within a variety of settings, including the home, freestanding hospice units, and hospice-based programs within hospitals in either discrete units or assigned beds (Zimmerman 1981, 10). Regardless, inclusion of family and friends is fundamental. This inclusion of family and friends, however, necessitates physical space, a commodity often overlooked in both the social science and nursing literature. This includes space in proximity to the patient, the site of the drama itself, as well as what Goffman calls "backstage" space. This latter is a place where "the performer can relax . . . drop his front . . . forgo speaking his lines, and step out of character" (Goffman 1959, 112).

In hospitals, the stage on which the drama is played out is commonly a very small stage when compared to a home with kitchens, dens, porches, and yards. In floor units, there may only be room for the patient's bed and one or two chairs. In the critical care unit, the space around the patient's bed is devoted to technology. The cost and complexity of this technology necessitates minimum space between beds of other patients. Thus, two or more dramas are often played out at the same time.

Backstage space for family and friends in both floor and critical care units is limited, and even when available afford little privacy (e.g., the family waiting room). Private areas are often at some distance from the stage itself (e.g., a chapel). This lack of backstage space precludes the release of emotions as an appropriate behavior. It also negates the opportunity to practice before the actual performance.

The Script

"Dying" has no place in the script being played out in the critical care area. The possibility of the patient dying may certainly occur to the patient, the nurse, or members of the family. However, as Chapple (1999, 25) notes, "Death is not the mission of any ICU." Indeed, the goal of everyone concerned is to prevent death. Thus, until the decision is made to discontinue treatment or to withdraw life support, death is a taboo topic. In contrast, the primary players in hospice care—the patient, at least one family member, and the hospice team—have agreed that death, although not the mission, is the prognosis. As such, dying is what the drama is all about.

In the institutional setting, then, the shift from an event-oriented drama to one of process necessitates a major shift in script—i.e., construction of reality for most, if not all, of the players. One or more members of the circle of family or friends may have already defined the patient as "dead" when he or she entered the hospital; others, however, hoped for continued life. Those who define the patient's situation as hopeless often avoid the hospital or spend their time in semi-backstage places such as the cafeteria or parking lot. Those onstage generally give lip service at least to hope.

With the shift from event-oriented to process-oriented drama, there may be greater inconsistency in construction of reality among those who are onstage. The nurse and the patient's mother, for example, may concur that the patient is dying; the father, on the other hand, may not. Multiple scripts demand more space onstage as well as greater access to backstage space, neither of which is available in the critical care unit and often limited in floor units as well.

One of my clients had been hospitalized for some weeks for treatment of an AIDS-related illness. As a result of the physician's decision to discontinue treatment and to provide palliative care only, the drama shifted. Both the mother and the young man's partner had questioned continued treatment for several days; the father, however, had continued to hope for a cure. I remember the moment that he walked into his son's room and suddenly realized that his child was dying. He began to shake uncontrollably, and the nurse suggested that I go with him to the nurses' break room. We had just entered this room when another nurse came in and demanded that we leave immediately, saying that this was where she ate her lunch. Fortunately I knew this hospital well and was able to guide the father out onto the fire escape where he sobbed for some 15 minutes or more. This is a good example of the lack of appropriate backstage space in institutional settings and the need for such space when the script changes.

Supporting Cast

The team approach is basic to hospice care. Physicians, nurses, clinical nurse practitioners, social workers, physical therapists, chaplains, and volunteers are all important components in a comprehensive approach to meet the social, physical, emotional, intellectual, and spiritual needs of the dying person. All the players share equal billing. It is also of importance to remember that this team is in place before the patient is defined as dying. They know each other; they have been through dress rehearsals together.

Although the various players mentioned above may be available in any given institutional setting, the coming together as a team for a specific person is problematic. In an event-driven drama, support staff are identified and called in as needed only. Trained to focus on event rather than process, the ability to work together in a process-oriented drama may take some time. These individuals may not know each other; they may not have ironed out any problems that could arise when boundaries between professional turfs are questioned, and some may still be using an event-oriented script.

The Lead Actors: Rights and Obligations

In the critical care area, the tasks of the primary actors are fairly simple. The patient is supposed to get well; the medical personnel are supposed to make this happen. Thus, the patient is supposed to relinquish his or her rights to dignity, privacy, and control to the medical personnel. In return, the medical personnel are obliged to make every effort to maintain, stabilize, and improve the patient's health. Although the role of the family is to be supportive in this endeavor, the primary task often becomes one of not interfering as the series of events resulting from the illness or trauma occur, are assessed, and treated. When the drama shifts to one that is process oriented, the rights and tasks of the lead actors shift dramatically.

The Patient. When death is inevitable, the task of the patient is to let go (not the same as giving up). Some thanatologists suggest that this is a conscious act on the part of the dying person. Certainly there are numerous anecdotal stories that support this notion (Callanan and Kelley 1992). Given this task, the patient's rights include comfort, respect, and above all, the right to make this decision to let go in his or her own time and not in accordance with someone else's need or preference. In addition, the patient has a right to choose companionship or privacy, both during the process and at the time of death.

Needless to say, the lack of space, proximity of other ill patients, and frequent reminders from other units (e.g., emergency or recovery rooms) that a transfer is imminent do not enhance the probability that the patient's rights will be honored.

Family/friends.   The primary task of the patient's significant other(s) is to say goodbye in such a way that the patient is allowed to die in peace and the family member or friend is able to look back on this time of farewell with a sense of fulfillment. In order to accomplish this task, family and friends have a right to information, guidance, and affirmation that they are doing what they need to do: play acceptable and appropriate roles in the drama.

The Professional Caregiver.   The professional caregiver has an obligation to define the situation (including providing information about the drama itself and expected role behavior), set the limits for the performance of both the drama and the roles within the drama, and to model the behavior expected of all of the performers. Professional caregivers also have the responsibility for taking care of themselves in order not to become an added responsibility for the other performers; coupled with these complex tasks is the right to feel good about themselves as professionals as well as human beings. This latter is especially important.

In contrast to a growing body of nursing literature that suggests critical care nursing is more stressful than nursing in other areas because of a variety of external factors (e.g., the need to assess and act quickly), a number of researchers have suggested that personality characteristics may be an even more important factor (Milazzo 1988). Thus, nurses may feel that they have provided the best possible nursing care and at the same time feel that they have somehow failed as a human being. The demand to shift quickly from an event-oriented drama to a process-driven one may exacerbate this feeling of failure as a human being. A closer look at the shift in roles required by the different dramas affords some insight.

THE PROCESS-ORIENTED DRAMA IN CRITICAL CARE AREAS

Chapple (1999) notes that although physicians, ethicists, and others may take an active role in making the decision to shift the drama from one of life saving to one of dying, it is often the nurse who is left to shift an event-oriented care plan to one that is process oriented. In Chapple's words, the nurse must now become "the referee and the coach" (p. 26). In Goffman's analogy, the nurse becomes the director of the new drama. The physician or the ethics committee may determine the shift in the drama; it is the nurse who will direct the players in this new performance. Chapple suggests that this shift in drama requires a shift in both objective and rules. The old objective was to aggressively treat the illness; the new objective is to attend to the dying process. The old rules were to watch, assess, and respond; the new rules are to invite participation of others into the process, which involves sharing both the power and the powerlessness, to allow time to pass, and to allow for unpredictability. These new rules are basic to hospice care. They may not be feasible or possible in the critical care unit. One type of behavior, however, is always possible. This is known in biblical terms as "the laying on of hands."

Touch

I often wonder if nurses are truly aware of their healing power. Given the traditional hierarchy in health care, I doubt it. The physician is traditionally thought of as the healer; nurses are assistants or perhaps associates in this process. Nurses, however, may have more opportunity than physicians to use their healing power both with patients and family or friends for at least two reasons. First, nurses are allowed to touch without asking permission. Second, nurses are afforded numerous opportunities to touch.

I have often watched nurses enter the room of an AIDS patient, adjust the infusion apparatus, assess the patient, and leave. In some cases, this attention evoked anxiety on the part of the patient. In most situations, the experience offered little more than a temporary diversion. In some instances, however, I have watched as the nurse removed his or her gloves following the adjustment of the apparatus and lightly touched the patient's shoulder. Sometimes a word or two is exchanged. Most often there is only the touch. Regardless, the touch takes only seconds, a minute at most. The nurse then leaves the room, and only I am there to observe what happens next. The breathing becomes more regular, shoulders relax, and often the patient drifts off into a restful sleep. I have witnessed this again and again in both alert as well as comatose patients. Nothing has been added to the infusion; the only difference is the touch.

Touch is also powerful when applied to family and friends. I have watched family members move from an agitated state to one of calmness, from aggression to cooperativeness, following the touch of a nurse as she or he left the room. I have often wondered if the nurse in question was actually aware of the volatile situation and his or her role in alleviating it with one simple touch.

My earlier work with bereaved parents prepared me for this phenomenon. As one of my counseling techniques, I often ask bereaved parents how they survived the trauma of witnessing or learning about the death of a beloved child. The usual response is, "There was this person." Occasionally, the person is a paramedic; more rarely, a physician. Most commonly, the person is a nurse. I ask what this person did that was so helpful at the time of the child's death. Sometimes it is some small act of kindness—a glass of water or a wet cloth. Most often, however, it is simply a touch. In the midst of chaos, this small touch was the means of survival for a person whose world was truly falling apart.

It is important to remember that touch implies just that, reaching out and touching another person. This is in sharp contrast to patting. While touch can be healing, patting is often interpreted as demeaning or deterring. I once knew a nurse who always patted the patient's head before leaving the room. Following such an event, one AIDS patient confided in me that he felt like a dog every time she did this. Indeed, he was thinking about biting her hand the next time it happened. I discussed with him the possible consequences that might follow such an action on his part, and he decided that the pleasure it might give him was not worth the cost. The next time that nurse entered the room, adjusted the infusion apparatus, and patted his head, however, he let out a low growl and then winked at me.

Patting is also used by both professional and laypersons to alter behavior. People who are crying or even sobbing often stop when patted on the shoulder. The pat is interpreted as a signal to "get a grip." Thus, patting demeans or corrects; the "laying on of hands" heals.

Invitation to Participate

Chapple suggests that the invitation to participate in the dying process involves sharing both the power and the powerlessness. Power includes both access to information and control of situation. Nurses can share information about the dying process in general as well as about particular cases that they have experienced. They can also invite the other participants to share experiences they may have had with both death and dying in the past, as well as contribute suggestions for the process that is taking place at this time. How do they define life and death? What do they think happens following death? Do they wish to be present during the process or the death? Are there religious or cultural norms that they wish to consider? Chapter 7, "The Kaleidoscope of Culture," explores the variety of attitudes toward dying and death across cultures. Sharing power means allowing cultural diversity to be acknowledged and affirmed. Sharing powerlessness means sharing lack of both information and control in the given situation. Acknowledgment of regrets, sadness, and fear is easier when these emotions are shared with and affirmed by others. This is a time for listening, not talking. A simple nod is often sufficient.

Allowing others to participate includes letting others share in immediate tasks. Knowing that you did something, however trivial, to assist your loved one in his or her last hours is a tremendous asset in grief work following the death of a loved one. I remember one occasion when a father was waiting for his son to die from AIDS. The young man was in no apparent pain but showed no evidence of being aware of the presence of others. His father paced the room, his hands clenched together. At one point I rose to adjust the damp cloth on the young man's head and the father asked if he could do that. As he stroked his son's face with the cloth, he told me about the times he had bathed his son when he was a little boy and prepared him for bed. I asked if he would like to do this now. At first he voiced concern that he might hurt him, but allowed me to bring a bowl of water, cloth, and towels to him. I asked if he wanted me to stay, and he said no but would I remain nearby "just in case." He then proceeded to bathe his son who died later that evening. At the wake, the father came up to me, smiled, and said proudly that his son died in clean pajamas. I do not believe that he will ever forget his son's dying; he will, however, always have the memory that it was he who made certain that his child died in clean pajamas.

An invitation to participate may not only be helpful to the family member or friend, it can also alleviate constant intrusion into the nurse's work by these persons. A few minutes spent teaching someone how to perform a simple procedure for the patient can avoid both repeated requests for this service as well as constant interruptions in the hall. Family and friends are often concerned about the cessation of feeding during the end-stage process. Feeding, after all, is how we show others that we love them. This is particularly true in some cultures, notably so in the Acadian ethos. Allowing family or friends to crush ice or popsicles and then place a small bit on the patient's lips can both provide immediate relief from the strain of watching a dying loved one and create good memories to draw on following the death. Sometimes participation of this type is not feasible, especially in crowded critical care areas. Changing the cool cloth, wiping the mouth, or moistening the lips, however, are small tasks that, although perhaps unnecessary or relatively unimportant, allow the family member or friend to actively participate in caring for the loved one.

Allow Time to Pass

In my experience, most participants want to know when death can be expected to take place. It is useful to acknowledge the wish to know this as normal and then draw attention away from the death itself to the process leading toward death. When cure is the goal, it is the professional who determines both procedures and the timing of these procedures. When death is imminent, it is the dying person who controls the process. Focusing on what is transpiring at the moment with the patient as well as those who wait with the patient—rather than the approximate time of a future event—helps to keep the drama flowing smoothly.

Encourage those gathered in attendance to talk *to* the patient rather than *about* the patient. This is the time to remember events that were important to all the participants. It is a time to forgive past omissions or commissions, a time to say thank you, a time to express the meaning that someone has for another. As death approaches, co-breathing can help family members, friends, and patient alike. The nurse can encourage those around the bedside to breathe in unison with the patient. If the patient's breathing is rapid, co-breathers can breathe with every other breath instead.

Allow for Unpredictability

Predicting when death will occur is often haphazard at best. I have often left a patient's bedside "knowing" that this would be the last time I would be with him or her before death occurred, only to return later that day or even a week or two later and find that person still alive or even improved. I remember clearly one night when the parents, the nurse, and I concurred that the end of a young man's life was near. I sat with the parents as we watched his breathing grow more and more labored and irregular. Just as dawn was beginning, he suddenly opened his eyes, looked out the window, and asked me why I was still at the hospital. I have to admit that I was at a loss for words.

Similarly, I have experienced the shock of learning that someone died when I thought death was days, weeks, or even months away. In the early months of my work with AIDS patients, I remember my surprise when a physician asked me if I thought death was imminent. It was then that I learned that dying was definitely not an exact science.

SHIFTING ROLES IN THE CRITICAL CARE UNIT

Shifting from the event-oriented drama of aggressive intervention to the process-oriented drama of letting nature take its course is tantamount to trying to produce grand opera on a stage designed for intimate supper theater. It's not going to work. The stage itself is too small, the supporting staff is unassembled, and few, if any, of the performers are reading from the same script. Time to plan, time to learn the script, and time to rehearse are essential if the process-oriented drama is to be successful. Hospice care professionals have learned that entry into hospice within hours or even days of death is problematic (Head 2000). It's unreasonable to pressure nurses in hospital settings, especially in critical care units, to provide hospice care at the end of the patient's life. Some aspects of this care, however, are possible; suggestions follow.

The Nurse As Director

It is important to plan ahead as much as possible. Locating available space for backstage use is best done prior to need, not as the result of need. Some hospitals have "family rooms" for this purpose, but these areas are often at a distance from the patient's room and/or lack essential privacy. Find out if there is a room on the floor that is not occupied. Locate a privacy screen for use in the waiting room or at the end of a hall. See if the nurses' lounge is available. These steps can alleviate having to disrupt other floor activity when the need for privacy is great and can help avoid the embarrassment of using the wrong backstage space at the wrong time.

Become acquainted with members of your social service or pastoral care staff. In an event-oriented drama, patients and families are referred to these areas of the hospital for services just as they are transported to other areas for specific procedures (e.g., x-ray, lab work). The focus in the event-oriented drama is on getting a task accomplished. Family members may simply be told where to go in order to meet with someone to discuss some issue, such as out-patient care. In this situation, it is the department and its service, not the specific person, that is important. In the process-oriented drama, the focus shifts. Continuity is important. Thus, being able to say that you have asked a particular person from social services or pastoral care to come by in order to talk about some of the things that were discussed earlier makes the occasion more personal. This support person is not expected to have answers, only suggestions. He or she also has time to sit and talk a few minutes; you may not.

The Nurse as Educator
In the past, most people experienced a death while still in childhood. It is not uncommon today for an adult to have had no prior experience with death. The nurse, then, serves as death educator. What are the signs of approaching death? What will take place as death occurs? What behavior is appropriate? What will happen following the death itself? What the nurse says at this time and the way in which it is said can have critical impact on the family member or friend both at time of death and thereafter.

Although we often use words like *death* and *dead* in ordinary speech—"death wish," "I laughed so hard I almost died," "deadbeat," "dead end"—we often use euphemisms when death actually occurs—"he passed away," "she left us." An expression traditionally used by nurses is "expired." The use of euphemisms by the professional is detrimental for at least two reasons. First, they support the notion that death is a failure, something that should not be mentioned openly. It thus adds to the stigma surrounding death. Secondly, it may lead to confusion about what has actually transpired. I have had people come to me following the death of a loved one who were distraught because they were concerned that their loved one felt abandoned or suffered physically while in the morgue. Statements such as, "They will be taking John down to the morgue to await the people from the funeral home" are misleading. John is dead. "Your son's body will be taken to the morgue" is much clearer.

Finally, the first task of grief work is to acknowledge that the person is dead. This does not mean that one accepts the death, just that one acknowledges that the person is no longer alive. The nurse as society's representative can promote this by using the correct words.

The Nurse As Role Model
The nurse directs the drama as well as provides the model for those who will take active roles. Touching the patient gives an example of how the family and friends may proceed. If the nurse treats the patient as an object, those who

witness this will probably do so as well. If the nurse, however, treats the patient as a human being with rights to dignity and respect, those in attendance will often follow suit. If the nurse can express feelings of regret, others may feel permission to do so as well.

As death approaches, the nurse's roles of director, educator, and model may commingle with that of co-participant. The relationship between the nurse and patient is coming to a close. It is time to give permission to die, and the nurse may be an important person in this ritual and a model of behavior for others. The moment of death may well be the most difficult time for the nurse, for it is at this time that the nurse must both step aside and set limits for the behavior of others.

Stepping aside is not always as easy as it sounds. I have to admit that I have often resented relatives who appear just before death occurs and take center stage with last-minute reconciliations, when I was the one who cared for this person during the long weeks or months that preceded the death. I have to remind myself that this is, after all, what I had hoped would take place. I need to step aside and give others the center stage. At the same time, it is the professional who must set the limits for final good-byes.

Removing any tubes that may still be present, wiping away secretions that may have occurred in the last moments of life, arranging the linens all attest to a shift in the drama. Allowing those in attendance time with the body is important. It is the nurse, however, who sets the limits for both behavior and length of time. Educating and modeling prior to the death can often make this much easier for everyone concerned.

SUMMARY

The nurse in the nonhospice setting is not going to be able to deliver hospice care. Even hospice workers cannot deliver all the services they want to when the patient is admitted shortly before death. In addition, the nurse in the institutional setting lacks the stage required to allow a full-scale process-oriented drama to take place, the backstage space for rehearsals, a pre-assembled supporting cast, and a consensus on script. Becoming aware of the need to shift from an event-oriented drama to a process-oriented one, however, may allow the nurse to facilitate end of life care for patient and family or friends. Head (2000, 5) suggests that when patients enter hospice care at the last moment, "expectations should be realistic and parameters for satisfaction of both patient/family and team must be redefined." This is good advice for the nurse in a nonhospice setting as well. It may not be possible to include all the persons in the end of life circle of care who want to be included or who would benefit from inclusion. It may, however, be feasible to include one or more to some degree. This in itself is quite an accomplishment when all is said and done.

REFERENCES

American Nurses Association (ANA). (1926). A suggested code. *The American Journal of Nursing, 26*(8), 599–601.

American Nurses Association (ANA). (1985). *Code for nurses with interpretative statements.* Washington, DC: American Nurses Publishing.

Aries, P. (1982). *The hour of our death.* New York: Vintage Books.

Barr, W. J., & Bush, H. A. (1998). Four factors of nurse caring in the ICU. *Dimensions of Critical Care Nursing, 17*(3), 214–223.

Callanan, M., & Kelley, P. (1992). *Final gifts: Understanding the special awareness, needs, and communications of the dying.* New York: Poseidon Press.

Chapple, H. S. (1999). Changing the game in the intensive care unit: Letting nature take its course. *Critical Care Nurse, 19*(3), 25–33.

Corr, C. A., Nabe, C. M., & Corr, D. M. (1997). *Death and dying, life and living.* Pacific Grove, CA: Brooks/Cole Publishing Co.

Goffman, E. (1959). *The presentation of self in everyday life.* New York: Doubleday Anchor Books.

Head, B. (2000, Winter). Short length of stay: Lessons learned. *The Hospice Professional,* 1–6.

Kalish, R. A. (1985). *Death, grief, and caring relationships.* Monterey, CA: Brooks/Cole Publishing Co.

Logue, B. J. (1994). When hospice fails: The limits of palliative care. *Omega, 29*(4): 291–301.

Milazzo, N. (1988). Stress levels of ICU versus non-ICU nurses. *Dimensions of Critical Care Nursing, 7*(1), 52–58.

Mother Teresa. (1983). *Words to love by . . .* Notre Dame, IN: Ave Maria Press.

Zimmerman, J. M. (1981). *Hospice: Complete care for the terminally ill.* Baltimore, MD: Urban & Schwarzenberg.

TAKING CARE OF YOURSELF

Dr. Sarah Brabant

Today I will affirm that I am a gift to myself and the Universe. I will remember that nurturing self-care delivers that gift in its highest form.

Melodie Beattie

INTRODUCTION

Nursing is generally acknowledged to be a high-stress profession (Jacobson and McGrath 1983) and the subsequent cost to the individual, the profession, and society is significant (Hudak, Gallo, and Morton 1998). Factors related to this high stress range from role responsibilities to organizational structure (Jacobson 1983a). Although other occupations may be similar in these regards, caring for ill or troubled persons creates an additional source of stress for those engaged in hands-on delivery of health care (Plante and Bouchard 1995–1996, Macks and Abrams 1992, Milazzo 1988). The hospice movement, coupled with "the good death" as a cultural ideal, adds yet another source of stress for nurses in nonhospice health care settings (Chapple 1999). This relatively new stress factor is the increasing demand for the nurse to shift from life-prolonging care to terminal care without benefit of clear regulations and oversight once the decision to terminate life support is made. In light of the increasing number of stressors associated with nursing, the need for self-care becomes an essential task for the professional, rather than merely a beneficial exercise. Before discussing self-care, however, we need to look more closely at three similar yet disparate concepts: stress, burnout, and compassion fatigue.

Stress

Stress can be defined in physiological, psychological, social, and situational terms; but regardless of the perspective, there are two fundamental components. First, stress is an event that takes place at a given time; second, the individual perceives the event as stressful. At its most basic level, stress is conflict between what individuals *want* to or *perceive* that they should do, think, or feel and what they *can* do, think, or feel in a given situation. Unlike trauma which can be defined objectively, stress must be defined subjectively. From a sociological perspective, stress as both an event and a subjective experience is best understood from the perspective of role strain theory (Goode 1960).

Role behavior consists of doing, thinking, or feeling with respect to another in accordance with the norms (blueprints for behavior) of a particular culture. Who we are in relationship to others, our social identity, rests on our ability to perform our roles in an acceptable and appropriate manner as defined by us or by our significant other(s). Difficulty in performing or failure to perform a role appropriately strikes at the very core of who we are. Two concepts, role strain and role conflict, provide insight into role-related stress. Role strain occurs in the performance of a particular role; role conflict pertains to problems that occur in the performance of two or more roles.

When we find it difficult to perform the obligations required by a particular role—due to lack of experience, inadequate training, or personal inability—role strain occurs. An individual may lack the skills or knowledge required to perform a particular role; stress can be alleviated by learning the skills or acquiring the knowledge demanded by that role. A role, however, may be difficult to perform because the individual lacks the physical, mental or emotional capabilities to perform the role. In this case, the role may have to be altered or even abandoned.

You have probably already experienced role strain in your professional training. A particular procedure may have been difficult for you. Practice, however, enabled you to perform this procedure with little difficulty or even with ease. You have alleviated this stress in your life. On the other hand, a severe back injury might render you incapable of performing the procedure, and thus negate your ability to perform adequately. In this instance, stress can only be alleviated by relinquishing the role. If the role is an important aspect of who you are, loss of that role can be devastating.

With role conflict, we are unable to perform a particular role adequately or appropriately because the performance of another role prevents us from doing so. For example, concern for our sick child (parent role) may intrude on the attentiveness demanded by our work role. In a world in which we play multiple roles, role conflict is a major source of stress. Given enough time, we could probably perform a multitude of roles successfully. As finite creatures, however, we are time limited. As a result, stress created by role conflict is an everyday occurrence; the possibility of role failure is ever present. We need to take a closer look at the roles we have assumed or had assigned to us and to let go of some of the roles we perform. It is an existential task, since the abandonment of significant roles inevitably alters our concept of who we are. This may necessitate time off for reflection or professional counseling.

Stress, then, is not just work related. It is inherent in the demands placed on us by ourselves and others in a complex society. Stress is not necessarily bad. Social scientists have identified a number of crisis or stress-evoking events that accompany the developmental process of the individual as well as the family. Although these crisis points may be painful, they also provide avenues for growth (McCubbin and Figley 1983). Remember that it was stress that caused you to perfect the techniques that render or will render you competent to engage in your chosen profession.

Burnout

Burnout, a term coined by Herbert Freudenberger in 1974, differs from stress in three important ways: (1) burnout is work related; (2) it is a process, not an event; and (3) unlike stress, it has no redemptive value. Burnout is a feeling state associated with mental and/or physical exhaustion (Freudenberger 1974). Although a number of factors may contribute to burnout, it occurs primarily as a result of a person's dedication and commitment to work. "We work too much, too long and too intensely" (Freudenberger 1974, 161). Burnout affects our ability to perform work roles adequately (leading to additional stress), and it impinges on our interpersonal relations both at work and elsewhere (Figley 1995). As a result of the exhaustion, individuals may leave or be forced to leave work that was very important to them.

Compassion Fatigue

Although health care professionals share the risk of burnout with people in other occupations, compassion fatigue is limited to those who work with troubled individuals. Originally identified by Figley as secondary victimization (1983, 7), compassion fatigue pertains to "the natural . . . behaviors and emotions resulting from knowing about a traumatizing event experienced by a significant other—the stress resulting from helping or wanting to help a traumatized or suffering person." Burnout is the result of overcommitment and dedication to one's work; compassion fatigue is related to an individual's capacity for feeling and expressing empathy with those in pain. There are other differences as well.

Burnout is a process that begins gradually and becomes progressively worse as one becomes increasingly detached from one's work. In contrast, compassion fatigue "can emerge suddenly with little warning" (p. 12). With burnout there is an increasing awareness of physical or emotional exhaustion. Compassion fatigue generally manifests itself in one of two distinctly different ways: over-identification with the client's traumatic event, or an intense distaste for the suffering of others.

In over-identification, the person's trauma becomes a viable possibility for you. To illustrate, I had been working as a support person with the local Compassionate Friends chapter, a self-support group for bereaved parents, for about a year when I became aware, quite suddenly, of a routinized behavior on my part. Following each meeting, regardless of the late hour, I phoned each of my children. This was not something I wanted to do; it was something I had to do. After months of listening to individuals talk about the deaths of their children, the possibility of one of my children dying had became a very real and frightening possibility. This over-identification is not uncommon. Persons who work with rape victims may begin to see all males as potential rapists; those who work with cancer patients may begin to imagine a variety of malignant growths in their own bodies.

In contrast to over-identification is an often sudden intense distaste for the pain of another. I remember returning from an AIDS workshop in Baton Rouge Louisiana. There had been so many deaths recently. The workshop had only accentuated the number of deaths to come. I was tired of losing people I cared about; I was tired of dealing with their issues. I slipped a Judy Collins tape into the slot, forgetting that one of the songs was "I've Had Enough Dying for Today." Suddenly I was screaming the words at the top of my voice. Until then, I had not realized how much I dreaded the thought of finding out that one more of "my guys" was either dead or near death. I did not want to deal with any more deaths.

Stress, burnout, and compassion fatigue, although related, are quite different phenomena. As such, each demands different strategies for both alleviation and prevention. Stress related to suddenly being asked to do two or more things at the same time can be alleviated relatively quickly. Repeated role conflict, burnout, and compassionate fatigue require additional steps.

QUICK FIXES

Three "quick fixes" that I find helpful are breathing, the quick vacation, and wringing the cloth.

Breathing

As strange as this may seem, simply focusing on our breathing may alleviate stress. Under stress, our muscles tense; we begin to take short, rapid, shallow breaths. As a result, we get less air into our lungs and, thus, less oxygen. Breathe deeply, hold your breath, and slowly release the air from your lungs. Focus on the air as it enters your nose; focus on the air as it moves out through your mouth. Be aware of your lungs filling and emptying and of your chest rising and falling. Do not try to push images, thoughts, or sounds out of your mind. Simply let them be and refocus on your breathing. Allow yourself (what you are thinking or feeling at the moment) to enter your consciousness. Take note of your thoughts and feelings. Do not try to change either. Simply become aware of them and then refocus on your breathing.

The Quick Vacation

Imagine a place where you might like to go or where you have been and found to be relaxing. An example would be a trip to the beach. Imagine the ocean.

Listen to the waves as they come ashore. Imagine the feel of the hot sand and the cool water on your body. Hear the cry of the gulls. Remain in this place for a few minutes. Then promise yourself that you will return to this place when your shift is done or before you go to bed. Remember to keep that promise.

Wringing the Cloth

Grip a washcloth or small towel in both hands and twist with all your strength. Hold the twisted cloth, count to five slowly, and release. Do this at least three times. If you are angry at a particular person, think of the cloth or towel as that person. This exercise is good for releasing both physical and emotional tension.

Although these exercises can alleviate temporary stress, burnout and compassion fatigue require more drastic steps. You may have to take time off from work in order to recover. In extreme cases, bed rest or therapy (both physical as well as emotional) may be necessary. If you have reached or are approaching this state of affairs, try to imagine that someone you care for has had major surgery and is coming to your home for a period of recovery. What would you do for this person? How would you treat this person? What resources would you make available for this person? You are an expert on how to take care of others; do these things for yourself! It could save your life. Burnout and compassion fatigue can be just as damaging as major surgery. If you are suffering from either or both, you will require the same care that a surgical or cardiac patient needs.

PREVENTATIVE MEASURES

Obviously preventive care is far less costly and time consuming than treatment after the fact. It is important to remember that as someone committed to caring for others and doing this within an institutional setting, you are at high risk for both burnout and compassion fatigue. They are not possible consequences; they are probable ones. Prevention, however, is not as simple as it sounds. A closer look at caregiving itself provides insight.

The word *caregiving* implies focus on "other." Further, it implies reaching out to others and assisting others. The person who needs this care is by definition the more vulnerable or fragile person in the relationship. Unfortunately, "vulnerable" and "fragile" get translated into "important." Think about this for a moment. Who is the most important, you or the person you are trying to help? If you answered that the most important person was the one you are trying to help, you are wrong. If you do not take care of yourself, you cannot take care of someone else. Thus, the first step in avoiding both burnout and compassion fatigue is to turn your attention away from other(s) and focus on you.

This is not an easy task for at least two reasons: First, society does not support us in this; we risk being called selfish. We risk thinking of ourselves as selfish, and many of us have been taught that selfishness is an undesirable trait. Second, we may not like what we see when we focus on ourselves. We may find a number of attributes that we do not admire in ourselves or others (e.g., the wish to control). Regardless, we have to begin with ourselves if we want to help others.

In order to get in touch with yourself, you may find it helpful to make a list of all the things you want in life. Your list may begin with global wants such as world peace. It is important, however, to become more concrete and particular. What is it that you want right now? Perhaps an ice cream treat comes to mind. If possible, indulge yourself in this treat as soon as possible. Identifying your wants is a first step in self care.

The next step is to do a personal support assessment. I call mine the "Support for Me Inventory," and there are five important areas that need to be considered if you are to avoid or mitigate both burnout and compassion fatigue. These are social support, physical care, emotional acknowledgment and release, intellectual development, and spiritual growth (Brabant 1992) .

Social Support

We are social creatures, which means that we need other people in our lives in order to be who we want to be. I cannot be a parent without a child, a teacher without a student, a nurse without a patient. We also need other people in our lives to affirm that what we do has value for others, that our pains are indeed painful, and that our joys are worthy of such joy. Have you ever had something wonderful occur in your life, a moment so beautiful you just had to share it with someone else and found that the sharing allowed you to relive the experience? Have you ever been in pain, emotionally or physically, and found that in the telling of this pain to another the pain became more bearable? You may be thinking that this is what family and friends are for. This may be true with respect to life in general. Working with troubled and traumatized people day after day is not an ordinary life event. Neither is trying to care for these people within an institutional setting that is focused on its own existence, not the people with whom you work. I think one of the most important things I have learned in my work is that my family was not and could not be my major source of support. Indeed, at some time or another each member of my family has bitterly resented the work that I do, for it takes my attention away from them. I finally came to realize that although I needed support, it really was not their responsibility to provide this for me. I choose to do the kind of work that I do. They did not. I have found that since I don't look to them for my basic support, they give it to me when I least expect it—and that's been like icing on the cake. However, I need to look for my "bread" support elsewhere.

I also felt at one time that the organization I worked for should provide this support for me. I even insisted that an AIDS agency start a support group for people like me. I soon found that others in the group looked to me for support, which only added stress rather than relieve it. I since have come to believe that support groups within the immediate work environment may not be the best source of support. First of all, it is difficult to support others when one is very needy. Second, a person may reveal information that is not appropriate for the work environment. Letting people you see only within the context of the support group know that you were sexually assaulted as a child may be a positive experience, giving this information to coworkers or a supervisor may be destructive. Thus, it is important to look for support outside of work.

I have also come to realize that I need different kinds of support from different people. I need to be able to complain about aspects of my work, to relieve tension by joking with someone who can share in-house humor, and I need to be able to share those wonderful, beautiful moments with someone who understands. I meet weekly with three other persons who share similar work with me but not in the same setting. Sometimes I need an additional type of support. These three other people are there for me when I need them, but I must be there for them as well. They are also biased in that I am a friend. I need someone who I do not have to take care of; someone who can be objective toward me. I think of this person as a paid friend. It's also called counseling. I have found that when I have these support systems in place for me, I can truly be there for others.

Physical Care

Kashoff (1982, 274) writes:

> There are some primary, basic requirements that human beings cannot function without. At the very least, these include rest, sleep, a reasonably nutritious diet, physical exercise, and some time for recreation and play. After long years of observation, I have learned that the worst offenders in these matters are those persons who dedicate their lives to the delivery of primary health care services. In short, they "do" it for everybody except themselves.

Are you getting enough sleep and adequate exercise? Do you eat properly or are you relying on fast-food machines for food and drink? Getting adequate rest, eating properly and engaging in planned exercise are critical to both your personal and professional life. Have you had a physical that was not work related? Are alcohol or other substances, legal as well as illegal, becoming ways of coping for you? If the answer is no to the first question and yes to the second one, you need to take immediate action.

Emotional Acknowledgment and Release

Do you allow yourself to feel? Are you able to express your feelings in a safe manner? Perhaps you were taught as a child that any expression of anger was a sign of lack of control. You were told that if you did not stop crying you would get something to cry about. You learned that feeling sad is not acceptable. Maybe you learned that fear was a sign of weakness. Anger, sadness, and fear are all natural emotions. We need to learn to acknowledge these emotions as well as others and to find ways to express them in healthy ways. It is all right to pull over to the side of the road and scream; it is all right to cry; and it is all right to be afraid.

Two emotions that are not natural but are learned in interaction with others, however, are guilt and shame. Anger, sadness, and fear, expressed freely in a way that does not hurt us or others, are avenues to growth. Guilt and shame are deadends. Although guilt and shame may be part of your personal history, they may also occur as a result of caregiving.

When we work with people who are experiencing physical or emotional pain, we put our own needs aside in order to focus on the needs of our patient. This is, after all, an important component in being a professional. Our professional life, however, is only one aspect of our total life. When we have completed our work, it is important to return to our own needs and concerns. When we work with people with multiple losses or intense physical or emotional pain, we tend to compare our own pain to their pain.

Some years ago the cancer on my nose reoccurred. I had done all the things that I had been told to do to prevent this reoccurrence and five years had passed. Everything seemed fine. Two years later I was facing more disfiguring surgery, and I was both frightened and angry. I also felt ashamed of myself. What is so bad about disfiguring surgery when compared to what the people I worked with were facing. Fortunately I shared my thoughts and feelings with a wise person. When I said, "It's just a nose," she replied, "But it's your nose." It was my nose and that made it important to me. This was a valuable lesson for me. We have losses and we have pains; maybe they seem minor in comparison to the losses and the pains of the people we're working with, but they are not minor because they are ours. We need to validate our own pains and reach out for comfort. In doing so, we affirm ourselves. When we affirm ourselves, we are better able to affirm others.

Intellectual Development

The fifth mandate in the Code for Nurses is the maintenance of competence (ANA 1985, 9):

> The nurse must be aware of the need for continued learning and must assume personal responsibility for currency of knowledge and skill. [This extends to] knowledge relevant to the current scope of nursing practice, changing issues and concerns, and ethical concepts and principles.

Professional development, however, is just one aspect of taking care of ourselves intellectually. I have found that I have had to give up certain childhood beliefs as well as certain cultural cliches and to explore alternative ways of looking at the world around me. I have had to look for books and workshops that address my questions, not necessarily those of others.

Spiritual Growth

Fortunato (1987, 7) refers to spirituality as the "journey of the soul—not to religion itself but to the drive in humankind that gives rise to religion in the first place." He writes (p. 13):

> If we want . . . to talk about achieving union with God, we must also want to experience ourselves as connected with all creation and all God's creatures. It means we must also come to know God within, experiencing our own inner connectedness and unity.

Spiritual growth, then, is the journey toward greater connectedness with ourselves, with others, and with our creator. This requires time to meditate, to become aware of the world around us, to think about life and death and the meaning these words have for us. We need time to be still and listen to our inner voice. It is the task of every human being to find ways to restore the connectedness that we often lose in our busy lives.

Although we have discussed the above dimensions as separate entities, they are interrelated. I have found, for example, that massage helps me to connect with myself both physically and emotionally. We often store repressed feelings in our bodies (our shoulders may be tense because we are angry). Massage can release this tension. If this sounds like something you think might be helpful, look for the right massage therapist for you. If money is short, consider having one at a local massage school or asking a friend to join you for a short course so that the two of you can trade massages.

We need to reconnect from time to time with the world in which we live. I have found that working with dirt is extremely important to me. I can feel like I am in a thousand different pieces, but when I get out into my garden and dig in the dirt, I feel better. I do not really have to accomplish anything; just digging with my hands is enough. The contact with the dirt heals me and restores me. Other people have shared that fire is healing for them. They find that lighting a candle and looking into the flame restores them. Still others use the sound of water, or the feel of wind against their face as ways of reconnecting. Bicycling, then, may be a means of reconnecting.

Play is something many of us need to learn more about. I did not learn how to play as a child, and to this day I'm not sure just what play is. However, I have decided that if some activity will not fit into my work evaluation or my resume, it must be play. Jumping in a pile of leaves and walking barefoot through mud are ways of playing. Join a dance class (you do not need a partner in line-dance classes), take an art course, or learn to play a musical instrument. Be careful not to turn "play" into "work." Give yourself permission to fail.

Find some time each day to be alone. You may want to sit quietly or engage in some activity such as running or walking. Do not engage in purposeful activity. Just allow yourself to be in the silence. Do not use this time to solve everyday problems. Just allow yourself to appreciate you.

SUMMARY

The above suggestions are just that, suggestions. If they seem useful, try them. If they do not, look for other ways to take care of yourself. What is important is that you recognize that stress is a part of today's world and that the demands of your chosen profession will result in both role strain and role conflict. You will also probably play out your professional roles in an institutional setting that hinders you or even prevents you from doing all that you want to do. Thus, you are at high risk for burnout. The people you will be working with are troubled people. You are, thus, also at risk for compassion fatigue. Taking care of yourself, then, is a mandate. You are responsible for both identifying your own needs and for finding the ways to meet these needs. Meeting your needs takes time. Make this time a priority. Self-care does not just happen. It is your responsibility as a human being and as a professional to make certain that it happens. The following rules are critical to those who are at-risk for both burnout and compassion fatigue:

1. It is my responsibility to take care of myself.
2. It is my responsibility to find the kind of self-care that is best suited to my particular needs.
3. It is important to see myself as part of a larger process; it is also important to see myself as a unique and important part of that process and, thus, deserving of self-care.
4. Only then can I be of help and comfort to others.

REFERENCES

American Nurses Association (ANA). (1985). *Code for nurses with interpretative statements.* Washington, DC: American Nurses Publishing.

Beattie, M. (1990). *The language of letting go.* New York: HarperCollins Publishing.

Brabant, S. (1992). Survivorship for the caregiver. *Illness, Crisis & Loss,* 2(3), 31–40.

Chapple, H. S. (1999). Changing the game in the intensive care unit: Letting nature take its course. *Critical Care Nurse,* 19(3), 25–34.

Figley, C. R. (1983). Catastrophe: An overview of family reactions. In C. R. Figley & H. I. McCubbin (Eds.), *Stress and the family: Coping with catastrophe* (pp. 3–20). New York: Brunner/Mazel.

Figley, C. R. (Ed.). (1995). *Compassion fatigue: Coping with secondary traumatic stress disorder in those who treat the traumatized.* Levittown, PA: Brunner/Mazel.

Fortunato, J. E. (1987). AIDS: *The spiritual dilemma.* New York: Harper and Row.

Freudenberger, H. J. (1974). Staff burn-out. *Journal of Social Issues,* 30(1), 159–165.

Goode, W. J. (1960). A theory of role strain. *American Sociological Review* 25(4), 483–496.

Hudak, C. M., Gallo, B. M., & Morton, P. G. (1998). *Critical care nursing: A holistic approach.* New York: Lippincott.

Jacobson, S., & McGrath, M. (Eds.). (1983). *Nurses under stress.* New York: John Wiley and Sons.

Jacobson, S. F., & Lawrence, L. (1983). An overview of stress. In S. Jacobson & M. McGrath (Eds.), *Nurses under stress* (pp. 3–25). New York: John Wiley and Sons.

Jacobson, S. F. (1983a). The contexts of nurses' stress. In S. Jacobson & M. McGrath (Eds.), *Nurses under stress* (pp. 49–60). New York: John Wiley and Sons.

Jacobson, S. F. (1983b). Burnout: A hazard in nursing. In S. Jacobson & M. McGrath (Eds.), *Nurses under stress* (pp. 98–110). New York: John Wiley and Sons.

Kashoff, S. (1982). Nursing your stress. In A. A. McConnell (Ed.), *Burnout in the nursing profession: Coping strategies, causes, and costs.* St. Louis, MO: The C.V. Mosby Company.:

Macks, J. A., & Abrams, D. I. (1992). Burnout among HIV/AIDS health care providers. In P. Volberding & M. A. Jacobson (Eds.), *AIDS clinical review 1992* (pp. 283–299). New York: Marcel Dekker, Inc.

McCubbin, H. I., & Figley, C. R. (Eds.). (1983). *Stress and the family: Coping with normative transition in the family.* New York: Brunner/Mazel.

Milazzo, N. (1988). Stress levels of ICU versus non-ICU nurses. *Dimensions of Critical Care Nursing, 7*(1), 52–58.

Plante, A., & Bouchard, L. (1995–1996). Occupational stress, burnout, and professional support in nurses working with dying patients. *Omega, 32*(2), 93–109.

Unit X

Caring for the Caregiver

Critical Thinking Activities

1. Discuss strategies to assist nurses with shifting roles in caring for dying patients in critical care settings
2. List realistic boundaries and limitations in caring for dying patients in critical care settings
3. List role conflict issues confronting nurses caring for the dying

Teaching-Learning Exercises

1. Examine the expectations and parameters for patient, family, and medical team satisfaction when death occurs in critical care areas
2. Write a one-page paper describing own crisis management skills
3. Write own belief statements about death including culture, spirituality, and societal aspects
4. Develop self-help strategies that enhance coping with the emotional stressors of working with the dying

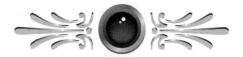

INDEX